LIGH
THERAPIES

"Plants use light effectively. Why not humans? Would Mother Nature take a strategy developed so effectively for the plant kingdom and wantonly squander it as she created the animal kingdom? In an articulate and beautifully illustrated book, physicist and long-term president of the International Light Association Anadi Martel authoritatively describes the therapeutic effects of light in a comprehensive, reader-friendly fashion, beginning with the nature of light and the ancient history of light therapeutics all the way to the modern, exponentially ———:—— £eld of science and medicine that uses light as a foundation. Th⌐   ⌐erally sprinkled with highlighted boxes containing little-knowı   ⌐ascinating insights. It's a joy to read. Highly recommended."

GERALD H. POLLAC⌐   ⌐OFESSOR OF BIOENGINEERING AT
THE UNIVERSIT⌐   ⌐IGTON, EXECUTIVE DIRECTOR OF
THE INSTITĮ   ⌐ITURE SCIENCE, AND AUTHOR OF
THE FOURTH PHASE OF WATER

"In this wonderfully detailed   ⌐ılly illustrated book, Anadi has thoroughly documented the pr⌐   ⌐ıf this rapidly advancing and very exciting field as has never been done before. Follow Anadi's remarkable scientific and spiritual journey as he uncovers the essence of light and its diverse therapeutic applications. Here you will find the fascinating physics of light described with accuracy that can only be provided by a physicist but also with the clarity that can only come from a person with a real love and passion for communicating science in ways anyone can easily understand. As we move toward the medicine of the future, all of us need to know how light and color can benefit us. Whether light therapy is a new or an old subject for you, this is the most valuable, enjoyable, and up-to-date book you can read."

JAMES L. OSCHMAN, PH.D., AUTHOR OF
ENERGY MEDICINE: THE SCIENTIFIC BASIS

"*Light Therapies* is brilliant, a star among books about light. It is a must-read for everyone interested in the field of light—beginners, experts, lay-people, health and wellness practitioners, teachers, and scientists. It covers the broadest spectrum of information about the historic, scientific, healing, and spiritual aspects of light's past, present, and future. . . . A spectacular achievement."

RAY GOTTLIEB, O.D., PH.D.,
DEAN OF THE COLLEGE OF SYNTONIC OPTOMETRY

"An important book that spearheads the new scientific paradigm in health and well-being. With profound insight, Martel explores how light lies at the very heart of our lives and outlines the effects of light on health, brain functions, cellular life, and our overall physical well-being. Here is a book that updates our understanding of physical reality—and how to benefit from it. *Light Therapies* will change the way we look at medical practice. Light medicine is the future, *now*. It will tell you everything you need to know—be informed!"

KINGSLEY L. DENNIS, AUTHOR OF *NEW CONSCIOUSNESS FOR
A NEW WORLD* AND *THE STRUGGLE FOR YOUR MIND*

"*Light Therapies* is the best book on the subject I have ever come across. Anadi Martel gives descriptions of ALL of the therapeutic techniques using light and color that he has personally investigated and experimented with. Anadi is also an expert in Buddhist culture which completes his concept of light having three aspects: the physical, the energetic, and that of consciousness."

DANIEL ASIS, M.D., AUTHOR OF *CHROMO-PSYCHOTHERAPIES*

"Anadi Martel has written a highly informative book on light therapies. It summarizes and explains the whole spectrum of light-based treatment methods and their broad applications in a beautifully illustrated manner. Surely, this volume will be very useful for beginners as well as for experts."

DETLEF SCHIKORA, PH.D., PROFESSOR OF SCIENCE AND
BIOPHYSICS AT THE UNIVERSITY OF PADERBORN

"The kind of light that Anadi brings to us is beyond alternative therapy; it is the healing power of light to restore alignment between the physical and emotional bodies with the reality of the spiritual Source of all light."

NISHANT MATTHEWS, FOUNDER OF SAMASSATI COLORTHERAPY

"For those who seek a deeper understanding of how light can heal our lives, this timely book is a must-read."

PAULINE ALLEN, PRINCIPAL OF
THE SOUND LEARNING CENTER (LONDON)

LIGHT THERAPIES

A **COMPLETE GUIDE** TO THE **HEALING POWER** OF **LIGHT**

ANADI MARTEL

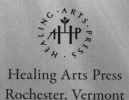

Healing Arts Press
Rochester, Vermont

Healing Arts Press
One Park Street
Rochester, Vermont 05767
www.HealingArtsPress.com

Healing Arts Press is a division of Inner Traditions International

Originally published in French under the title *Le pouvoir de la lumière: À l'aube d'une nouvelle médecine* by Guy Trédaniel éditeur
Translated from the French by Vidhan Carroll Guerin, Deva Boersma, and Anadi Martel
First U.S. edition published in 2018 by Healing Arts Press

Note to the reader: *This book is intended as an informational guide. The remedies, approaches, and techniques described herein are meant to supplement, and not to be a substitute for, professional medical care or treatment. They should not be used to treat a serious ailment without prior consultation with a qualified health care professional.*

Library of Congress Cataloging-in-Publication Data
Names: Martel, Anadi, author.
Title: Light therapies : a complete guide to the healing power of light / Anadi Martel.
Other titles: Pouvoir de la lumière. English
Description: First U.S. edition. | Rochester, Vermont : Healing Arts Press, 2018. | Includes bibliographical references and index.
Identifiers: LCCN 2017038372 (print) | LCCN 2017038989 (e-book) | ISBN 9781620557297 (paperback) | ISBN 9781620557303 (e-book)
Subjects: | MESH: Phototherapy | Light
Classification: LCC RM666.P73 (print) | LCC RM666.P73 (e-book) | NLM WB 480 | DDC 615.8/31—dc23
LC record available at https://lccn.loc.gov/2017038372

Printed and bound in the United States by Versa Press, Inc.

10 9 8 7 6 5 4 3 2 1

Text design and layout by Virginia Scott Bowman
This book was typeset in Garamond Premier Pro, Gill Sans, Futura, and Avenir with Cocomat, Helvetica, and Futura used as display typefaces

Original drawings and charts by Jocelyn Garder

To send correspondence to the author of this book, mail a first-class letter to the author c/o Inner Traditions • Bear & Company, One Park Street, Rochester, VT 05767, and we will forward the communication, or contact the author directly at **www.sensora.com.**

*

To my beloved Deva—
Without her unconditional support
this book would not have seen the light of day

CONTENTS

FOREWORD

Jacob Liberman, OD, PhD, DSc (Hon)

IT WAS 1971, and I was beginning the clinical portion of my optometric training. One of my first patients was an eleven-year-old boy who'd been diagnosed with "lazy eye," amblyopia. Even though his eyes were healthy and he didn't require prescription glasses, he was only able to see the big *E* on the eye chart. Having never worked with someone with this condition, I spoke with one of the clinic doctors, and he suggested I have the boy look through a yellow filter at a light bulb that was slowly flashing on and off. The technique the clinic doctor recommended supposedly stimulated the part of the eye dealing with the ability to perceive color and see details clearly. Even though I had no idea how or why this might work, it did. In fact, I measured improvement after the first session, and this continued for weeks, resulting in a 300 percent improvement in the boy's visual acuity.

Three years later, I used a photographic strobe light to pulse a flash of light into the better eye of another patient with the same condition, and then allowed the energy created by the light to travel through the brain to the other eye. Since both eyes are neurologically connected, I reasoned that the better eye would then train its counterpart to see more clearly. To my amazement, the patient's visual acuity improved by 200 percent in less than thirty minutes.

A year later, I attended a conference on behavioral optometry in Miami. As chance would have it, the keynote speaker, Dr. John Ott, a pioneer of photobiology, shared his discoveries about the effects of light on health. Dr. Ott's research demonstrated that light profoundly affects plants, animals, and humans in ways I had never even considered. Over the next twenty-five years, Dr. Ott and I developed a friendship and communicated often. In fact, I was invited to his Florida home on many occasions, spending countless hours talking about light.

During the years that followed, I conducted research about the therapeutic use of colored light via the eyes and reached out to experts worldwide who were also researching or using light and color to alleviate physical and emotional disorders. Because the internet and email had not yet been developed, I spent a great deal of time doing obscure research in libraries, writing letters, and calling the doctors, scientists, and laypeople who were investigating this field.

I traveled to Germany at the invitation of Dr. Fritz Hollwich, professor of ophthalmology at the University of Muenster, West Germany. Later I spent time with Dr. Fritz-Albert Popp, a leading researcher in the field of biophotons, at his laboratory in Neuss, Germany. I also visited the National Institutes of Health to meet with Dr. Norman Rosenthal, a South African psychiatrist who was the first to describe seasonal affective disorder (SAD) and pioneered the use of light therapy for its treatment. I introduced Dr. Rosenthal to syntonic phototherapy and shared my discoveries concerning the relationship between color and unresolved emotional issues. I then proceeded to Philadelphia, to Thomas Jefferson University, to discuss my findings with Dr. Bud Brainard, professor of neurology. From there I went to the University of Texas Health Science Center to learn more about the pineal gland from neuroscientist Dr. Russel Reiter. I later invited these three scientists, along with Darius Dinshah, Harry Wohlfarth, and other pioneers in the field of light therapy to be keynote speakers at the annual College of Syntonic Optometry meeting. By now I was so inspired to share my discoveries with others that I sold my optometric practice and moved to Colorado, where I founded the

Aspen Center for Energy Medicine* and began writing my first book.

Around the time my book *Light: Medicine of the Future* was published over twenty-five years ago, I tried to create a historical, scientific, and clinical foundation for the biological and therapeutic effects of light and color. What began as a dream launched me on a worldwide speaking and teaching tour and inspired me to develop the Color Receptivity Trainer and Spectral Receptivity Systems I and II. However, I was not alone on this mission. I was graced to share the journey with dear friends and colleagues such as Dr. John Downing, Dr. Larry Wallace, Dr. Ray Gottlieb, Dr. Brian Breiling, and Dr. Roberto Kaplan, among others. All of our contributions, along with those of others already mentioned, and many more, resulted in the emergence of a new science and medicine that uses light as its foundation, as well as many novel light-based healing technologies, and an industry and architecture devoted to healthy environmental lighting. Since then, practitioners from all walks of life have been using light and color therapeutically.

In the foreword to my book *Light: Medicine of the Future,* John Ott compared me to a member of a relay team to whom he had passed a baton that would eventually be taken up by others. It is now my turn to pass the baton that John entrusted me with, as light finally *is* the new medicine. Over the years, *Light: Medicine of the Future* has introduced tens of thousands of people to the science and art of light and color therapy. Like me, some of those people were deeply touched and have gratefully accepted the mantle of responsibility for carrying the light forward. Among those, Anadi Martel stands out, for he has been blessed with a brain and heart of equal size. He is not only intellectually brilliant, technologically gifted, and spiritually evolved, he has integrated those gifts to create *Light Therapies,* an encyclopedia of light and color therapy unique in the depth and breadth of information and knowledge it shares. Having had the pleasure of contributing to this emerging science, I could not be more delighted to support Anadi Martel in the launch of this absolutely incredible book. Without

---

*The Aspen Center for Energy Medicine has since closed.

hesitation I can say that it is the best book on the subject of light and color that I have read in many years.

There is one light and many lamps—shine on!

JACOB LIBERMAN holds a doctorate of optometry, a Ph.D. in vision science, and an honorary doctorate of science. He is a Fellow Emeritus of the American Academy of Optometry, College of Optometrists in Vision Development, International Academy of Color Sciences, and past president of the College of Syntonic Optometry. Recipient of the H. R. Spitler Award for his pioneering contributions to the field of phototherapy, he is the author of *Light: Medicine of the Future, Take Off Your Glasses and See, Wisdom from an Empty Mind,* and *Luminous Life: How the Science of Light Unlocks the Art of Living.* He is the inventor of several light therapy devices and the only FDA-cleared medical device that significantly improves overall visual performance.

PREFACE

TRAINED AS A PHYSICIST, I had been conducting research on sound and light almost entirely on my own for fifteen years until one day in 1998, in Marin County, near San Francisco, I met Dr. Brian Breiling, a clinical psychologist and ayurvedic specialist. In the heady days preceding the dot-com crash, my companion Deva and I found ourselves in California, where I served as research and development director for a local sound company. Two years earlier, in 1996, Brian had edited an extraordinary anthology of the most innovative research in light therapy, titled *Light Years Ahead: The Illustrated Guide to Full Spectrum and Colored Light in Mindbody Healing*. This collection opened a window to perspectives previously quite unimaginable.

Brian and his wife, Jennifer, herself a therapist well versed in light applications, invited us to their home, where we were given a warm welcome. The sharing of information was mutually beneficial. I spoke to Brian about my multisensorial system called Sensora; he showed me the recently developed Photon light therapy unit. From then on ensued an agreeable and valuable connection that endures to this day.

Some years later, I received an invitation from Brian. He and several others were organizing a large meeting with the goal of bringing together all those researchers interested in the dissemination of information on therapeutic light. The meeting, which attracted about a hundred participants from all over the world, was held in October 2003 in Antwerp, Belgium, and it led to the formation of the International Light Association (ILA). For the majority of us, it was a revelation to find that we were no longer alone as individual researchers, and that there were others who shared the same passion that gave life to our work. Most significant was the all-important scientific confirmation of the fact that light can heal. Since then the association has created an annual meeting, and each time it has provided a very enriching occasion for all of us not only to hear the presentations of some of the most notable researchers in the field, but also to renew our connection with this new "light family."

I was very happy to propose and then organize the ILA conference in October 2011, held in the Québec village of St. Adele, where, in the forest bordering the lovely little Lake Violon, I have established my home and laboratory. Along with the scientific meeting, we were able to offer the participants an opportunity to experience the vibrant colors of autumn in the Laurentians, which were then at their peak.

Subsequent to this event I became president of the association, a role I still hold at the time of this writing. This task gives me the precious privilege of meeting the most knowledgeable and forward-looking researchers of our era, whom we invite each year to our conference. In the following pages I have the pleasure of introducing several of them, as their contributions become relevant to the unfolding story.

After outlining the background and ancient origins of light therapy, the first half of this book focuses on the new light medicine, with an emphasis on recent scientific and technological developments that are not only transforming our knowledge of light, but also bringing it into greater service for the purpose of health in an unprecedented way.

We will first examine how science has understood light throughout history, leading up to the latest insights in contemporary physics. Next, we will explore the new discoveries that have transformed our knowledge about how light affects our biology, opening the door to revolutionary medical applications and treatments. Since light can have a beneficial effect on our health, this implies that it can have an equally negative effect when used improperly. I will therefore touch on important questions regarding the health risks of light, including the appropriate use of light both from the sun and from the new sources of

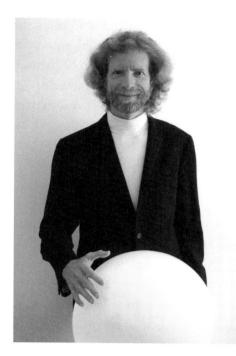

Author Anadi Martel
with the SensoSphere

artificial lighting, such as compact fluorescent light bulbs (CFLs) and LEDs.

We can easily intuit that light not only has an effect on the body, but also on the psyche. Therefore, the second half of this book investigates this more speculative dimension of the power of light, wherein the different facets of its effects on the energetic and cognitive dimensions of life are outlined. Here I touch on the subject of energy medicine, a science that is still young but growing rapidly. Energy medicine expands on the purely biochemical concepts of allopathic medicine, since it takes into account the close relationship between the living being and its energy fields. These of course include light, an energy field par excellence because of its electromagnetic nature. This knowledge will help us understand the workings of color medicine, called *chromotherapy,* an alternative light medicine still almost unknown to the general public. I introduce fascinating contemporary methods, many of which are a meeting ground for modern technology and older therapeutic traditions in which color is used, some dating back thousands of years.

The last part of this book concentrates on the cognitive influence that light has on the emotional, mental, and spiritual aspects of life. The vibrational nature of light brings us to a discussion of the universal phenomenon of resonance and its role in the healing power of light.

Following this, a few pages are devoted to an original subject connected to my own personal research in this domain, which I call *subjective light*. To conclude I offer certain considerations about the relationship between light and consciousness, by which light bestows on us its most precious gifts.

Light has a unique status in our reality. It belongs as much to the material dimension, as a source of energy that we all depend on, as it does to the nonmaterial plane, as a symbol of all that is most uplifting in our consciousness. An examination of these themes is to be found in both halves of this book, reflecting the double nature of light. In writing these lines, my sincere wish is that these two fundamental dimensions of light, one as much as the other, will awaken your interest.

ACKNOWLEDGMENTS

Special thanks to my friends Robert Purnam Dehin and Michel Saint-Germain for their precious guidance and support all along the writing process;

to Jacob Liberman for generously paving the way to the publication of this book;

to my translators Vidhan Carroll Guerin and Deva Boersma, who patiently endured my word-by-word revisions of their work;

to Lyn Doole, who reviewed the text with hawk-eyed precision;

to my close collaborator Ma Premo, who never ceased inspiring me to keep digging more deeply during our thirty-year exploration of light;

and to all my colleagues at the International Light Association for turning the discovery of light into an ongoing adventure.

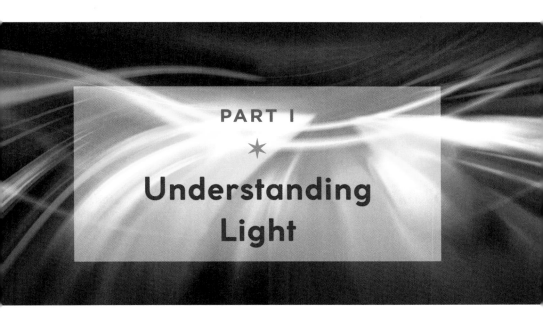

PART I

✳

Understanding Light

1

THE ORIGIN OF LIGHT THERAPY

Ancient and Modern Uses, Advancements, Controversies

You rise beautiful from the horizon on heaven, living disk,
origin of life.
You are fine, great, radiant, lofty over and above every land.
Your rays bind the lands to the limit of all you have made,
you are the sun, you have reached their limits.
You are distant, but your rays are on earth.

GREAT HYMN TO THE ATEN
(EGYPT, 14TH CENTURY BCE)

ALMOST ALL THE ENERGY that gives life to our planet comes from the light of the sun; thus it is only natural that this light has played an essential role for humankind since the beginning of time. Until just a few years ago I was unaware, however, of all the different aspects of this fascinating and close relationship. Some remarkable encounters with researchers I have met through the International Light Association changed this for me.

The ILA has many members who are exceptional historians of light therapy, and it is they who initiated me into this aspect of the field—Brian Breiling to be sure, the editor of the pioneering 1996 anthology *Light Years Ahead,* but also Jacob Liberman, Alexander Wunsch, and

Karl Ryberg, whom we speak of later. As they conducted their search, they accumulated a collection of rare documents and ancient books on light, a veritable treasure trove of information and anecdotes on the subject. Much of what follows has been inspired by their words.

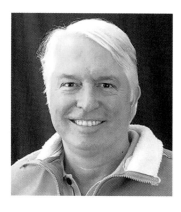

Figure 1.1.
Dr. Brian Breiling

LIGHT THERAPY IN ANTIQUITY

Few ancient civilizations are without a cult involving the sun, the importance of which is primordial in any hierarchy of gods. The sun is the source of life, abundance, eternity, wisdom, and, of course, light. We find gods of the sun everywhere we look, whether it be ancient Egypt, Babylonia, India, China, Greece, Rome, or the Celtic and Aztec civilizations. In some rare cases very precise facts have come down to us with regard to *heliotherapy*, practices involving the use of sunlight for medicinal purposes. It is quite likely that the majority of these ancient peoples had similar knowledge.

From Cults of the Sun to Heliotherapy
One of the oldest extant testimonials comes from the Egyptian Old Kingdom and dates from approximately 2600 BCE. It was attributed to the great sage Imhotep, the legendary architect of the Saqqara pyramids, and contains medical formulas that indicate a profound understanding of the effects of light. The importance accorded each moment of the day with regard to the appropriate treatment suggests an understanding of *chronobiology*, the science of biological rhythms controlled

by the cycle of the sun. The use of solar rays for the sterilization and drying of food is also mentioned, together with the photochemical activation of pharmaceutical preparations. Imhotep even practiced a technique known today as *photodynamic therapy* (discussed in chapter 5) through the application of photo-activated tar and resins.

The ancient Greeks were also fervent practitioners of heliotherapy. In 450 BCE, the great historian Herodotus described the use of solariums, areas of healing based on the light of the sun, stating that "being exposed to the sun is highly recommended for those people who need to regain their health." Hippocrates of Kos (460–370 BCE), the "Father of Medicine," insisted on the importance of light and the heat that emanates from it to fortify the bone structure as well as treat a multitude of ills, including rickets, obesity, and diverse metabolic disorders. He would cauterize scabs with the aid of light focused though crystal and quartz, which transmitted the photoactive ultraviolet rays. For the Greeks, the connection between light and health was clear: Asclepius, god of medicine and healing, is none other than the son of Apollo, god of the sun. The Greeks' cultural successors, the Romans, perpetuated this awareness. Their legal code contained "right to light" clauses guaranteeing people's access to sunlight in their homes, buildings that frequently featured a solarium. One of the great second-century physicians, Soranus of Ephesus, a Greek who practiced in

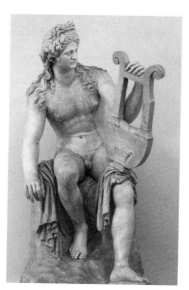

Figure 1.2. Apollo, god of light, music, and prophecy (photo by Marie-Lan Nguyen)

Rome, recommended exposing jaundiced newborns to the sun, thereby fore-shadowing modern neonatal jaundice treatments that use blue light.

From Heliotherapy to Chromotherapy

Another form of light medicine even more specific than heliotherapy is chromotherapy, the therapeutic use of color.

From the very beginning, humankind has demonstrated a great deal of ingenuity with regard to the creation and manipulation of color. Seventeen thousand years ago the artists of the Lascaux Caves knew how to prepare an attractive palette of colored pigments to accomplish their extraordinary work. The Egyptians demonstrated great respect for the power of color, as demonstrated in the very precise and codified iconographic use of various hues that can still be seen in Egyptian bas-reliefs and works on papyrus. Temples and statues were painted in the liveliest tones. The extraordinary monochromatic iridescence of the scarab gave it a divine status in its representation of Khepri, the solar aspect of the great god Ra. The Egyptians also had a highly refined cosmetic art, the products of which, including extravagantly colored powders and creams, were exported throughout the ancient world. Precious stones, objects of the purest and most translucent colors to which they had access, were used in sacred rituals and for healing.

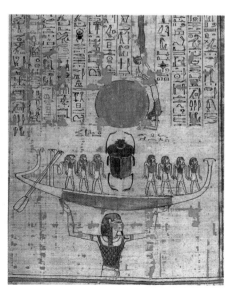

Figure 1.4. The sacred scarab Khepri, a solar deity

The "Evolution" of Color

Our extreme sensitivity to color is encoded in our genes as a result of an evolutionary process dating back hundreds of millions of years that informs our sense of vision. Zoologist Andrew Parker (2003) has developed a hypothesis known as the *light switch theory*. This theory concerns the enigma known in paleontology as the Cambrian explosion; 543 million years ago, at the beginning of the Cambrian era, a 3-billion-years-long evolutionary process had led to the appearance of only three animal phyla (the highest level of taxonomic rank below kingdom). Barely five million years later—a mere wink in the geological scale of things—thirty-eight phyla were in existence, a number that has hardly changed since that time. This fact has not been properly explained by the larger scientific community; however, Parker says the explanation is directly linked to the appearance of the sense of vision. Until that time many creatures had been well equipped with photosensitive cells in their organs (even bacteria had some) that were capable of distinguishing between light and dark. But the first creature known to have possessed a real eye—that is, a system of vision capable of perceiving an image—is the trilobite (Schoenemann et al. 2017), a little arthropod no longer in existence today, but whose appearance on the evolutionary scale corresponds exactly to the beginning of the Cambrian explosion. Because vision gave such an advantage to those creatures who had managed this step forward, it produced a veritable "arms race" among all animal life of that era, resulting in a hitherto unseen acceleration of the evolutionary process.

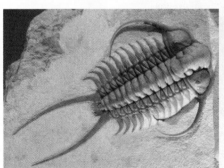 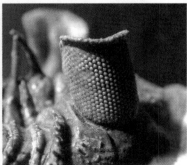

Figure 1.3. Left, the trilobite (photo by Tim Evanson) and right, its eye
(photo courtesy Moussa Direct Ltd.)

Whatever happened exactly, there is no doubt that as a result of the emergence of vision a multitude of vegetal as well as animal life-forms adorned with an infinite variety of colored features began to appear. Whether to attract or to threaten, the more intense a color in terms of standing out from the background environment, the more chance it had to be perceived by this extraordinary new sense of vision.

Life-forms responded by developing a great number of *chromophores*, which are portions of biological molecules absorbing or reflecting light in a selective manner to produce a variety of different colored pigments. Also emerging were regular networks at the microscopic level that interfered directly with light rays to obtain structural colors that are of a perfectly pure iridescence, such as those in the feathers of a peacock or a hummingbird. Simultaneously occurring within this dance of evolution, the eyes and their interconnecting visual brain structures refined their sensitivity in such a way as to enable them to detect with ever greater precision the whole spectrum of visible color and beyond.

And so it is for humans. The most brilliant colors fascinate us and inevitably attract us. For some civilizations these colors acquire properties that are almost supernatural. For example, those objects considered most essential and precious in the afterlife were carefully laid out in the tombs of the Cro-Magnons: next to food, arms, and talismans, one finds vividly colored beads.

India possesses an ancient and rich tradition of chromotherapy dating from at least 1500 BCE, according to the Atharvan Veda, which emphasizes the healing power of the colored rays of the sun. The very sophisticated traditional curative system known as ayurveda considers color to be a key element in its therapeutic arsenal—of the same importance as food and medicinal remedies—and it is to be applied as much to the skin as to the visual system.

In the encyclopedic *Canon of Medicine,* completed in 1025, the great Persian physician Ibn Sīnā (known as Avicenna) gave much importance to the role of color for both diagnostic and treatment

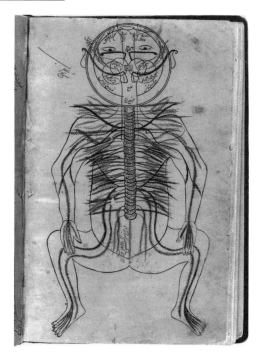

Figure 1.5. Page from Avicenna's *Canon of Medicine*
(photo courtesy Wellcome Images)

purposes. For example, he says that red stimulates the circulation of the blood, blue cools it, and yellow reduces inflammation and muscular pain.

My colleague Karl Ryberg, in *Living Light: On the Origin of Colours* (2010), a historical treatise on light therapy, points out that Avicenna benefited from the unsurpassed expertise of the glass workers of the Arabian world, who succeeded in creating panels of tinted glass of an unprecedented chromatic purity and translucence, far superior to the more opaque glasswork that had been made in an earlier time by the Egyptians or Babylonians. Of special interest is that Avicenna devised a treatment alcove that allowed his patients to bathe in the rays of the sun that were filtered by glass panels of these new crystalline colors.

To have perfected the technique of producing such colored glass was significant because it gave impetus to the healing potential of colored light. The Venetians, whose commercial empire held a monopoly on this technology imported from the Orient, jealously guarded their privilege. The artisans of Murano, who still create their celebrated Venetian glass, were held to secrecy under pain of death with regard to their technique. Inevitably, the secret got out, and from the twelfth century on the most stunning stained glass windows made their appearance in the churches and cathedrals of Europe. The incomparable purity of their light was considered to be of heavenly origin, and they became an essential element in the great Gothic cathedrals, offering grandiose masterpieces such as the rose windows of Chartres, or Notre-Dame in Paris. It is said that when people suffering from physical or mental ailments were exposed to the rays filtered through the stained glass, they experienced peace and harmony, which brought unparalleled healing.

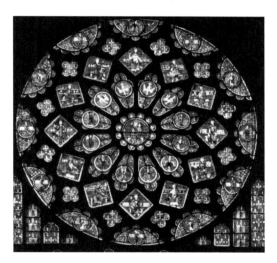

Figure 1.6. The Great Rose Window of Chartres Cathedral
(photo by Harmonia Amanda)

The Cultural Role of Color

Colors have had widely different interpretations and uses around the world depending on the era and the culture. Take, for example, the caste system of the Hindus, among the world's oldest forms of social stratification, where the priest or Brahman class would be robed in white, the Kshatriya warrior class in red, the Vaisya merchant class in yellow, and the Sudra, or untouchable class, clad in black or blue.

In ancient times, the exclusive color of the Roman emperor and his consuls was purple. Among Celtic people, the naked warrior would smear himself with a layer of blue dye, which purportedly offered invincible protection, whereas the Druids wore pure green. In China, only the emperor had the right to use yellow, a color reserved for the descendants of the sun. In Islamic countries, the color of the Prophet Mohammed is green, a symbol of fertility and victory in a desert culture.

There are also wide variations in the use of color in funeral customs: whereas black is the accepted color in the West, white is the appropriate color in China. In Mexico it is yellow, and for the Native American it is red. It is the same with regard to colors associated with the primordial elements. For the Greeks, fire, air, water, earth, and ether are red, yellow, white, black, and transparent or clear, respectively; for the Tibetans these colors are, respectively, red, green, white, yellow, and blue.

Can one therefore conclude that because of all the differences these time-honored interpretations of color have no real validity? Certainly not! The interpretations and associations are perfectly intelligible within the specific cultural context in which they arise, though the ancient systems of chromotherapy can appear incoherent or fragmentary at first. Emerging entirely from purely empirical observation and necessarily limited by their cultural and historical context, they offer in general an inextricable mixture of elements coming from the multiplicity of ways in which light influences us. This leads to muddled models in which science and superstition overlap—a circumstance which no doubt has always been connected with the human condition but, from our point of view as contemporaries, was more pronounced in ancient times.

To better understand this, it's useful to look at the three distinct types of therapeutic influence of light, a subject we'll consider in greater detail throughout this book.

THE THREE TYPES OF THERAPEUTIC INFLUENCES EMANATING FROM LIGHT

* The first type of influence color exerts is biophysical in nature; that is, connected to the effects of light on the biochemistry of

cells and on the overall visual and hormonal systems. This type of action is the one most readily investigated by science, and today the new field of light medicine is elucidating this influence with ever greater clarity.

* The second type of influence is of an energetic nature and relates to the interaction between light and the systems of subtle energy ascribed to life. This can, for example, be described as interactions with the system of meridians found in acupuncture or, more generally, as interactions with the internal network of energy fields that keeps us alive. This way of viewing living processes as being connected to fields will be described in greater detail in chapter 7.

* The third type of influence is of a psychological and symbolic nature, which derives from ancient associations with light and color proceeding from millions of years of human evolution, from our specific cultural environment (with its different conventions relative to color, as we have seen), and also from our personal history, including our individual preferences and aversions with regard to color. Although this kind of influence is admittedly subjective, it nonetheless represents a profound influence on our health, both physical and mental. A good example is what science calls the placebo effect; that is, the influence of mind on matter. It suggests a psychology of color and in a larger sense informs us of the relationship between light and consciousness.

LIGHT THERAPY IN MODERN TIMES

The advent of the Age of Enlightenment in eighteenth-century Europe, followed by the birth of modern science, sparked interest in defining the effects of therapeutic light in a more objective, systematic way. Building on a better understanding of the properties of light, as well as on advances in medicine taking shape at this time, new methods were introduced that were more clearly delimited within the three types of influence of light we've just described, lifting some of the overlap between science and superstition found in antiquity.

In 1810, poet Johann Wolfgang von Goethe published his *Theory*

The Many Names of Light Therapy

Various words have been used to designate the application of therapeutic light, but the definitions are often unclear, which can lead to some confusion. The following list defines the terminology used in this book.

Light Therapy: A general term that encompasses all forms of therapy that use light

Phototherapy: Therapy that depends on artificial sources of light

Heliotherapy: Therapy that employs the light of the sun

Chromotherapy: Therapy that uses the specific influences of different colors from the visible spectrum

Bright Light Therapy: Therapy that uses relatively intense light sources to influence one's chronobiology (often erroneously identified as *light therapy* in common literature)

Low Level Laser Therapy (LLLT): Therapy that uses red and near-infrared light to boost cellular metabolism (now called **photobiomodulation**)

Actinotherapy: Therapy that uses the ultraviolet part of the light spectrum

Thermotherapy: Therapy that uses the infrared part of the spectrum through its calorific effect

---

of Colours, in which he made a study of color from the perceptual point of view rather than the physical, opening the way for the development of a psychology of color. One of his most important contributions is the symmetrical color wheel, wherein the deep reds and violets at both ends of the rainbow that correspond to the limits of our visual perception are joined and fused in magenta, a *synthetic color* that does not match with any actual physical color within the rainbow.

In the nineteenth century, the Industrial Revolution and the development of new manufacturing processes led to previously unknown problems of public health. These were oftentimes the result of a chronic, long-term lack of light experienced by people living in the smog of manufacturing cities who worked long hours in factories without seeing the light of day. This contributed to a host of maladies, among them rickets, arthritis, tuberculosis, paralysis, and scurvy, all

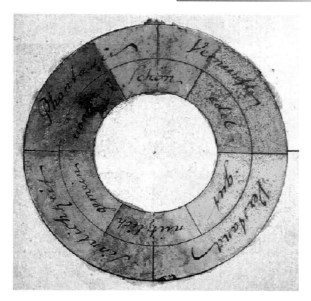

Figure 1.7. Goethe's color wheel

stemming from chronic deficiencies, including light, such that many doctors resorted to a renewal of the ancient practice of heliotherapy.

A Return to the Sun

In 1860, when the Florence Nightingale School for nurses first opened, the institution's by then well-known British namesake taught nurses the importance of being exposed to sunlight, as well as the significance of fresh air and of cleanliness in hospitals. In 1869, the German ophthalmologist Hermann Cohn established the relationship between the lack of light in schools and the development of nearsightedness in children. And in the early 1900s, at a time when Europe was ravaged with tuberculosis, Swiss doctor Auguste Rollier, known as "the Sun Doctor," opened therapeutic centers located at high altitudes, where he exposed his patients to controlled doses of ultraviolet light emitted by the sun. At a time when the only existing medical treatment consisted of surgery, where fewer than 50 percent of patients survived, Dr. Rollier performed miracles. In 1916 he published a treatise titled *La Cure de soleil et de travail à la clinique militaire suisse de Leysin* (The Sun Cure).

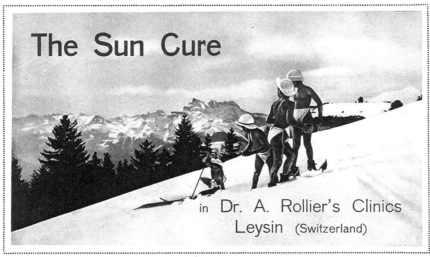

Figure 1.8. Rollier's Sun Cure (from a 1921 brochure)

Contemporary to Rollier, Danish doctor Niels Ryberg Finsen, called the "Father of Phototherapy," began in 1890 to explore the effects of the different portions of the light spectrum in a systematic way. Finsen himself suffered from a metabolic disorder, Niemann-Pick disease, which inspired him to sunbathe and investigate the effects of light on living things. Working in Scandanavia, where there is very little sunlight during a major portion of the year, Finsen developed different types of artificial light sources for use in his healing procedures. His method of treating Lupus vulgaris, a form of tuberculosis of the skin resulting in lesions of the nose, eyelids, lips, cheeks, ears, and neck, was to use blue filters to concentrate the short waves of the light spectrum. Finsen thought that the curative properties were due to a sterilization effect of the ultraviolet light, but in a notable recent discovery, research has shown that Finsen's filters in fact blocked the ultraviolet rays, and that it was rather the blue light that functioned in the treatment. Whatever the case may be, Finsen's success for those patients who would otherwise have had no hope was such that he was chosen in 1903 to be one of the very first to receive the Nobel Prize in Medicine.

In 1910, American physician John Harvey Kellogg (creator,

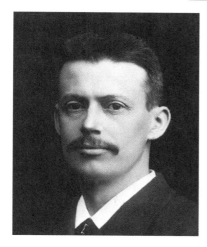

Figure 1.9.
Niels Ryberg Finsen

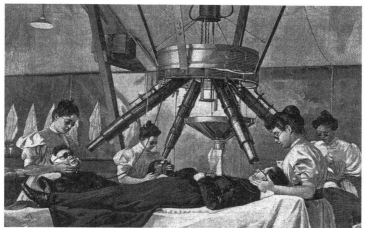

Figure 1.10. Finsen's "light elves" applying a treatment

together with his brother, of the popular cereals that bear his name) published his book *Light Therapeutics*. He designed a wide range of phototherapeutic inventions, including visible, infrared, and ultraviolet light sources, to treat different maladies. One such invention was an ultraviolet lamp that could be "swallowed" to treat problems of the throat (see fig. 1.11). Another of his inventions was his incandescent light bath, designed in the early 1890s, which was partly motivated by the overcast skies of Michigan, and which he used to treat thousands of his patients at his Battle Creek Sanitarium (see fig. 1.12).

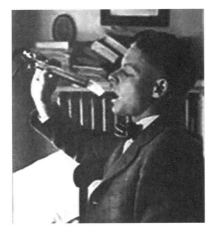

Figure 1.11. Kellogg's "swallowed" ultraviolet light

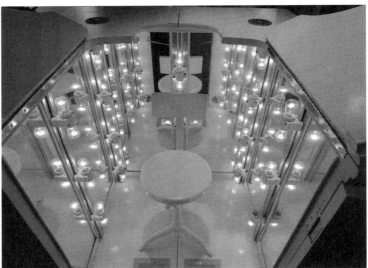

Figure 1.12. John Harvey Kellogg's radiant heat bath, patented in 1896, on display at the United States Patent and Trade Office (photo by Fuzheado)

The Rediscovery of Chromotherapy

Around this same time, American researchers rediscovered the value of the ancient practice of chromotherapy, the specific healing influences of different colors from the visible spectrum. In 1876, Augustus James Pleasonton, a militia general during the American Civil War, published *The Influence of the Blue Ray of the Sunlight and of the Blue Colour of the Sky,* in which he describes his experiments dealing with the effects of different colored lights on plants, animals, and humans. Pleasonton accomplished some of these by means of hothouses equipped with glass of blue and green hues, which tripled the growth rate of grapes.

Influenced by the work of Pleasonton and others at this time, Dr. Seth Pancoast published his *Blue and Red Light; or, Light and Its Rays as Medicine* in 1877. But the most eminent of all light therapists using chromotherapy in the nineteenth century is surely Dr. Edwin Babbitt, whose comprehensive volume *The Principles of Light and Color,* published in 1878, would influence a whole generation (see fig. 1.14). In it Babbitt expounds on a complex theory of the effects of light by extrapolating the fragmentary facts available in that era with regard to the nature of atoms and electromagnetic waves. Babbitt was able to produce, at minimal cost, items that could be sent by post, such as the Chromolume, a device that could project colored light by using interchangeable tinted glass panels. There was also a smaller version, called a Chromo-Disk, as well as a Chromo Lens, a flask made of colored glass used for "charging" drinking water.

The various theories of these early light-therapy pioneers were often based on the spiritualist notions then in vogue, the relevance of which has not survived in modern times, so their work is now of greater interest more from a historical perspective than from a therapeutic

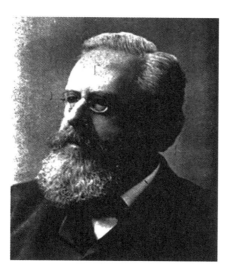

Figure 1.13.
Dr. Edwin Babbitt

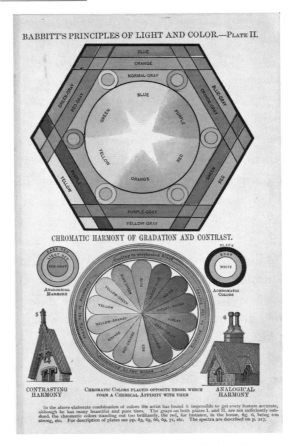

Figure 1.14. A page from Babbitt's
The Principles of Light and Color

point of view. Nevertheless, they opened the door to more modern and still-relevant research, such as that carried out by Dinshah Ghadiali (1933) and Harry Riley Spitler (1941).

In 1897, while he was still in India, his native land, Dinshah Ghadiali conducted research on the healing power of color following a remarkable experience that was to change the course of his medical career: through applications of indigo light, he was able to save a young woman who was severely ill with advanced dysentery. By 1920, after Dinshah had relocated to the United States, he created a sophisticated system of chromotherapy that he called *Spectro-Chrome*. He based his system on more scientifically solid ground than his predecessors had, having benefited from the new science of spectroscopy that revealed how the various elements of the periodic table each emitted specific colors (see chapter 10). He could then associate each color with properties connected to those of physical compounds that spectroscopically emitted similar colors. He defined a set of twelve principal colors covering the visible spectrum and matched them to standardized filters of tinted glass, from which he established different procedures appropriate to the treatment of many different illnesses. As this technique became well known, it was adopted by a number of physicians and remained available until the beginning of the 1940s.

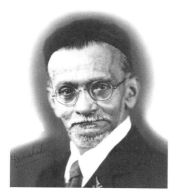

Figure 1.15.
Dinshah Ghadiali

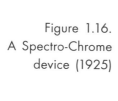

Figure 1.16.
A Spectro-Chrome
device (1925)

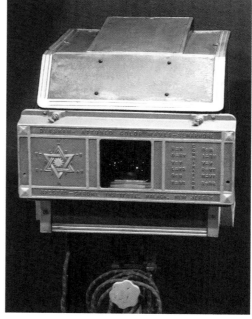

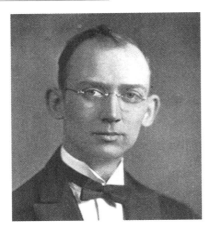

Figure 1.17.
Harry Riley Spitler

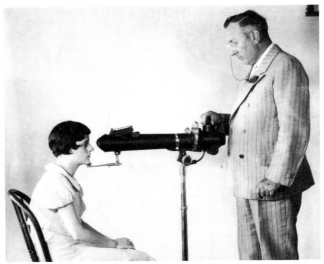

Figure 1.18. Spitler's Syntonizer (shown here with a patient
and the device's co-inventor, Dr. Alex Cameron, 1935)

The American medical doctor Harry Riley Spitler, in the 1920s, developed his method of syntonic optometry. *Syntony* means "to bring into balance." Spitler used a technique based on the direct application of colored light to the eye. He was the first researcher to give major importance to the use of color in reestablishing the equilibrium of the autonomic nervous system, the lack of which, according to his syntonic principle, was the origin of many chronic illnesses (a subject covered in greater detail in chapter 9). He developed his Syntonizer device for ocular light stimulation (see fig. 1.18). His system was of particular interest to eye-care professionals, and by 1933 more than a thousand optometrists were using it with great success.

The Golden Age of Light Therapy

As a result of the work of the pioneers just mentioned, by the beginning of the twentieth century different methods of light therapy were being routinely used in Europe and the Americas. These methods were offered in the context of a host of medical specialties, including psychiatry, optometry, and chiropractic. Many clinics that used heliotherapy were opened, and Auguste Rollier alone was the director of fourteen hospitals totaling more than a thousand beds. Many psychiatric hospitals were equipped with colored rooms—a red one to treat "chronic melancholy" (including depression and insomnia) and a blue room to benefit those suffering from mania and alcoholism.

Psychologist Brian Breiling (1996) calls the period from 1860 to 1938 "the golden age of light therapy," while he dubs the period that succeeded it, from 1938 to 1980, "the era of darkness" with respect to widespread acceptance of light therapy. The year of demarcation, 1938, was when the first antibiotic, penicillin, appeared on the medical scene. The subsequent pharmaceutical revolution, with its miracle drugs that healed the worst illnesses in a few days, was soon to completely overshadow other, more natural therapeutic approaches such as light therapy, which took longer to show healing effects, and which were also less reliable in producing the desired results.

There is no doubt that the development of pharmaceutical medicine has been beneficial beyond measure to public health. A large number of otherwise fatal illnesses have effectively disappeared from the world, and most people can look forward to a much longer life span. And now genetic medicine, the latest carrier of the scientific flame, encourages us to look forward to an even more spectacular future.

Darkness Descends

The rise of pharmacological approaches after 1938 quickly eclipsed the use of light therapy in medicine, a process that did not happen in a completely reasonable way. Light therapy is based on a holistic approach to healing. This is at odds with the mechanistic approach of orthodox science that now controls modern medicine. The witch hunt by the medical establishment began in earnest in the 1930s.

In the United States, the magnates of the new industrial pharmaceutical companies that were cropping up financed the publication of the *Flexner Report* in 1910. The aim of the report was to discredit all therapeutic approaches its publishers considered unscientific, including naturopathy and homeopathy and, by extension, light therapy. Throughout the early to mid-1900s the U.S. Food and Drug Administration, under pressure by the pharmaceutical industry's already powerful lobbying groups, gradually succeeded in rendering illegal the majority of practices involving light therapy, systematically assailing its principal representatives. Harry Riley Spitler was forced to close his school, and his Syntonizer light devices were declared illegal and banned from being transported from one state to another (although the syntonic optometrists cleverly got around this interdiction by transporting their instruments in detached pieces). Dinshah Ghadiali, who was pursued in American courts in 1931, narrowly escaped condemnation thanks to the eloquent testimonies of some physicians using his technique, such as that of surgeon Kate Baldwin (1927), who stated, "After 37 years of active hospital and private practice in medicine and surgery, I produce quicker and more accurate results using Spectro-Chrome than with any other methods, and there was less strain on the patient." However, Dinshah was not so fortunate the next time. He was charged again in 1947 and was forced to close his institute and destroy all his books, documents, and research papers (only one copy survived). In 1958, the FDA served him with a permanent injunction, which even by the time of his death in 1966 had not been lifted. In fact, it is still in place today, and because of this many of his original publications have been out of print for decades.

There is no doubt that Dinshah was not entirely innocent in attracting the wrath of the medical establishment: he had never hesitated to criticize it vigorously, and his scientific method was certainly not entirely beyond reproach. But it would have been far wiser to try to understand the basis of the beneficial effects of light that he had started to uncover than to set about destroying and erasing all traces of his life's work.

By the beginning of the 1950s, the majority of outlets for the practice of light therapy had disappeared from hospitals and clinics throughout the world, and those who still dared to practice this technique had to do so more or less undercover. What a change in just a few short years, as illustrated by the following: An advertisement in a 1927 edition of the *Journal of the American Medical Association* (the official publication of the American Medical Association) contains the praiseworthy statement, "Light is to Health and Happiness as Darkness is to Disease and Despair." A February 2000 edition of the same journal offers the following: "The therapeutic efficacy for infrared, ultraviolet and low energy laser therapies has not been sufficiently established to permit recommendation" (Bello and Phillips 2000).

One hundred and fifty years of medical treatments using therapeutic light were thus obliterated.

THE NEW AGE OF LIGHT

Luckily for our story, a new starting point began with the emergence in the 1980s of what Brian Breiling (1996) calls "the new age of light." It had already been foreseen through the work of those like photobiologist Dr. John Nash Ott, who in the 1970s was able to establish the importance of biological considerations when evaluating the quality of artificial light sources. Ott showed that artificial lights often have a deficient spectra, thus provoking what he called *malillumination,* an environmental condition characterized by the absence of full-spectrum light. Other significant research included that of Dr. Fritz Hollwich, a German ophthalmologist who published a trailblazing book in 1979 titled *The Influence of Ocular Light Perception on Metabolism in Man and in Animal*. Norman Rosenthal et al. (1984) studied the relationship between the lack of light and depression, coining the term *seasonal affective disorder,* or SAD, to describe this condition. And Michael Terman et al. (1988) explored the use of *bright light therapy* as a treatment of SAD, which opened the door to a renewed interest in research on chronobiology.

Today's syntonic optometrists, who now number more than

1,300 professionals worldwide, are continuing the work of Harry Riley Spitler, reexamining the work of the past to promote the worldwide diffusion of this technique.

Meanwhile, the son of Dinshah Ghadiali, Darius Dinshah, continues the work of his father, whose institute he has reopened. Some therapists, such as Dr. Alexander Wunsch, a German physician of holistic medicine and *photobiology*, are reviving the Spectro-Chrome system, but with more efficient and proficient means based on modern light sources that are far more effective than those that were available to Dinshah himself.

In 1986, American optometrist John Downing developed a new pulsating light device, the Lumatron (see fig. 1.20), which later on led to the development of the Photron light therapy unit—the very same device that Brian Breiling demonstrated to me in his home in California. Both these devices can help reestablish the equilibrium of the autonomic nervous system according to Downing's theory of neurosensory development.

Finally, in 1990, Dr. Jacob Liberman published his book *Light: Medicine of the Future,* which has since become one of the most popular books of all time on vision and chromotherapy.

Key Discoveries

Scientific research on the biophysical influence of light has led to some of the most prominent discoveries in recent years. In 1995, biologist Tiina Karu, head of the Laboratory of Laser Biology and Medicine of the Russian Academy of Sciences, published her discovery of the main component in the regenerative action of light on our cells, the cytochrome c oxidase enzyme. Her undeniable evidence for the existence of this regenerative process, which she calls *photobiomodulation,* has rekindled a global interest in the biological effects of light. In 2002, Samer Hattar et al. announced in the journal *Science* their discovery of a new type of photosensitive cell in the retina, until then unknown, revealing the missing link that explains the influence of light on our hormonal system.

Beginning in the 1990s, the American space agency NASA, as well as its Russian counterpart, has been showing great interest in the

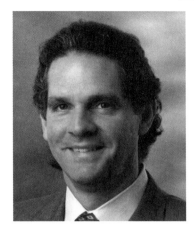

Figure 1.19.
Dr. John Downing

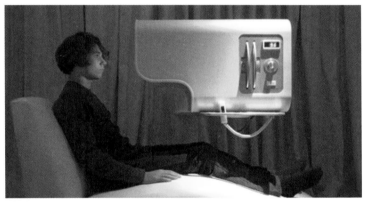

Figure 1.20. The Lumatron Light Stimulator (1986)
(© Dr. John Downing)

medical potential of light for astronauts undergoing space travel. The goal is to produce devices for healing and regeneration that are small and lightweight enough to be operable in space. The initial financial investments that have been made in this area have contributed significantly to stimulating the new wave of research.

Recently, curious to know the magnitude of actual research being done on therapeutic light, I conducted a small inquiry using Google Scholar, which indexes a repository of scientific articles published all over the world. One finding was particularly relevant: the number of articles in the "Medicine and Pharmacology" category containing the keywords related to my search: *light, health, color,* and *therapy.* It was of particular interest to me to note that although only a few dozen articles or so per year could be found from the 1980s, we are suddenly confronted with an acceleration in publications in this area beginning in 1995, with consistent progression increasing to some 10,000 articles per year at this present time. Furthermore, this number represents 5 percent of the total for the entire "Medicine and Pharmacology" category—a remarkably sizable proportion. So we are now witnessing a veritable explosion of scientific research in this field, heralding a new "medicine of light" that is unfolding before our eyes.

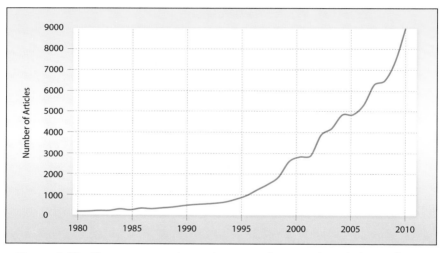

Figure 1.21. The exponential acceleration of research in light medicine

The Future of Light Medicine

A new generation of researchers is pressing up against the old boundaries zealously imposed by the medical establishment, delving into what is broadly known as *energy medicine* and opening vast new domains of study previously rejected by the mechanistic and reductionist approach that dominated institutionalized science for the last century. These researchers are often found at the forefront of their specialty and have been incorporating such fields as bioelectronics, quantum mechanics, and neurophysiology in their exploration of the interaction between living organisms and energy fields such as light (more on this in chapter 7). They have been uncovering a level of sensitivity and complexity in these interactions hitherto unimaginable.

This emerging paradigm naturally faces great resistance. The medical establishment is one of the largest enterprises of our society. Its sheer size generates enormous inertia that is driven by economic and political interests that very few people continue to consider impartial. The pharmaceutical industry behemoth—Big Pharma, as it has come to be known—behaves according to its nature and therefore does everything in its power to maintain the status quo, investing some $230 million a year in the United States for lobbying purposes alone, more than any other industry.

Apart from the economic pressures brought by the pharmaceutical industry, scientists have a very human tendency to reject that which goes beyond their conditioning, acquired from a long and arduous formal education. And since scientists have become the priests of our modern world, public opinion and the media can do nothing other than obey their wise counsel.

Regardless, even this kind of resistance cannot stop the inevitable. Biologist James Oschman (2015), author of the groundbreaking book *Energy Medicine: The Scientific Basis,* expresses this eloquently. He says the amount of research carried out on the energetic properties of life has already attained such critical mass that it has now become impossible for any reasonable scientist to ignore this field of inquiry, so the scientific world is gradually being forced to shift. The energetic influence of light, an essential aspect of its nature, although still largely ignored by conventional medicine, is destined to assume a place of growing importance in the near future. The story behind some of these new and wonderful developments will be told in the chapters that follow.

2

A SHORT HISTORY OF THE SCIENCE OF LIGHT

Revelations from Crucial Experiments

All these fifty years of conscious brooding have brought me no nearer to the answer to the question "What are light quanta?" Nowadays, every Tom, Dick, and Harry thinks he knows it, but he is mistaken.

ALBERT EINSTEIN, IN A LETTER TO
HIS FRIEND MICHELE BESSO, 1954

PRECISELY ONE THOUSAND YEARS AGO, the great Arab polymath Ibn al-Haytham (aka Alhazen) was the first to propose a coherent scientific theory of light in his *Book of Optics*. Based on the ancient works of Euclid, Ptolemy, and Aristotle, he conceptualized light as linear rays, the trajectories of which he studied in detail using mirrors and lenses.

Alhazen's works, translated into Latin, inspired generations of researchers in Europe, including Galileo. The latter, in 1609, created his first telescope based on models that two Dutch glassmakers had tried to patent the year before.

It was in 1666 that Isaac Newton, while attempting to improve a similar sort of optical instrument, obtained a magnificent spectrum of colors, like a rainbow. This he achieved by passing plain white light through a prism. Others had done this before, but Newton was the

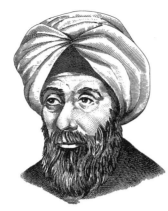

Figure 2.1.
Ibn al-Haytham

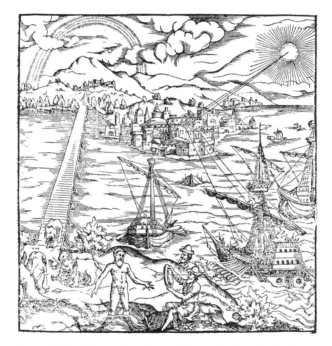

Figure 2.2. Illustration from Alhazen's *Book of Optics*

first to show that all these colors were actually contained in white light, a discovery he confirmed by sending the colored spectrum through a second inverted prism to reconstitute the white light. This demonstration is so pertinent in science that it is referred to as his *experimentum crucis,* his "crucial experiment" (see fig. 2.3).

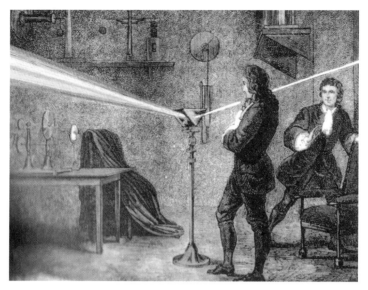

Figure 2.3. Isaac Newton and his *experimentum crucis*

LIGHT HAS LENGTH

Though he found that each color as it passes through a prism bends at a different angle, Newton could not explain this fact within the context of the model he had devised, in which light is composed of small particles. We must wait till 1801, when English physician and physicist Thomas Young demonstrated experimentally that light is a wave, with peaks and valleys of intensity, like a ripple on the surface of water, and that the length of the wave varies according to the color. Remarkably, Young was able to measure that length: it goes from 0.0004 millimeters in the case of violet to 0.0007 millimeters for red. Young further deduced how, when going through Newton's prism, a light wave is deflected according to its wavelength.

In his most famous experiment, Young had light from a single source pass through two narrow slits while he examined the effect of the projections on a screen placed beyond the slits. He observed a surprising result: alternating patterns of lighter and darker bands. Only one conclusion was possible: the waves from the two slits overlapped, combining their peaks and valleys in what is called an *interference*

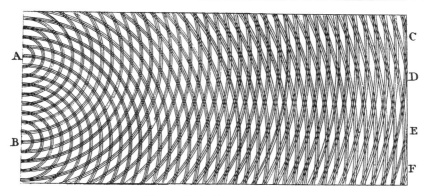

Figure 2.4. Young's slits

pattern. One can easily visualize this phenomenon with the analogy of waves on water. Imagine a calm lake into which two stones are dropped near to each other: circular waves will expand from the point of impact until they meet and overlap—just as light waves did when passing through Young's slits. Later we will come back to this experiment, which in its great simplicity reveals more than just one secret.

LIGHT HAS SPEED

By synthesizing and building on the research of his contemporaries, including Charles-Augustin de Coulomb, André-Marie Ampère, Michael Faraday, and Carl Friedrich Gauss, Scottish physicist James Clerk Maxwell published in 1861 his equations describing the behavior of electric and magnetic fields. In the years that followed, Maxwell came to realize that these equations reveal that these fields propagate in the form of waves, and furthermore that electric and magnetic fields can become associated in such a way that they are perpendicular to one another to form a joint wave called an *electromagnetic wave* (see fig. 2.6). The orientation of the two fields determines the direction of *polarization*, which is always perpendicular to the direction in which the wave is traveling.

Maxwell was even able to calculate the speed of these waves, in the order of 300,000 kilometers per second.* As it happened, a few years

---

*The precise value of the speed of light in a vacuum is 299,792,458 meters per second.

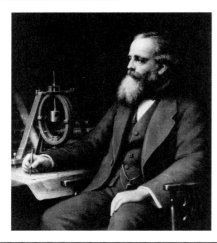

Figure 2.5.
James Clerk Maxwell

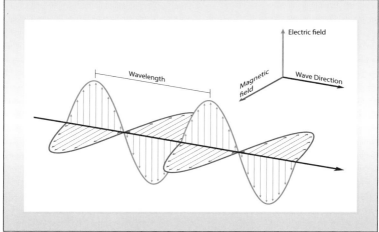

Figure 2.6. The electromagnetic wave

earlier, in 1850, French physicist Léon Foucault had measured the speed of light with greater precision than had ever been achieved previously and had obtained the same value. So it was revealed that light had to be a form of this new kind of electrical wave!

With regard to this remarkable discovery Einstein wrote the following in 1940:

> The precise formulation of the time-space laws was the work of Maxwell. Imagine his feelings when the differential equations he

had formulated proved to him that electromagnetic fields spread in the form of polarized waves, and at the speed of light! To few men in the world has such an experience been vouchsafed . . . it took physicists some decades to grasp the full significance of Maxwell's discovery, so bold was the leap that his genius forced upon the conceptions of his fellow workers.

For nineteenth-century physicists, light waves, like waves that travel on water, had to have a static surrounding medium in which to move. They called this hypothetical substance filling space *ether,* but research on its mysterious nature brought up more and more contradictions. The final blow was struck by an experiment by American scientists Albert Michelson and Edward Morley. In 1887, they attempted to measure the speed of the "wind" created as Earth moves through this ether,* which is assumed to be stationary. No ether was detected, and the speed of light remained constant regardless of the movement of its source. This absolute constancy has since then been confirmed to the extreme precision of one part per 10^{17}.

LIGHT IS ENERGY

Drawing inspiration from this paradoxical property of light, Albert Einstein published his first theory of relativity in 1905. Rather than look for a cause for this behavior of light, Einstein considered it to be a fundamental law of nature, and he imagined a model of the world from this perspective. In doing so he had to take into account another empirically confirmed fact: namely, that the laws of physics remain constant regardless of the speed of an observer. Thus a physicist making

---

*To attain this the two scientists built a device with two perpendicular arms on which they shined the light from a single source that then recombined to make an interference pattern (as Young had done). If one arm is aligned with the direction of Earth moving though ether, and the other is perpendicular, their rays of light would take slightly different times to reach the target, and this minuscule difference would be detectable in the interference fringe pattern. But regardless of how they rotated their device (which was floating on liquid mercury), the light always traveled at the same speed in both arms.

a measurement pertaining to a particular system will obtain the same result whether he is moving in relation to that system or not.

Focusing on just these two postulates—the constancy of the speed of light and the invariance of the laws of nature with regard to the movement of an observer—Einstein made a series of crucial deductions. Time and space as perceived by an observer can become compressed or stretched, and the mass of moving objects tends toward infinity as they approach the speed of light—a speed that henceforth can never be surpassed. A few months later, Einstein further deduced the extraordinary relationship between energy and mass at rest, a discovery now known as the famous $E = mc^2$ equation.

It is hard for us to conceptualize this peculiar constancy of the speed of light. For example, in our world if two trains are hurtling toward each other, both traveling at speed v, they will collide at twice the speed of v, or $2v$. But if two rays of light, each traveling at speed c—the symbol used to denote the speed of light in a vacuum—are heading toward each other, then time and space are modified in such a way that their relative speed will remain at c (see fig. 2.7). This strange behavior indicates the extent to which light, even if it is so familiar and ever present around us, arises out of a very different reality from our material world.

In fact, the speed limit c is not as much a property of light as it is of space itself. An analogy can be made if we imagine a slope along which a current of water will spontaneously flow; this natural movement at the

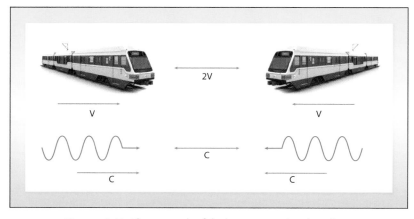

Figure 2.7. The speed of light, c, an absolute limit

speed c is that which all particles unencumbered by mass (such as light photons, which have zero mass) will flow freely in the vacuum of space-time. In the Earth's atmosphere light slows down by about 90 kilometers per second and in water by as much as 200,000 kilometers per second. It is even possible to stop it completely in a superfluid, an environment composed of magnetically confined atoms, as Danish physicist Lene Vestergaard Hau managed to observe in 2001.

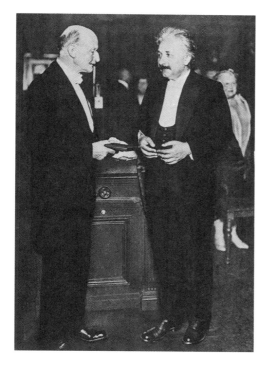

Figure 2.8. Max Planck offering the Planck Medal to Albert Einstein, 1929

THE BIRTH OF THE PHOTON

The year 1905 was a very fertile one for Einstein,* as it was also then that he published his explanation of the photoelectric effect, which says that light is composed of small packets of energy. Already in 1900

---

*It was in this *annus mirabilis*—Latin for "wonderful year"—that Einstein, age twenty-five, published four articles that changed the course of physics; besides the theory of special relativity and the photoelectric effect, the other two are concerned with the Brownian motion and the mass-energy equivalence $E = mc^2$.

his mentor, German theoretical physicist Max Planck, had introduced the idea that light behaves as if it is formed from a stream of separate, individual packets, called *quanta*. He arrived at this conclusion by analyzing the theoretical radiation emitted by a *black body*, an idealized object that reflects no color (hence its name), the emission of which is entirely produced by its own heat. Such an object is of great interest to physicists, as it is a good approximation of thermal sources of light, which are objects with temperatures sufficiently hot to make them glow. Examples would be fire, the sun itself, and, in our homes, incandescent light bulbs.

To describe the emission coming from a luminous object we must examine the *intensity* of all the individual colors that it is radiating. The result is a curve of the light intensity versus its wavelength, called an *emission spectrum*. Quite precise empirical measurements had already been obtained from the emission spectra of black bodies, and Planck realized that the only way to explain these results was to conceptualize light in the form of a multitude of particles, the energy of which can only be delivered in discontinuous or quantified values. He was even able to calculate the factor of proportionality in the equation that describes the size of these packets—a factor that has since been referred to as *Planck's constant*. For Planck, this was simply a mathematical technique enabling him to solve his problem. But Einstein saw it as a reflection of a physical reality: in fact, light is indeed composed of such quanta, and each carries an amount of energy proportional to its frequency, which is to say, its color. The quanta of light thus behave like true particles, just as Newton conceived them. But what about the wavelike behavior of light that had been so well established for over one hundred years? How could light be both a particle and a wave? Needless to say, Einstein's proposal was met with great resistance by the scientific community at that time.

It was not until 1922, with experiments such as those of American physicist Arthur Compton on X-rays, another form of electromagnetic radiation, that it was proven beyond a doubt that the quanta of light do indeed exist. That same year Einstein received the Nobel Prize "for his services to theoretical physics, and especially for his discovery of the law of the photoelectric effect."* In 1926, these newly found light quanta were named *photons* by American chemist Gilbert Lewis.

THE QUANTUM REVOLUTION

All of this contributed to the second great scientific revolution of the twentieth century (along with Einstein's theory of relativity): the birth of *quantum mechanics*. In 1926, Austrian physicist Erwin Schrödinger published his now-famous eponymous equation, a mathematical formulation for studying quantum mechanical systems that was to become one of the main pillars of this extraordinary new science.

Until then, equations in physics were meant to calculate the state or the trajectory of material objects. But Schrödinger's equation instead describes a wave function, a sort of mathematical construct representing the probability of a particular state appearing in time and space. Particles no longer have a precisely defined existence; they can only be described by a probability distribution (also known as a *probability cloud*) that represents them. This way of describing the material world is so radically different from the previous classical understanding that even today, almost a hundred years later, we are striving to fully understand its implications.

For the fathers of quantum mechanics such as Schrödinger, Niels Bohr, and Werner Heisenberg, the wave/particle duality of light (as, in fact, that of all elementary particles comprising matter such as electrons and protons) becomes a fundamental aspect of its manifestation: one should therefore no longer try to figure out which form is the right one since both forms exist simultaneously, though only one form will appear according to the particular conditions in which the light is

---

*An amusing anecdote: We now know that the Nobel committee was biased against Einstein and his theory of relativity and refused to honor it. As they had received a flood of requests to nominate Einstein, they had to acquiesce, but they only mentioned his discovery of the photoelectric effect. Einstein, who was traveling at the time the prize was awarded in 1922, made no effort to attend the ceremony and therefore was not present when it was awarded. It was only in the following year, 1923, that he gave his Nobel speech, which he dedicated entirely to relativity!

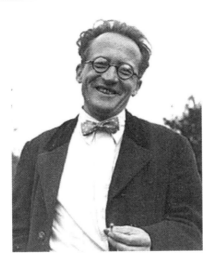

Figure 2.9.
Erwin Schrödinger

observed at any given time. This twofold reality, virtually incomprehensible at the macroscopic scale in which we live, reminds us once again of the mystery surrounding the true nature of light.

Many physicists now consider the most fundamental aspect of light to be its wave form. Recent experiments, such as those conducted by Iranian-American physicist Shahriar Afshar in 2004 using an improved version of Young's slits, demonstrate that even when light manifests as particles, that is, photons, these photons conserve the properties of a wave. This was the same conclusion that Schrödinger came to at the end of his life.

Some Key Concepts in Quantum Mechanics

The following concepts of quantum mechanics are especially significant for the rest of our exploration of light.

The Observer: Quantum mechanics is a description of the world of elementary particles in terms of their *wave functions*, which define the probability distribution of all possible states within a given system. But at our macroscopic scale, particles are very real and precisely localized in space. How is the link between these two dimensions established? Through the "collapse," or reduction, of a quantum wave function, which represents the instant when a particle emerges from the virtual world of probabilities into our world of the observable. This reduction is normally provoked by the act of observation, which in itself forces the particle to "materialize" in a particular state among all the possible states in which it can exist. Essentially, this implies that a new component must be added to our physical reality: that of the observer who, by his or her very presence, transforms the quantum world.

But who can observe, apart from a conscious being? For the first time in the history of science, the role of consciousness seems to be intimately linked to the manifestation of the material world. This concept is of major importance in the interpretation of quantum mechanics, but at the same time it is so radical that it is still not unanimously accepted by contemporary physicists. We will come back to this subject in chapters 11 and 12.

Nonlocality: *Quantum entanglement* is a phenomenon by which two or several particles remain connected, even when they are separated from each other in time or space. The famous EPR paradox (a *thought experiment** named after its three authors, Einstein, Boris Podolsky, and Nathan Rosen) proposed in 1935 was the first to highlight the apparent contradictions inherent in quantum mechanics. Einstein never accepted quantum mechanics' indeterminacy, and he summed this up by saying, "God does not play dice."

The EPR thought experiment consisted of taking two particles issuing from a common source and in interlinked quantum states described by a shared wave function, then separating the particles at a distance, such that they could no longer interact. Observing one of the particles, and therefore identifying its quantum state, instantly determined the state of the other particle, however far away it may have been. But this seemed to imply a link that is faster than the speed of light, an impossibility according to relativity. Physicists name this strange property *nonlocality,* as it seems to mock the physical separation of objects in space.

It was not till the 1980s that French physicist Alain Aspect managed to actually carry out this thought experiment with real photons, and his results were unequivocal: quantum entanglement and nonlocality were very real and exhibited a synchronization at more than twenty times the speed of

---

*A thought experiment considers some hypothesis, theory, or principle for the purpose of thinking through its consequences. Given the structure of the experiment, it may not be possible to perform it, and even if it could be performed there need not be the intention to perform it.

light between the two tested particles. More recent versions of the experiment, such as the one performed by Swiss physicist Nicolas Gisin in 1997, brought this synchronization to at least 20,000 times the speed of light. The nonlocal link of entanglement appears to be essentially instantaneous. Remarkably, this entanglement has been shown to happen whenever particles interact with one another at any moment in their history; they do not even have to originate from a common source, as was originally thought.

Coherence: Coherence between particles is another important aspect of the quantum world. Coherence comes into play when a group of particles are unified from a quantum point of view; that is to say, their wave functions remain synchronized, or one common wave function can describe them all. This coherence is in play when light waves create patterns of interference, as in the case with Young's slits. This can only happen if the waves are in phase, which is when their peaks and valleys are aligned and overlapping in a stable and continuous fashion.

In recent years, some physicists have attributed a much bigger role to quantum coherence. According to the big bang theory, the universe was a single point at its origin, with all its components therefore being linked by cosmic-scale quantum coherence. This would imply that all phenomena in the universe are in a way interrelated.

More concretely, the most common example of coherence around us is that of a laser (the term *laser* is an acronym for *light amplification by stimulated emission of radiations*), now used in a multitude of devices ranging from CD players to printers. First built in 1958, the laser generates a ray of photons with wave phases all in perfect coherence. This gives it certain distinctive properties such as a reduced divergence, an immense spatial range, and potentially enormous intensity. As we will see later on, these properties offer great possibilities for certain therapeutic applications.

We use light in myriad applications, and we can appreciate it fully with our senses, which gives us the illusion that we know it well, but let us never forget that in fact we do not ultimately know what it is . . .

3

WHAT IS LIGHT?

Physical Properties

Light, my light, the world-filling light,
the eye-kissing light,
heart-sweetening light!
Ah, the light dances, my darling, at the centre of my life;
the light strikes, my darling, the chords of my love

RABINDRANATH TAGORE

HERE, THE MAIN PHYSICAL PROPERTIES OF LIGHT as they are understood by contemporary science will be examined. If the reader finds the descriptions overly technical, a summary at the end of this chapter lists the main qualities of light, which will be helpful in understanding the rest of this book.

Since the discoveries of physicist James Clerk Maxwell we know that light is a wave and as such is part of the immense range of electromagnetic waves. It is of the same nature as all other waves in that range, going from (in increasing frequency order) radio waves, to microwaves, to infrared rays, to visible light, to X-rays, and finally to higher-energy gamma rays.

Waves play a major role in our world; we are familiar with a variety of other wave types, most notably sound waves. Sound waves are of course of a completely different kind from light waves. They propagate though mechanical compression of air molecules rather than as

41

electromagnetic waves and have greatly reduced frequencies compared with those of light (by a factor of one to a trillion). But some universal laws governing waves remain valid throughout all of these dimensions.

A TINY OCTAVE OF LIGHT

One of the laws governing all types of waves is that of the equivalence of the octave, which is a frequency multiplied by a factor of 2; a wave one octave above another wave will possess similar properties. This is the basis of music, where the scale of twelve notes covers precisely an interval of one octave; a C an octave above and below a given C will still sound like a C to the ear. And waves at an octave interval from one another can become coherent, a subject that will be further discussed in chapter 10.

An octave is thus a useful standard for evaluating ranges of frequencies of any description, including electromagnetic waves. What we call light corresponds to one single octave of frequencies in the middle of a vast electromagnetic expanse that contains over seventy octaves at the cosmic scale (see fig. 3.1). A very special octave to which our sense of vision is sensitive is perceived as color.

To help us get a sense of this vast range we should note that the frequency of light is about a million times higher than the radio frequencies of a cell phone, and a thousand times lower than those of X-rays.

WAVE LENGTH

Light can be characterized either by the energy of its photons (in its particle form), or by the *frequency* of its wave (in its wave form); these two descriptions are equivalent and proportionally related to each other by Planck's constant. The unit used to designate a frequency is the hertz (Hz), representing one cycle per second and named after German physicist Heinrich Hertz, who in 1887 was the first to test Maxwell's theory and to produce an electromagnetic wave.

In practice, when we are describing light we usually speak of its wavelength rather than its frequency. The *wavelength* is the distance

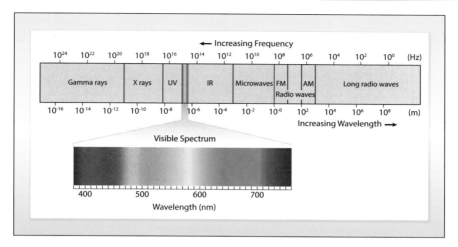

Figure 3.1. Seventy octaves of electromagnetic waves

between two peaks in the undulating wave that light generates as it moves through space, the very same length that Young measured for the first time in 1801.

Wavelength and frequency are inversely proportional: as the frequency of the wave increases, the wavelength shortens, since its speed (that of the speed of light at approximately 300,000 kilometers per second) remains constant. The unit most commonly used to measure wavelengths of light is the nanometer (nm), which is one billionth of a meter. Using this unit, the octave of visible light extends from about 380 nm to 760 nm.*

COLORS, PRECISELY, AND BEYOND THE VISIBLE SPECTRUM

As our visual system perceives each wavelength of light as a color, we can equally refer to a color or to a wavelength to designate a particular frequency of light. However, it is more precise to speak in terms of nanometers because our eyes have a limited capacity when it comes to distinguishing colors: they can at most differentiate a hundred hues

---

*The extreme limits of our perception are from 310 nm to 1,050 nm—but only in rare, special circumstances.

within the rainbow. Moreover, our vocabulary is rather vague when it comes to describing color; how many types of blue do you know?

The table below lists the wavelengths of the main colors.

TABLE 3.1. THE WAVELENGTHS OF THE MAIN COLORS, EXPRESSED IN NANOMETERS

COLOR	WAVELENGTH
Red	760–635 nm
Orange	635–590 nm
Yellow	590–560 nm
Green	560–520 nm
Turquoise	520–490 nm
Blue	490–460 nm
Indigo	460–430 nm
Violet	430–380 nm

The frequencies immediately above and below this octave of color are by convention considered to be part of the domain of light. Even if they are no longer visible to our eyes, we can still perceive them indirectly.

In 1800, British astronomer William Herschel was the first to explore the range of frequencies just below red, the infrared. He produced a rainbow by projecting sunlight through a prism and then placed a thermometer just beyond the red limit of the rainbow. Though no light was visible, he could observe a calorific effect on the thermometer. The following year, inspired by this experiment, German chemist Johann Wilhelm Ritter detected ultraviolet at the other end of the rainbow, this time by observing the effect on a solution of silver chloride that turned black when placed in that range.

Below infrared lies the range of radio waves starting with microwaves (that of our cell phones), with wavelengths around 1 million nm (1 millimeter). Wavelengths beyond ultraviolet (shorter than 10 nm) can be found in the gamut of X-rays. These transitions are gradual, so the limits given to the infrared and ultraviolet ranges are more or less arbitrary.

PURE COLORS, MIXED COLORS

Until now we have examined colors that are called *pure* or *saturated*. These are composed exclusively of photons of a single frequency, and they are thus intense colors, like those in a rainbow. In most applications of chromotherapy pure colors are favored, as their individual frequency can have a precise effect both physiologically and perceptually.

When we view several frequencies of light simultaneously, our visual system processes this information in such a way as to extract a "virtual" average of all the frequencies, which are then perceived as colors that are more diluted or pastel. These mixed colors are called *nonsaturated*. It is estimated that we can distinguish up to a million distinct shades of nonsaturated colors in all the possible combinations of frequencies. The best example of nonsaturated light is that of the sun. Our visual system interprets as white the average sum of all the colors of the rainbow simultaneously contained. When studying the properties of a light source it is always very informative to examine the profile of the intensity of each frequency being emitted, which is called the *emission spectrum* (see fig. 3.2). The solar spectrum is very close to that of the black body that Planck had calculated in 1900, indicating that this mathematical model corresponds well to the conditions of the sun: a nonreflecting object that shines from its own heat.

COLOR TEMPERATURE

According to Planck's equation, the spectrum emitted by a black body does not depend on its particular shape or composition, but solely on its temperature. The profile of the sun's spectrum corresponds to that of an object at a temperature of 5,700 K,* and we can deduce that this is

---

*The kelvin (K) temperature unit, named after William Thomson, the 1st Baron Kelvin, an eminent Scots-Irish physicist of the nineteenth century, is favored by physicists and is conventionally used to specify color temperature. Kelvins have the same scale as the familiar degrees C (centigrade) but take their point of origin at −273° C, the temperature of "absolute zero," the lowest that can be attained, which Kelvin was the first to calculate. Thus 0° C is equal to 273 K.

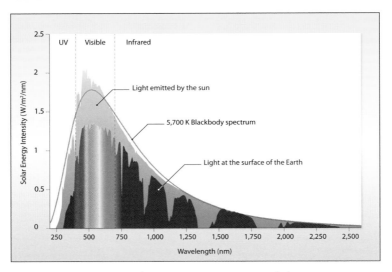

Figure 3.2. The emission spectrum of the sun

the temperature at its surface, known as the *photosphere*. That may seem hot, but it is not so hot when one considers that the nuclear fusion taking place at the sun's core generates temperatures of around 15 million degrees. The extremely energetic photons that are produced by these core reactions travel from atom to atom for more than 100,000 years, losing a little energy each time. By the time they reach the photosphere, their temperature has cooled to the 5,700 K temperature just mentioned. This journey would take light barely two seconds if it were traveling in a straight line. From the surface of the sun, the photons take only another eight minutes to reach Earth. Earth's atmosphere filters certain wavelengths (in particular, those in the ultraviolet and infrared bands), the result being that the spectrum of the light reaching us on the surface of planet Earth is somewhat different from the black body profile emitted by the sun.

When describing the quality of different light sources, lighting professionals often refer to the temperature of the black body spectrum closest to the light source spectrum (see fig. 3.3). We use the term *correlated color temperature* (CCT), or more simply, *color temperature,* to indicate that the light source appears to our visual system as a black body of that temperature would. This mathematical analogy can even be applied to nonthermal light sources that generate light through processes not related to the hot glow of black bodies. That's why an LED can be spoken of as having a temperature of, say, 6,000 K, even though we know very well that it gives off little heat. Though it is not a black body, it emits a light that looks closest to a black body of that specific temperature. This is the temperature that you will see marked on the packaging of some of the newer CFL and LED bulbs.

Higher color temperatures correspond to spectra with more energetic photons and look more bluish. Lower color temperature spectra look more reddish or amber. For example, the color of the temperature of a candle flame is 1,850 K. Artificial light sources typically have a color temperature ranging from 2,000 K to 10,000 K. (Such variations can have significant physiological impacts, as we shall see in chapter 6). Light spectra at these various color temperatures appear as different shades of white. Thus the bluish white of a 6,000 K light bulb is commonly called "daylight white" or "cold white" (depending on manufacturers), while the yellowish white of a 2,700 K bulb is known as "warm white." It may seem paradoxical that the highest color temperatures are considered to be cold, while the lowest are considered warm. These terms simply reflect the fact that we usually associate blue colors with cold objects (such as ice), and red, orange, and yellow colors with warm objects (such as fire).

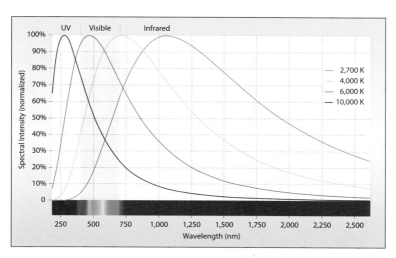

Figure 3.3. Emission spectra for black bodies at various temperatures

LIGHT AS EXPLAINED BY
PARTICLE PHYSICS

This part of the book is geared to those readers who may be interested in understanding how modern *particle physics* describes light within its model of physical reality. Obviously, a complete explanation is beyond the scope of this book, so the following is a basic overview of the most up-to-date contemporary science.

Particle physics is a branch of modern physics that studies the elementary constituents of matter and radiation and the interactions between them. It says that everything in our world is ultimately composed of elementary particles. The current theory that explains the interaction of these particles and the quantum fields that govern their interactions is what is known as the *Standard Model* (see fig. 3.4). This model recognizes two key classes of elementary particles: *fermions,* the particles that constitute matter, and *bosons,* the particles that carry the forces acting between these particles of matter. As one might suspect, light is associated with the bosons, as it is more energy than matter. Let's take a closer look:

Fermions are divided into twelve types: the six quarks that make up the atomic nucleus with its protons and neutrons, and six leptons, which are lighter particles (one of which is the electron). There are four fundamental interactions, or forces, acting between fermions:

* **Two forces that act over large distances** and therefore are familiar to us at the macroscopic level: 1) gravitation, which affects all forms of matter; and 2) the electromagnetic force, which affects all particles having an electric charge, such as electrons and protons.
* **Two forces of very short range** that we cannot perceive directly and that intervene only at the scale of the atomic nucleus: the 3) strong interaction that ensures the cohesion of the nucleus; and 4) the weak interaction that is responsible, among other things, for nuclear fission.

In *quantum field theory* (QFT), these four forces are understood as being transported by mediator particles, called *gauge bosons*. Each of the four fundamental interactions obeys different laws of varying complexity and therefore requires a different number of bosons.

The strong interaction, the most complex, requires eight kinds of bosons called *gluons*. The weak interaction has three, one called a *Z boson* and two *W bosons*. Quantum understanding of gravity remains incomplete, but the existence of a boson called *graviton* is hypothesized. As for the electromagnetic force, its mediating boson is none other than the photon, the particle of light with which we are already familiar.

One final mediator boson apart from the rest is the enigmatic Higgs boson that gives rise to mass in the other particles. It is a very large particle that was postulated by, among others, British physicist Peter Higgs, in 1964, and was finally identified in 2013 at the giant CERN particle accelerator.

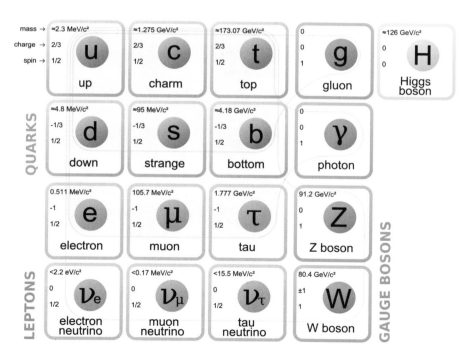

Figure 3.4. The Standard Model in modern particle physics

Light and Electricity, Indissolubly Linked

According to the Standard Model there is an indissoluble link between electricity and light. Photons, carriers of the electromagnetic force, are emitted and absorbed by electrically charged fermions of matter, such as electrons. In so doing they add or remove the energy that they carry to and from the fermions. These gains and losses of energy determine the orbital layer at which the electron will be positioned around the atomic nucleus. All of molecular chemistry, therefore all of life, is based on the interplay of electrons occupying energetically stable layers around atomic nuclei and jumping from one layer to another under the influence of nearby photons.

Among the four fundamental interactions, the most powerful is the strong interaction acting at the heart of atomic nuclei. Next comes the electromagnetic interaction, approximately 100 times less strong, but still far surpassing the two weakest forces, that of the weak interaction by a factor of 10,000, and that of gravity by a huge factor of 10^{37}. To get an idea of what this implies, let's imagine two bags located one meter apart from one another, each containing 1 kilogram of electrons. The electromagnetic force repelling them would be equivalent to the gravitational force exerted between two planets the size of Earth at the same distance! It is therefore not surprising that the electromagnetic force, and consequently light, is key to the existence of our material world.

In *quantum electrodynamics* (QED), the modern theory of electromagnetic interaction developed notably by American physicist Richard Feynman, the attraction or repulsion between electrically charged particles is caused by the pressure of virtual photons, evanescent particles that emerge from the surrounding vacuum only to disappear into it just as quickly. When a photon does not return to the vacuum immediately, it is freed, and at that point it ceases to be virtual and becomes light as we know it. If this strange vision of things may seem exaggeratedly complex, it is reassuring to know that QED theory explains numerous quantum phenomena with unequalled precision and is thus a good description of reality.

THE KEY PROPERTIES OF LIGHT

For reference, here are the most important features that characterize light sources:

Intensity corresponds to brightness and thus to the quantity of photons emitted at each instant.

Color refers to the wavelength (or the equivalent frequency) of the emitted photons. In visible light, wavelengths range from 380 nanometers (violet color) to 760 nanometers (red color).

Saturation refers to the purity of a color. A fully saturated light contains photons of a single frequency and is called *monochromatic;* these are the pure colors of the rainbow. The more a color is non-saturated, containing a mix of light frequencies, the more pastel it will appear. In the extreme case of light containing all frequencies, such as daylight originating from the sun, it will appear as white.

Color temperature (sometimes called *correlated color temperature,* or CCT) is used to describe the quality of nonsaturated light. It does not necessarily refer to the actual temperature of the light source but serves rather to characterize its tint. Higher color temperatures appear more blue, whereas lower color temperatures look more red or amber. Color temperature is expressed in kelvin (K). Artificial light sources typically have color temperatures ranging from 2,000 K to 10,000 K.

Coherence refers to the degree of synchronization to be found in the waves of the multitude of photons comprising the light. A laser is an example of highly coherent light. Natural light is seldom coherent.

Polarization refers to the orientation of the electric and magnetic fields that make up the electromagnetic wave that is light. This orientation can be linear (in a specific axis) or circular (constantly rotating). A familiar example of polarization is that of polarized sunglasses, which manage to reduce glare by filtering out light with horizontally oriented polarization. Certain types of light therapies make use of the special effects of polarized light.

Now that we have a better understanding of the properties of light and its governing principles, we are ready to explore light's pervasive influence on our body and its health.

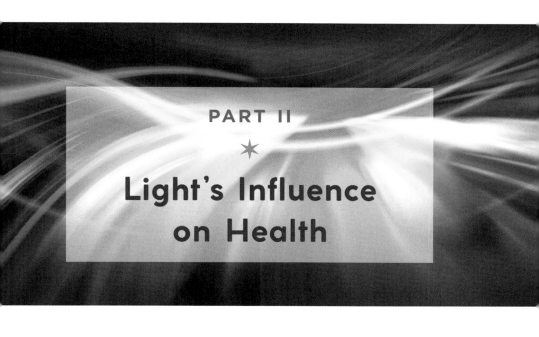

PART II

✳

Light's Influence on Health

4

THE THREE BIOLOGICAL PATHWAYS OF LIGHT

Entry and Influence

We can talk to the cells, but we must first learn their language.

TIINA KARU

LIGHT AFFECTS US in multiple ways. The most obvious way is through the organ of vision, the eye, which is miraculously sensitive to the tiniest subtleties of light. Vision is the sense that brings by far the most information to the brain; thus, it is our first pathway of light.

But vision is not the only function of the optic system. We now know of the existence of a separate and equally vital function that occurs when light enters the eyes: it has a direct effect on the central region of the brain, the *hypothalamus*, which contributes to regulating our basic hormonal balance. This *nonvisual optic pathway* is the second pathway of light, complementing the *visual optic pathway* of vision.

Aside from these optical effects, light has a surprisingly profound effect on the rest of the body. Only recently have we begun to understand how it influences each cell, stimulating its metabolism and reaching all the way to the DNA in the nucleus. This is the phenomenon of photobiomodulation, the modulation of biological processes by light, and it constitutes the third pathway.

In this chapter we will examine these three principal pathways by which light influences us, and this will help us understand why light plays such an essential role in our health and well-being.

FIRST PATHWAY: VISION

Our sense of vision necessitates two components: the eyes, capable of transforming photons of light into bioelectrical signals compatible with our nervous systems, and the brain, which analyzes and interprets these signals to recreate in the mind an image of the observed reality. Of all the organs of the body it is the eye that medicine has studied the most, and of all brain functions it is those of the visual cortex that neurology has explored most deeply.

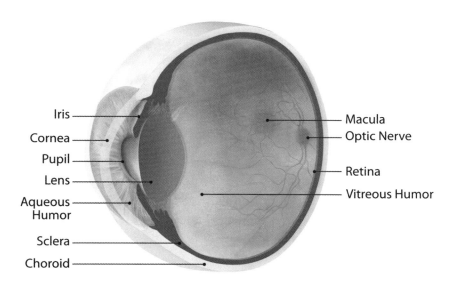

Iris
Cornea
Pupil
Lens
Aqueous Humor
Sclera
Choroid

Macula
Optic Nerve
Retina
Vitreous Humor

Figure 4.1. The human eye

The eye is a marvel of evolution, an instrument of exquisite precision amalgamating these four functions: optics (through the geometrically variable lens), photosensitivity (via the retina, a complex network of cells that captures various wavelengths of light), mechanics (by means of a set of minuscule muscles able to move the eye with great speed), and an autoregulatory function (with the pupil, a system to adjust to the intensity of light). In the 1840s, the perfection of the eye confounded Charles Darwin as he was elaborating his theory of evolution of the human species. How could all these interdependent functions of the eye have evolved gradually when they only make sense as a unit? This dilemma is still unresolved today, though evolutionary biologists have various hypotheses.*

Our eyes are extraordinarily sensitive and flexible: they can adapt to an extreme intensity of 100,000 lux, which is the typical brightness of a sunny day. On the other end of the scale our eyes can perceive all the way down to 0.0001 lux, the dark of night—an incredible range of a billion to one!†

The Retina, the Key to Vision

Without a doubt the most critical component to vision is the retina, a network of photosensitive cells covering the back of the eye. The retina is remarkably complex, and we have yet to elucidate all of its mysteries. In fact, it is essentially a projection of the brain into the eye, made up of a series of successive layers:

* At the surface, facing the light, is a layer of ganglion cells from which optic nerve fibers travel to the center of the brain.
* At the back are the photoreceptors that are made up of photo pigments that can absorb individual photons and, in an extraordinary feat of photomultiplying biochemistry, convert these photons into electrical impulses.
* Between these two layers other cells (amacrine, bipolar, horizontal) perform a preliminary organization of the visual information by relaying the electrical impulses of about a hundred photoreceptors to each ganglion cell.

---

*By means of simulations, researchers have demonstrated that a sequence of 60,000 generations over a few million years (a short span on the evolutionary scale) would suffice for a primitive photosensitive surface to evolve into a whole functioning eye (Nilsson and Pelger 1994)—but only if the mutations of each generation are in the right direction.
†A *lux* is a unit quantifying the amount of illumination shining on a surface.

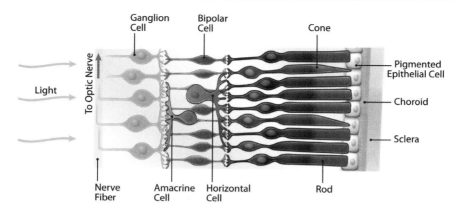

Figure 4.2. The structure of the retina

The optic nerve is composed of about a million neural fibers that go across the brain to reach the visual cortex, in the occipital region. This massive cerebral structure takes up a large part of the brain. It is comprised of multiple zones that decode the complex signals coming from the retina into different types that are analyzed in parallel. We are not conscious of most of this immense processing of information; we only perceive the final result—an image filtered and reconstituted from an ocean of photons.

Rods and Cones for Night and Day

The electromagnetic spectrum is vast, but we call only a small part of it light. It is the photoreceptors that determine this according to the range of wavelengths to which they are sensitive. We call the profile of this sensitivity for each photoreceptor its *action spectrum*. We have two kinds of photoreceptors: the *rods*, which are very sensitive to low light intensities but are slow; and the *cones*, which are less sensitive but quicker. The rods are numerous (there are from 60 to 90 million) and cover the whole surface of the retina. They are largely responsible for our peripheral and nocturnal vision. The cones are fewer in number (from 3 to 5 million) and are concentrated in the central portion of the retina, the macula. They make up our central field of vision and allow us to see details with precision.

Each of these two types of photoreceptors use photopigments, the molecular properties of which are optimized for their specific functions: *rhodopsin* for rods and *photopsin* for cones. Their sensitive components belong to the larger family of chromophores, which are living molecules capable of interacting with light. We possess other types of chromophores in other parts of our bodies, which will be described later in the chapter.

The Gift of Color

Cones come in three distinct varieties, each with an action spectrum covering a different part of the light spectrum: one is sensitive to red, another to green, and the third to blue (see fig. 4.3). It is this trichromatic assortment of cones coupled with the brain's wonderful process of reconstruction that gives us the capacity to perceive color.

According to its wavelength, a photon will stimulate to a different degree each of the three types of cones. A specialized part of our visual cortex recombines these signals to arrive at the original wavelength of the photon and translates these abstract impulses into the sensation that we call *color*. The precision of this process is limited, as we can differentiate at most about a hundred monochromatic colors across the whole rainbow spectrum. If we include mixed colors (pastels and gradations in intensity), our register increases to around a million different tints.

When we observe the continuous palette of colors in a rainbow it is good to remember that what we are seeing is a construct of our perception synthesized in the color center of the brain, based on composite signals from the retina.

Tetrachromacy and Other Marvels

Do other species perceive color? It depends on the number of different types of cones the eye possesses. Like us, primates are trichromatic, but most other mammals, including dogs and cats, have only two cones, the red and the blue. That would reduce the number of colors that can be seen by a factor of 100, limiting the total range to 10,000 tints. Since the green cones are missing, the perception of the fine gradations around this color is notably reduced.

Many other species are trichromatic, but their vision does not

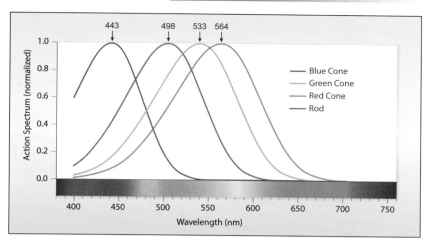

Figure 4.3. The action spectra of the red, green, and blue cones (photopsins) and the rods (rhodopsin) (adapted from Dowling 1987)

necessarily have the same range of colors as ours. For example, in bees the red cone is replaced by an ultraviolet one, allowing the insect to see up to 300 nanometers, thus making accessible a world of subtle details in flowers, elements invisible to our human eyes (see fig. 4.4c). Geckos, on the other hand, have cones so sensitive that their nighttime vision is in full color, while we, reliant after sundown on our rods, discern only shades of gray.

Some species among birds, insects, and fish go further, as they possess four types of cones, expanding their visible register from red to ultraviolet. Yet other species, such as some pigeons and butterflies, have five cones. The record seems to be held by the mantis shrimp, whose eyes have twelve cone types, making it impossible for us to even imagine the extraordinary subtlety of this creature's chromatic universe.

There are certain humans who have a fourth type of cone, the sensitivity of which is situated between red and green, in the orange range. Though this is relatively common in women,* it is estimated that only in about 1 percent of the population (comprising 2 to 3 percent of

---

*Jameson, Highnote, and Wasserman (2001) find that the figure varies from 10 percent to 50 percent of all women, compared to fewer than 8 percent of men.

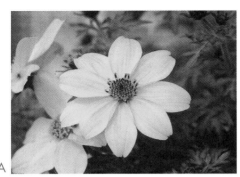
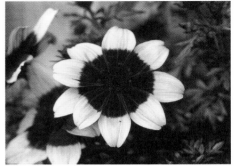
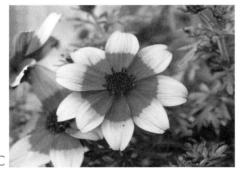

Figure 4.4. (A). A spring flower (*Bidens ferulifolia*) seen through a UV filter (B), and in simulated bee vision (C); the central part of the flower stands out in sharp contrast, attracting the bee toward it
(© Dr. Schmitt, Weinheim Germany, uvir.eu)

women) is this fourth cone sufficiently different from the regular red cone to make the eye truly tetrachromatic. (Neitz as quoted by Roth 2006). Color refinement is superlative for those lucky people who are capable of distinguishing up to 100 million tints.

Living Fiber Optics

The complexity of the retina is such that we are constantly surprised by new discoveries as we unravel its mysteries. It was only in 2007 that one particular paradox was solved: Generations of biologists have wondered why it is that the structure of the retina is seemingly inverted, with the photo-receptors at the very back layer in such a way that light is filtered and diffused by the layers in front. Is this an artifact of evolution, one of those "errors" that sometimes seem to make their way into the web of life? As one might imagine, such is not the case. . .

Researchers have discovered that there is a network of glial cells called Müller cells that spread across the retina and act as living fiber optics, carrying the light to the photoreceptors (Franze et al. 2007). More recently it has been confirmed that not only does this arrangement focus the light in the right places, it also modifies the spectral composition (favoring the transmission of red and green) in such a way that day vision is optimized without degrading night vision (Ribak et al. 2015). There certainly is no mistake of nature here!

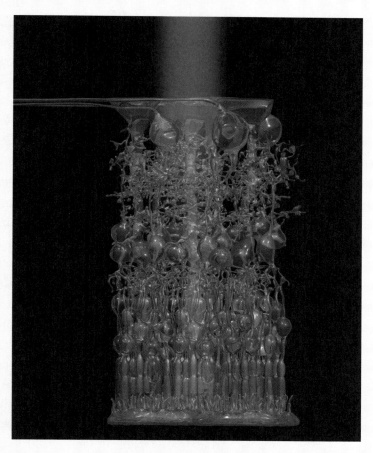

Figure 4.5. Müller cells, living fiber optics
(© Dr. Jens Grosche)

SECOND PATHWAY:
THE NONVISUAL OPTIC PATHWAY

It was only recently that a startling discovery occurred that shook the scientific community. Scientists had known about cones and rods for over 150 years, so it was completely unexpected when a new type of photoreceptor was observed. In 2000, American neuroscientist Ignacio Provencio and his team identified a new photopigment, which they named *melanopsin* (Provencio 2000). Melanopsin first appeared in invertebrates and is therefore more ancient than the opsins in our rods and cones, which evolved later in vertebrates. To their surprise, the researchers found this new photopigment in certain ganglion cells, first in mice, and then in humans. These cells are evenly distributed throughout the retina but are relatively few in number, comprising only 1 to 3 percent of all ganglion cells. It was further found that these cells react to light in an autonomous fashion, independently of the rods and cones to which they are connected (remember that the primary function of the ganglion cells is to serve as a neural relay to these photoreceptors) (Berson, Dunn, and Motoharu 2002).

At around the same time, it was found that the neural fibers coming from these ganglion cells containing melanopsin do not go to the visual cortex, as is normal, but to a central region of the brain, the *suprachiasmatic nucleus* (SCN), the area of the hypothalamus that governs our internal clock (Hattar et al. 2002). This direct link with light is highly significant. Many neurologists consider the hypothalamus to be the most important area of the brain, a "brain within the brain," as it manages the coordination and regulation of most of our vital functions. Located at the core of the brain, it integrates the information originating from our nervous, endocrine, and immune systems.

These successive discoveries elucidated a long-standing mystery. A basic regulating factor for life on Earth is the *circadian* rhythm, the ability of living organisms to synchronize their biological patterns with daylight, the light of the sun. For almost a century biologists had known that even when deprived of vision, animals are capable of such synchronization (Foster et al. 1991), though they could not understand the mechanism by which it happened. Pioneers such as Dr. Fritz Hollwich (1979) had earlier deduced that there must be a direct link between the eye and the pituitary (which Hollwich called the *energetic circuit* of the optic nerve in his 1948 inaugural dissertation), but this remained hypothetical until these new neural fibers were identified.

In a parallel achievement, the teams of Brainard et al. (2001) and Thapan, Arendt, and Skene (2001) found that light suppresses the secretion of melatonin, a key hormone involved in our circadian rhythm. They were able to measure the action spectrum driving this effect; centered on 460 nm (in the blue color range), it did not match the spectra of the rods and cones but was nearly identical to that of the new photopigment melanopsin (see fig. 4.6). Melatonin is secreted by the pineal gland according to a sequence of neurological events originating in the SCN under the influence of light.

All these findings make it clear that an important and once-missing link in our understanding of the visual system has now been found. The new cells have been given an edifying name: *intrinsically photosensitive retinal ganglion cells,* mercifully abridged to the acronym ipRGC (see fig. 4.7). The part of the optic nerve that is connected to the hypothalamus has been given various names: *retinohypothalamic tract, nonvisual optic pathway,* and *non-image-forming (NIF) pathway.*

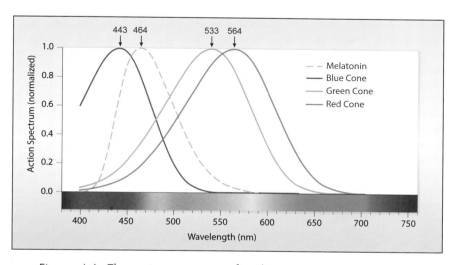

Figure 4.6. The action spectrum of melatonin suppression at 460 nanometers, compared to those of other photoreceptors in the brain

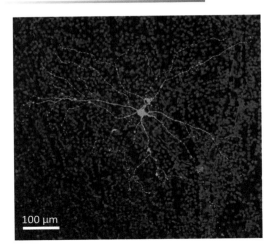

Figure 4.7. Intracellular dye fill of an intrinsically photosensitive retinal ganglion cell (ipRGC) in a flattened piece of rat retina (© Dr. Kwoon Y. Wong, University of Michigan)

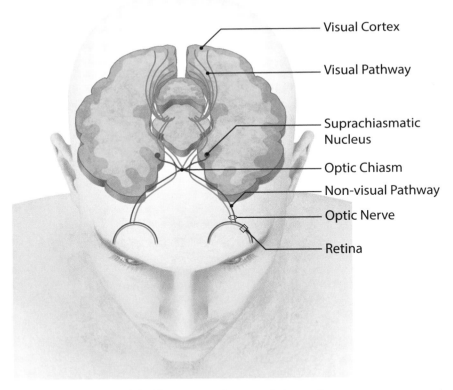

Figure 4.8. The two pathways of the optic nerve: visual (in red) and nonvisual (in blue)

Opsin Tales

Well before vision appeared, living creatures had ways of synchronizing their activities with the natural cycles of day and night and the seasons. They developed a multitude of proteins that are sensitive to light, and these are categorized under the general term *opsins*. Opsins are found in most animals and distributed in various body parts. They allow numerous metabolic functions such as reproduction, growth, temperature, blood pressure, immune-system fluctuations and the like to adapt to the daily (circadian) and seasonal rhythms.

The eye may be the most refined photosensitive organ, with its multiple opsins such as the rhodopsin, photopsin and melanopsin in the rods, cones, and ipRGCs (intrinsically photosensitive retinal ganglion cells, discussed earlier in this chapter), but it is not the only organ that is photosensitive. For example, Nissilä et al. (2016) recently found that melanopsin is present in neurons in most central brain areas, a fact that calls into question whether ambient light could have targets in the brain outside the optic tract. Other nonvisual opsins such as panopsin and neuropsin are found in numerous organs, including the brain, the heart, the testicles, and the skin, though their function is still poorly understood.

The suprachiasmatic nucleus (SCN) in the hypothalamus may contain our master clock, but most other organs have their own internal clocks as well. It was recently discovered that the retina uses neuropsin to regulate circadian functions independently of the SCN (Buhr et al. 2015).

The neuropsin action spectrum is centered at 380 nanometers, in the violet and near-ultraviolet (UVA) range. These short wavelengths are heavily filtered in the eye, with the lens blocking most photons below 400 nanometers because their higher energy would cause photo-oxidative damage in the retina. This might explain why the cornea itself uses neuropsin to drive its local circadian rhythm: since UV does not penetrate inside the eye, it makes sense to detect it at the very front of the eye.

With the discovery of the ipRGCs we have learned to take into consideration the role of the blue portion of light spectrum on our health. Perhaps we will soon have to consider the role of violet as well.

The Third Eye

One of the organs with the most photoreceptors is the pineal gland, situated in the middle of the brain. It has several opsins, including those found in the rods and cones as well as other nonvisual opsins. The function of these endogenous receptors is poorly understood, but it is probably an evolutionary phenomenon, the pineal gland having served as an additional eye in the past. Some species of reptiles, amphibians, and fish still have an external projection of the pineal gland, called a *pineal eye*. Our own pineal gland, even though it no longer has an external eye, nevertheless receives a certain dose of light that penetrates through the skull. It is thus not impossible that it still has a photosensitive function. It is therefore not surprising that the third eye, a mystical source of inner vision in some spiritual traditions, is sometimes associated with the pineal gland.

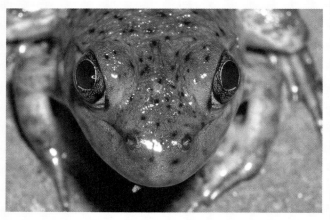

Figure 4.9. The pineal eye is still present in the juvenile frog

The Deeper Influence

The nonvisual optic pathway, which Fritz Hollwich describes as an "energetic circuit," allows light to directly influence the hypothalamus, the core of the limbic brain, master of our hormonal system, our autonomous system, and our most fundamental internal equilibrium. It was discovered quite quickly that dendrites (the branching extensions of nerve cells that receive and transmit impulses) from the optic

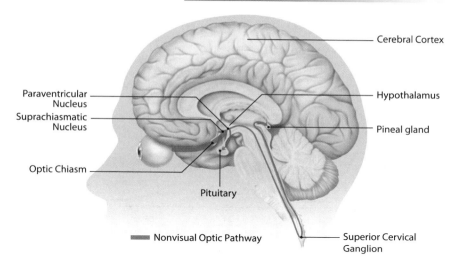

Figure 4.10. The nonvisual optic pathway, reaching multiple core brain areas, including the hypothalamus and our master glands

nerve reach into multiple hypothalamic zones, beyond the previously mentioned suprachiasmatic nucleus (SCN).* Thus the influence of light extends much farther than previously thought. By a complex network of neurons, light reaches all the way to the master glands (the pituitary and the pineal glands) and regulates their secretions.

The effect of light on suppressing the secretion of melatonin, the "darkness hormone," by the pineal gland is much studied by researchers, as it is one of the clearest and most easily quantified influences of the non-visual pathway. The presence of melatonin determines the quality of our sleep, and the long-term consequences of its depletion as a result of over-exposure to light (particularly artificial light) may be as serious as cancer.

Less studied but perhaps more essential is the influence of light on the pituitary gland that regulates the circadian variations of numerous vital hormones such as the ACTH (adrenocorticotropic hormone), which in turn regulates cortisol, the "stress hormone" implicated in a wide variety of diseases (see fig. 4.11).

---

*Notably, to the IGL (intergeniculate leaflet) implicated in the circadian clock, and the OPN (olivary pretectal nucleus), which manages the pupil constriction reflex

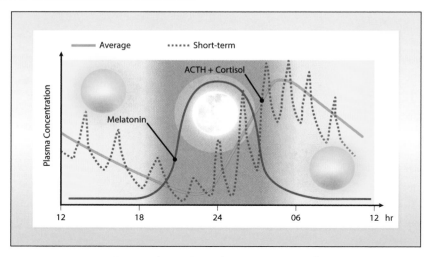

Figure 4.11. Circadian variations of
melatonin and cortisol, two essential hormones
(© Alexander Wunsch)

The influence of light on circadian rhythm and hence its effects on health cannot be overstated. It is clearly established that the blue part of the light spectrum plays a major role in influencing circadian rhythm through its stimulation of the ipRGCs. It is more important than ever to understand this nowadays because new sources of artificial lighting such as LEDs and CFLs have substantial amounts of blue in their emission spectra and therefore pose an increased risk of interfering with circadian rhythm—a subject we'll take up in depth in chapter 6.

The Circadian Plot Thickens

After the relatively simple view that we had of the nonvisual pathway in the early 2000s, we are only now beginning to discern its complexity. Since its discovery, it has been the subject of intensive research, with hundreds of scientific papers being published each year.

It is impossible to do it justice with the brief summary presented in this chapter, but to demonstrate the effervescence in this area of research I will mention just a few of the latest findings:

• We now know that there exist several subtypes of ipRGCs: at last count, five have been identified, each having a different action spectrum and a different network of dendrites (Ecker et al. 2010).

- The reaction speed of these ipRGCs as well as that of the traditional rods and cones connected to them varies considerably. It is now suspected that complex temporal dynamics take place within the retinal neuronal matrix (Gooley et al. 2012), leading to nonvisual effects that are dependent on the duration of light exposure.
- The clear division between the visual and nonvisual pathways is no longer so clear. It is now thought that the ipRGCs project their connections beyond the hypothalamus and toward all the major areas of the visual cortex in such a way as to influence certain aspects of visual perception (Lucas 2013).
- The light action spectrum that controls the circadian rhythm is constantly being updated since it was first measured (Brainard et al. 2001, Thapan et al. 2001). The most recent models (Rea et al. 2012) take into account nonlinear antagonistic interactions between the various photoreceptors involved, and this leads to surprising variations of around 500 nanometers (corresponding to the color turquoise).

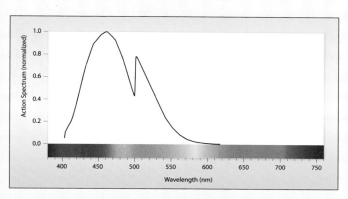

Figure 4.12. The circadian influence action spectrum
as evaluated today (from Rea et al. 2012)

Waves among the Experts

Certainly the period when light was considered solely for its utilitarian and artistic properties is over. Lighting professionals and the light and design industry must now take into consideration lighting's impact on health, and that is causing quite a stir. Furthermore, our understanding of the nonvisual optic pathway is still fragmentary, and consequently the regulatory standards in the lighting industry are constantly changing. The situation is such that fourteen leading scientific experts in the field recently concluded that "simple prescriptions are as likely to do harm as good, and even experts may have divergent ideas about best practice under some situations" (Lucas et al. 2014).

THIRD PATHWAY: PHOTOBIOMODULATION

Ultimately, almost all of the energy necessary for life on planet Earth is derived from the sun. This is achieved through the process of photosynthesis, in which plants use light to convert carbon dioxide (CO_2) and water into high-energy glucose molecules, releasing oxygen in the process. Essentially, photosynthesis is the biochemical means of capturing solar photons.

In a mirror process, animals combine the oxygen they breathe and the glucose they consume to extract the energy needed for their own metabolism, releasing CO_2 and water. This cellular respiration takes place in each of our cells and is a veritable key to life that is found in almost every species, and thus must have developed very early on in evolution. The final result is the synthesis of a molecular fuel that can be directly assimilated by the cells: adenosine triphosphate, or ATP, the "molecular unit of currency" in the transfer of energy between cells.

Cellular respiration is extremely complex, and analysis of its multiple facets occupied biologists during the whole of the twentieth century, resulting in several Nobel Prizes, in both medicine* and chemistry, along the way. Surprisingly, it has been found that the final step of the process takes place in the mitochondria, organisms that evolved separately from animals but that live in complete symbiosis with them.

---

*Notably, the great physiologist Albert Szent-Györgyi , whom we will speak more of in chapter 7, won the 1937 Nobel Prize.

Mitochondria, the Powerhouse of the Cell

Mitochondria are organelles* that reside in most of our cells but are, however, quite distinct from them. They possess their own DNA, separate from that of the cell's nucleus, and they divide independently from their host. It is believed that they originated from bacteria and that they fused with eukaryote cells (cells like ours, with a nucleus) around 1.5 billion years ago. Mitochondria are literally the powerhouses of the cell because they generate ATP, the fuel essential to its survival. There are up to a few thousand mitochondria in each cell, according to its energy needs.

Okay, but what do mitochondria have to do with light?

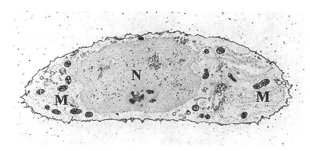

Figure 4.13.
Mitochondria (M)
inside a cell
(photo by
Robert M. Hunt)

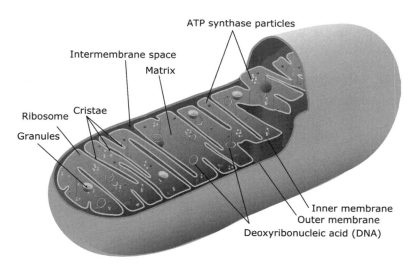

Figure 4.14. A single mitochondrion cross-section

---

*An organelle is a specialized subunit within a cell, about a micrometer in size, that has a specific function.

Mester's Laser

The first commercial laser appeared in 1960, and just three years later surgeons began using lasers to replace scalpels. Hungarian physician Endre Mester (who passed in 1984) was a pioneer in their use in medicine, beginning only a few years after their invention. At his hospital in Budapest, he wanted to explore the applications of this previously unknown, mysterious new light source. As early as 1965 he began in vivo experiments aiming to destroy tumors, which seemed to be the most obvious application at that time. The primitive ruby laser at his disposal was not as powerful as he had expected it would be;* it had little effect on the tumors he implanted in the skin of unfortunate laboratory mice. Nevertheless, Mester observed something completely unexpected that proved to be significant: the incisions he made seemed to heal more quickly in the mice he treated with the laser—the complete opposite of what he thought would happen. He began a series of experiments on the healing effects of the low-intensity lasers, work that he pursued for the rest of his life. Mester observed that the laser could accelerate the healing of burns, ulcers, and infected wounds and encouraged the regrowth of hair on mice he shaved. All of these effects seemed to imply that the laser had a biostimulatory effect.

Mester's sons, Andrew and Adam, took over their father's work

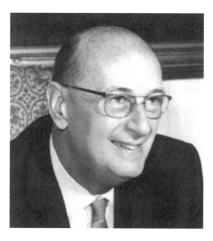

Figure 4.15.
Dr. Endre Mester
(photo courtesy
Dr. Adam Mester)

---

*Its power was about 1 J/cm² (joules per square centimeter, a joule being a unit of energy released by one watt during one second).

after he passed away, and when I met Adam Mester at the 2006 ILA conference he showed us the extent of progress accomplished since the time of his father's discoveries. But this progress was not easy. In fact, Mester's research in the 1960s, which was published behind the Iron Curtain, had been largely overlooked in the West. The main obstacle to the acceptance of his work was that no one could understand *how* such a biological stimulation could be possible. After all, conventional thinking goes that plants may feed on light, but animals cannot.* As no mechanism then known could explain the effects of lasers, Mester's observations were not accepted by the medical establishment until the work of another exceptional researcher emerged.

The Lady of Light

It rarely happens in the history of science, especially in our day, that an entire field is revolutionized by one person. But that is exactly how our story unfolds . . .

In the early 1980s, the Estonian biophysicist Tiina Karu was the head of the Laboratory of Laser Biology and Medicine in Moscow. There she conducted the first systematic investigation of the biostimulation

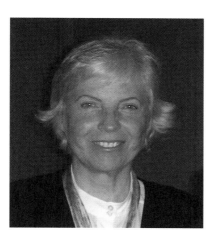

Figure 4.16.
Tiina Karu

---

*There is, however, an enduring tradition that says that certain humans in an appropriate state of consciousness are capable of living on light alone (or on ambient vital energy)—but this is another subject. For more on this see the 2010 documentary *In the Beginning There Was Light* (Straubinger 2010).

phenomena documented by Mester. For the next twenty years she persevered in this arduous task.

Karu first examined the effects of light on several aspects of cellular metabolism,* including the levels of synthesis of DNA and RNA and other indicators of vitality. Whereas Mester only had one light frequency at his disposal (the red of his helium-neon laser at 633 nm) Karu irradiated her cultures with a wider spectral range (from 300 to 900 nm, so from ultraviolet to near-infrared) and was thus able to establish detailed action spectra. She observed clear effects at specific frequencies.

Early on she noted that the action spectra of very different vital aspects are almost identical, with the same frequencies having the greatest effect. This could only mean one thing: a single root phenomenon must be driving these various effects. In 1988, after more years of research, she was finally able to affirm that the mysterious biostimulation phenomenon occurs (as you may have guessed) in the mitochondria of the cells. In so doing she was the first to demonstrate that light interacts with the cellular respiratory chain, the energy-producing engine of life.

About this she wrote: "A surprising circumstance is that the photoacceptors for this phenomenon in eukaryotic cells and in prokaryotic cells (*E. coli*) appeared to be natural components of the respiratory chain, and not specialized photoreceptor molecules. This is different from the classical photobiological phenomena which utilize specific photoreceptors (chlorophylls, rhodopsins, etc.)" (Karu 2008).

Pursuing her extraordinary biophysics detective work, in 1995 Karu finally isolated the long-sought-after key to the photobiological mystery. It lies precisely in one of the last links in the mitochondrial respiratory chain, that driven by the enzyme cytochrome c oxidase. This enzyme, a considerably complex protein, can exist in multiple states in which it absorbs photons of the various peak frequencies of the action spectrum that she had already mapped.

Throughout this research Karu (1980–2015, 1998, 2007) published an impressive body of scientific articles by which she established

---

*She used cultures of HeLa cells, the oldest and most common line of human cells used by biologists for in vitro investigations.

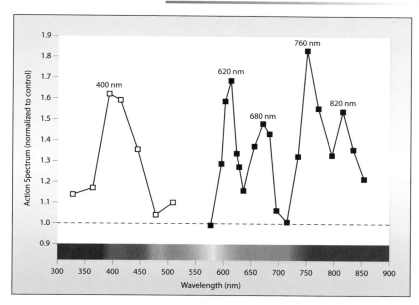

Figure 4.17. The generalized action spectrum of photobiomodulation according to Tiina Karu. The main peaks are at 400 nm (violet), 620 nm (red), 680 nm, 760 nm, and 820 nm (infrared).

beyond a doubt the existence of the phenomenon that she named *photobiomodulation*. The scientific and medical world finally woke up to this reality, leading to a surge of research in photobiology, starting in the 1990s.

From Mitochondria to DNA

One of the findings that most surprised Karu was the occurrence of certain cellular effects taking place well beyond the boundaries of the mitochondria. One expects that photobiomodulation, by stimulating the respiratory chain, will increase the amount of energy available to the cell in the form of ATP. But how to explain other observed effects, such as an increase in DNA synthesis happening in the insulated nucleus of the cell? To resolve these questions Karu persevered until the 2000s, when she identified multiple cascades of biochemical reactions, all originating in the mitochondria with the photonic stimulation of cytochrome c oxidase, then continuing to spread throughout the entire cell after light exposure to the point of stimulating the expression of genes in the DNA. It was known that the DNA in the nucleus is capable of sending messages regulating all the components of the cell, but this was a new means of communication in reverse, from the mitochondria to the nucleus, now known as *mitochondrial retrograde signaling.*

So light increases metabolic energy by the production of ATP; it increases motility and cell division; and it regenerates DNA. Considering such a range of biostimulating effects, it becomes much easier to understand the healing benefits of light observed from Mester onward.

How Deep?

Light biostimulates living cells—that is, if it can reach them. Can light penetrate our skin and irradiate the deeper parts of our body? That depends on its color. The longer its wavelength, the deeper it can penetrate. For example, blue light does not go much beyond the epidermis (just 0.5 mm), while red can reach depths of several millimeters. Penetration

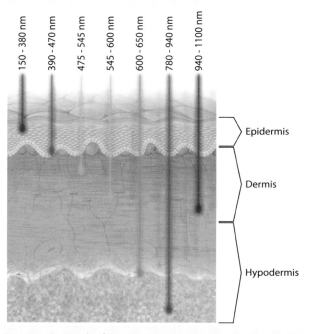

Figure 4.18. Depth of penetration into the skin of various colors

is at its maximum with near-infrared (between 650 and 940 nm), and then diminishes with the far-infrared spectrum.

Fortunately, the most important peaks in photobiomodulation are in that range of maximum penetration. With relatively intense sources of red and infrared light we can reach organs and muscular areas several centimeters deep, and we can actually treat the brain through the skull. Yet even shallow penetration with blue light can be of great significance. Recent research has shown that key immune T cells present in the upper dermis layers are activated by blue photons, which increase cells' ability to move throughout the body (Phan et al. 2016). Sunlight, with its ample blue content, is therefore an immunity booster when shining on the skin.

We can easily observe how light traverses our own body by taking a flashlight and putting it on our palm to see how the red part of the spectrum lights up the back of the hand a few centimeters away.

Autoregulation of Biostimulation

Another of Tiina Karu's observations is that the effect of light depends largely on the initial state of the living tissue.* Healthy cells already in an optimal state react less, whereas it is mostly cells that are sick or in need of oxygen that are stimulated. This highly beneficial system of auto-regulation also tends to reestablish the acid-base equilibrium of the cells.

This then explains how light can accelerate the regeneration of cells in a wound without affecting the healthy cells around it. It also explains why light therapy has so few undesirable side effects.

Coherence or Monochromaticity?

Laser light was used in the first studies on biomodulation, and it was known that it has two properties that distinguish it from ordinary light: *coherence*, where all photons are in phase; and monochromaticity, where all photons are of the same wavelength (see "What Is Light," chapter 3). It was not initially clear whether one or both of these properties were

---

*In scientific terms: the reaction of cells to light depends on their oxidation-reduction potential (redox), a measure of the tendency of their chemical constituents to acquire electrons.

essential for biostimulation. This is another of the mysteries unraveled by Karu: she demonstrated that light needs to be monochromatic for biostimulation to occur. In some of her experiments the effects of biostimulation disappeared when a white light was superimposed on a monochromatic light. As for the coherence of laser light, it deteriorates quite quickly at the surface of the skin and is not a determining factor.

It follows from this that LEDs, far more economical than lasers, can be used in many photobiomodulation applications. They are not coherent sources of light, but they are relatively monochromatic and thus are widely used in light therapy today.

A Meeting with Tiina Karu

Biophysicist Tiina Karu has a quasi-mythical status in the light therapy community, and it was therefore with some trepidation that I first met her in 2011, at an ILA conference I had organized in my hometown, St. Adele, Quebec. She had been invited by Karl Ryberg, one of the founders of the ILA, who had known her for a long time and who met with her often in Russia and Sweden. With her kindness and her lack of affectation, it didn't take this eminent scientist long to put us all at ease. In fact—and perhaps not surprisingly—I realized that this pioneer of light was herself radiant. I

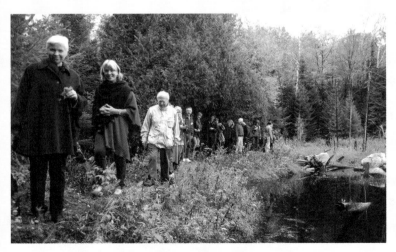

Figure 4.19. Tiina Karu (in the foreground) with members of the ILA
on the beaver dam on our property in St. Adele.

have had the opportunity to meet Tiina often since then and have had many captivating exchanges with her, during which she has shared some of the lesser-known aspects of her research.

At the conference she related how it all began for her:

Her husband, physicist Vladilen Letokhov, was already in 1980 one of the most respected scientists in the Soviet Union. A laser specialist, he had heard of the strange experiments of Mester and was skeptical of the results. He suggested that Tiina run a few lab tests to prove Mester wrong. She accepted the challenge, thinking that this would be a short-term project—though we now know how the rest of the story unfolded. Tiina's first papers were so controversial that she believes they would not have been published had her husband not been so influential. In the beginning she was often criticized and ridiculed for being interested in such an absurd area of research.

Even if she expresses no regrets concerning the passing of the Soviet era, she is somewhat nostalgic for the freedom enjoyed by the scientific community at that time. Research was not dominated by commercial or institutional interests as it is in the West,* and audacious projects could be undertaken. Otherwise her work may not have seen the light of day.

In 2012 the International Light Association awarded her the Frances McManemin prize in recognition of her major role in the development of phototherapy. And in her honor we held the 2015 ILA conference in Tallinn, capital of her native Estonia.

Perhaps the most precious moment that I have had the pleasure to share with her is when, coming out of her first experience of my Sensora chromotherapy system, she confided: "I have studied light for thirty years, but I had not till now realized how we can be so moved by its beauty."

---

*Even since the demise of the Soviet Union, researchers in the Eastern bloc remain more advanced than we in the West are in many aspects of energetic and vibrational medicine.

Now that we've learned about the various biological pathways of light, we are ready to explore how medicine can make the best use of them to restore health and balance.

5

LIGHT MEDICINE

The Modern Use of Phototherapy

We are still on the threshold of fully understanding the complex relationship between light and life, but we can now say, emphatically, that the function of our entire metabolism is dependent on light.

FRITZ-ALBERT POPP

AT THE DAWN OF THE TWENTY-FIRST CENTURY, the importance of light for our health and well-being has been confirmed by modern science. Today there is a great confluence of discovery and invention. Two extraordinary discoveries in biology have been brought to the study of light: the nonvisual optic pathway and photobiomodulation. At the same time, technological advancement is leading to new types of light sources, more powerful and more flexible than ever, and to new biomedical measuring devices that can assess the effects of light in minute detail.

A new era of light medicine has arrived.

In this chapter we will take a look at the main areas of its application and mention some of the most recent and promising developments in this exciting new branch of medicine. As I see it, there are two main categories of *phototherapy:*

* There is the type that makes use of the interactions that light already has with the body. We call this *endogenous phototherapy.* It includes therapies based on photobiomodulation and chronobiology, and it usually has regenerative properties and

tends to reestablish the natural order in a noninvasive way.

* Then there are therapies of the type that use light as a catalyst in novel, custom-made biological processes. This we call *synthetic phototherapy*. These therapies arise from our increasing understanding of the biochemistry of chromophores, those molecules capable of absorbing or emitting light, enabling us to make use of them in completely new ways. These therapies are generally more invasive and radical and are used for more aggressive interventions. For example, dynamic phototherapy excels in the destruction of cancer cells, and ultraviolet phototherapy can heal certain infections and serious diseases through the sterilization of pathogens. In this category I also include the fascinating field of optogenetics, in which photosensitive genes are inserted into the DNA of various cells, which then emit light or are activated by light. For the time being, optogenetics is essentially only used in medical research and will not be examined here.

These two categories of phototherapy employ very different principles and mechanisms, and their only common denominator is the use of light. Yet they are complementary and together constitute a formidable arsenal for the field of light medicine.

PHOTOBIOMODULATION THERAPY

Photobiomodulation is without a doubt the most impressive form of phototherapy because it intervenes at the very source of the cell's regenerative abilities. All traditional peoples in times past—as well as the light-therapy pioneers of the last century—have used it intuitively. But it was not until the spread of the laser in the 1960s that its use in medicine began, followed by a surge in its popularity as a result of the discoveries of Tiina Karu in the 1990s. It is one of the most active fields in photomedicine today, involving thousands of researchers throughout the world.*

---

*Several important international conferences on the subject are held each year, notably the International Society for Medical Laser Applications and the American Society for Laser Medicine and Surgery.

The Tools of
Light Medicine

Lasers: Due to their ability to generate light with very precise wavelengths and almost no divergence, lasers allow for a very fine and intense focal point. Several types of medical lasers are now in use:

- Ablative lasers, often in the infrared range and very powerful, can vaporize layers of the epidermis and are used in dermatology. Other types emit green light to vaporize vascularized tissue (since red blood best absorbs green light) and are used in tumor excision.
- Fractional lasers fracture their rays into tiny microbeams, making it possible to treat the skin without harming it. These are commonly used in aesthetic dermatology.
- Pulsed lasers emit light in very intense but very short bursts in the range of a nanosecond (10^{-9} s) to a femtosecond (10^{-15} s). They are used as scalpels in surgery.
- Excimer (or exiplex) lasers produce ultraviolet light and are used in the treatment of psoriasis and vitiligo.
- Laser diodes, low-intensity semiconductor lasers, are more compact and economical than other types of lasers. They're used for photobiomodulation to reach specific spots in deep tissue.

Intense Pulsed Light: IPLs are flashing lamps fitted with colored filters that emit several powerful pulses per second. They are increasingly used in dermatology and aesthetic medicine. The best ones have an integrated cooling system to improve comfort.

LEDs: These can replace lasers in certain applications, particularly in photobiomodulation. Medical LEDs come in a wide variety of strengths and optical beam widths. Different colors are used for different purposes—infrared and red for photobiomodulation, amber for aesthetics, green and blue for acne and chronobiology, ultraviolet in dentistry and for sterilization.

Fluorescent lamps: These are mostly used in the treatment of depression and for other chronobiological applications.

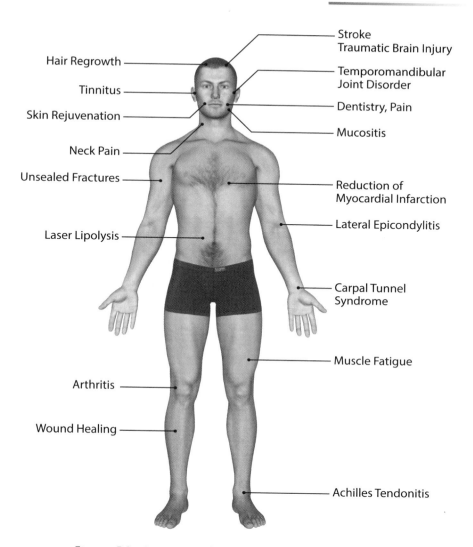

Figure 5.1. Current applications of photobiomodulation
(according to Hamblin and Huang 2013)

This field has gone by numerous names in the course of its development, and this has led to a certain amount of confusion: it has been called *low-level laser therapy* (LLLT), *cold laser therapy, laser phototherapy, low-level light therapy* (since a laser is not essential), *photobioactivation,* and almost seventy other names. There is a growing

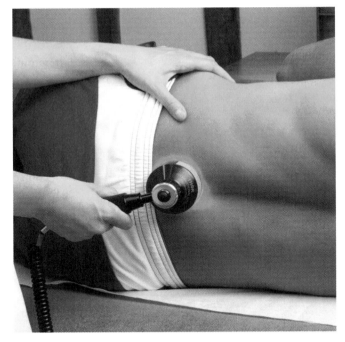

Figure 5.2. A typical photobiomodulation treatment
(© Thor Photomedicine Ltd.)

consensus that it should be called *photobiomodulation therapy,** and that is how we shall refer to it in this book.

Given the fundamental nature of the cellular processes involved in photobiomodulation, it is not surprising that the scope of possible applications keeps expanding, as one can see from the illustration on page 83 (fig. 5.1) that enumerates some of its current uses.

Photobiomodulation can bring about the following effects:

* Repair and regeneration of tissues by the biostimulation of cellular metabolism (for wounds, muscle trauma, hair loss, macular degeneration, regeneration of internal organs such as the heart, liver, and kidneys)
* Stimulation of the immune system, resulting in a lowering of

---

*This is the term adopted by the United States National Library of Medicine in November 2015.

inflammation (for dermatitis, eczema, asthma, arthritis)
* Pain relief (for postoperative pain, dental treatments, mucositis)
* Neurological effects, both physiological and cognitive (for brain trauma, stroke, depression, memory problems, dementia)

A Well-Kept Secret?

Photobiomodulation is already being used by many specialists. High-performance athletes (for example, in the Tour de France) and the military have used it for several years now to treat muscle trauma and tendinitis, and astronauts have been using it longer still. Why then, apart from a few exceptions in sports medicine, would photobiomodulation not be more prevalent? This can partly be explained by the fact that many of the applications of photobiomodulation are still experimental. Even if numerous clinical studies have shown convincing results, protocols still need to be established and the necessary clinical experience acquired before it can be put to general use. It will therefore probably take a few more years before the remarkable treatments of photobiomodulation become readily available to all of us. Even after purely technical issues have been resolved, there is the matter of the basic inertia of the medical system, which delays the practice of treatments that are radically different from those that are commonly accepted.

The implementation of photobiomodulation varies greatly from one country to another. Russia, with its history of discoveries in laser medicine, is often at the forefront in this field. There, phototherapy treatments are relatively common, including innovative applications such as for the prevention of heart problems (angina, cardiac arrest, and others). In the United States, some devices have already met the standards established by the U.S. Food and Drug Administration (FDA). The first such device, which appeared in 2002, was designed to treat carpal tunnel syndrome. In 2008, the World Health Organization endorsed photobiomodulation for the treatment of cervical pain. And in 2010, the American Physical Therapy Association recommended it for the treatment of injuries to the Achilles tendon.

So, slowly but surely, photobiomodulation is being integrated into our health habits.

How Much Is Too Much?

In phototherapy there are a considerable number of variables that need to be adjusted in order for treatment to be effective. Not only the wavelength, but also the spectral bandwidth, the intensity, the total energy delivered, the surface and depth of exposure, as well as the duration, frequency, and number of treatments have to be established. There are also more subtle factors such as the pulsation or coherence of the light source, or the time of day at which the treatment is administered.

At the root of this complexity is a key phenomenon of phototherapy: while a low dosage may be ineffective, too high a dosage will not necessarily be better, and an excess of light can actually inhibit the process that we are trying to stimulate. This is called a *biphasic reaction* to the stimulation. This phenomenon follows the Arndt-Schulz rule that is widespread in biology and was named after the two medical doctors who described it in the nineteenth century: For every substance, small doses stimulate, moderate doses inhibit, large doses kill. We can therefore understand the difficulty of establishing optimal dosages for photobiomodulation.

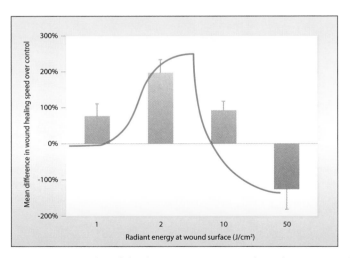

Figure 5.3. An example of biphasic reaction in phototherapy as shown by the duration of wound healing in a mouse after exposure to various intensities. We clearly see the optimal dose (here around 2 J/cm², or joules per square centimeter), above which results are even worse than an absence of treatment (from Huang et al. 2016).

Transcranial Infrared Therapy

One of the most fascinating prospects of photobiomodulation therapy is the healing of the brain by way of transcranial *near-infrared laser transmission* (NILT). Since neurons are the most energy-consuming cells of the body, they contain a high density of mitochondria (see the previous chapter's discussion of mitochondria) needed to produce their main fuel, ATP. Neurons therefore are ideal candidates for photobiomodulation therapy, which primarily enhances the activity of mitochondria.

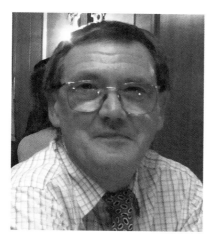

Figure 5.4. Michael Hamblin

But how can therapeutic light reach inside the skull? Dr. Michael Hamblin of Harvard Medical School, one of the main researchers in this field, has an explanation. His team observed that 2 to 3 percent of the near-infrared favorable to photobiomodulation (at 820 nanometers) penetrates the skull, thus enabling the use of relatively intense and focused light sources to stimulate the cerebral cortex. Hamblin's team has been conducting a remarkable series of studies on the use of NILT in the treatment of several different brain pathologies, with often surprising results in applications such as the following:

* Traumatic brain injury (Wu et al. 2010)
* Acute ischemic stroke (Lapchak 2010)
* Clinical recovery of neurodegenerative disease (Lapchak 2012)
* Alzheimer's (Sommer et al. 2012) and Parkinson's diseases

Hamblin told me that he expects ambulances will eventually be equipped with NILT devices because an application of light can play a critical role during a stroke, especially if it is administered early on, preferably within an hour.

More surprising still, the researchers obtained positive results using NILT for cognitive issues such as:

* Memory loss (Rojas, Bruchey, and Gonzalez-Lima 2012)
* Chronic cognitive dysfunction (Naeser 2009)
* Mild to moderately severe dementia (Saltmarche 2017)
* Anxiety and depression (Schiffer et al. 2009)
* Academic performance of university students (Barrett and Gonzalez-Lima 2013)

In some studies a single irradiation, barely a few minutes long, was sufficient to produce clinically measurable results—something with potential to dream about . . . All of this intrigued me to such an extent that I decided to engineer my own source of the appropriate infrared light and start my own experimentation with NILT.

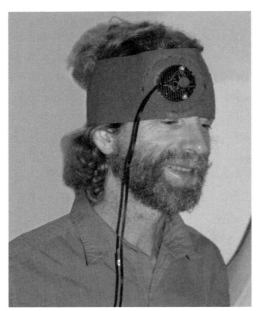

Figure 5.5. The author boldly experimenting with NILT

Recent Developments in Photobiomodulation

Researchers are now exploring a variety of avenues to optimize the effects of photobiomodulation. One of these is the application of a phenomenon called *quantum optically induced transparency,* or QIT, in which two light sources of slightly shifted wavelengths create a *resonance* that increases their penetration of the tissues of the body. Dr. Detlef Schikora, head of the biophysics research group in the faculty of science, Paderborn University, Germany, has developed photobiomodulation devices based on this principle, which he calls *medlouxx* (a word loosely derived from *mitochondrial excitation due to lowering of light absorption*).* These devices carry the effects of photobiomodulation deeper into the tissues. This could be particularly valuable for transcranial phototherapy, where the reduced penetration of light is a limiting factor.

Dr. Schikora has also developed a powerful combination of photobiomodulation and acupuncture in a device he calls the Laserneedle (Schikora, Klowersa, and Suwanda 2012) (see fig. 5.6). In this technique, the traditional acupuncture needle is replaced with a light source that is transmitted through an optic fiber.† His recent versions combine two light sources, one red for its effect on tissue regeneration and the other blue to activate local systems of pain inhibition (Litscher 2009). His team has found an increased effectiveness, particularly in pain treatments.

Another improvement in photobiomodulation has been explored since the 1970s by Russian researchers using magnetotherapy. This technique, which involves the application of magnetic fields, pulsed or not, is now recognized in therapeutic applications as diverse as bone repair, chronic pain management, and inflammation reduction. The combination of this modality with photobiomodulation brings about a synergy in which the therapeutic effects surpass what would be obtained from either treatment alone (Friedmann, Lipovsky, Nitzan, and Lubart 2009). In the 1990s this led to the development of the first *magneto-infrared*

---

*See www.medlouxx.com
†This technique is different from other acupuncture-related approaches used in chromotherapy such as Colorpuncture because it relies on the biochemical properties of photobiomodulation rather than on the effects of color (see chapter 9's discussion of Colorpuncture).

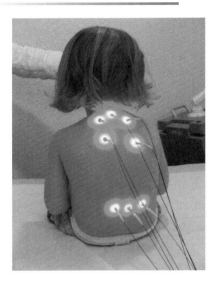

Figure 5.6. Laserneedle
therapy session
(© Dr. Detlef Schikora)

laser (MIL) therapy devices (Illarionov 2009). Variations of these MIL-therapy instruments are commonly used in Russia to treat diverse pathologies. More recently, other international researchers have widened this approach by adding a chromotherapeutic component (such as the coMra and Milta therapies described in chapter 9).

Light in the Service of Beauty

One of the most obvious signs of the progress that light medicine has made is the multitude of light-based treatments now being offered in aesthetics and dermatology. The number of beauty salons providing such treatments are increasing so rapidly that at least two have appeared in my rather modest village of St. Adele within the last year. In this, photo-therapy has found its first truly profitable commercial application.

Many different techniques that use a wide range of LED or laser instruments at diverse wavelengths are now on offer. The field is still so new, with so few established standards, that it can be difficult to find one's way around. It is essential to consult an experienced and reliable professional for proper guidance. This arsenal of ablative, fractal, or pulsed lasers can eliminate spots, firm up the skin by stimulating the production of collagen, and reduce fine lines and scars. Intense pulsed light devices (IPLs) are ideal for treating acne and removing unwanted hair as well.

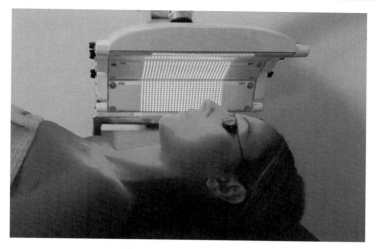

Figure 5.7. LED beauty

Amber, red, and infrared LEDs bring the regenerative qualities of photobiomodulation to the skin. They are used either as a complement to laser treatments, to reduce inflammation and accelerate healing, or on their own, to firm up and rejuvenate the skin. Blue LEDs are sometimes added in the treatment of acne, but opinions on their effectiveness in this application are divided. All these treatments require patience and perseverance, particularly in the case of photobiomodulation due to its gentle and noninvasive nature. A typical course of therapy would require a dozen treatments at a rate of two per week.

SHINING A LIGHT ON CHRONOBIOLOGY

Since the discovery of the nonvisual optic pathway, the science of chronobiology has been in full swing. Whatever the exact mechanisms underlying the circadian influence of light are, their effects are profound. The team of chronobiologists led by John Hogenesch discovered that nearly half of all the activity of our genes is influenced by the circadian rhythm (Zhang et al. 2014)—a much higher proportion than previously thought.

Photobiomodulation at Home

When it comes to photobiomodulation, the expertise, experience, and equipment of a qualified professional practitioner is irreplaceable. However, anyone can experiment with the benefits of this healing light by buying a therapeutic device intended for home use. A quick search on the internet for "LED therapy" will turn up an overwhelming number of products. Here are a few selection criteria to keep in mind:

LED color: Red and infrared are the most important for photobiomodulation, especially if their wavelengths are close to the peaks of its action spectrum at 620, 680, 760, and 820 nm. Some models add blue LEDs (around 470 nm; studies show their usefulness in the process of cell regeneration, for example in healing wounds) or amber LEDs (at 590 nm, considered optimal for the formation of collagen and the firming up of skin).

Power: Most of these products have relatively low power and so require proportionally longer exposures if they are to have a significant effect. Choose units with a higher number of LEDs or with higher power LEDs.

Laser diodes: Some products offer laser diodes instead of LEDs (or a combination of the two)—they are usually more powerful but also more expensive. They may be interesting for certain specialized uses but are not necessary for general use.

Treatment area: Some devices are designed to irradiate a small focused area (for example, for the treatment of tendinitis or small wounds), while others have a wide emitting surface to treat larger skin areas.

The quality of the construction and ease of operation: Units equipped with a timer are more practical.

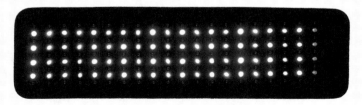

Figure 5.8. A typical example of a phototherapy light pad with red, blue, and infrared LEDs (© INLight Medical Polychromatic Light Therapy Systems)

Some products are designed for specific applications: treating facial skin, muscle relaxation, and so forth. One popular application confirmed in scientific studies is for stimulating hair growth (Avci et al. 2014). The FDA has actually approved several devices for this purpose. One can find a variety of brushes, helmets, and other devices in the most singular configurations.

An example of a professional-quality instrument for general use is the Bioptron,* made in Switzerland. It uses a halogen light source that supplies 10,000 lux. Its wide spectrum (480 to 3400 nm) contains an abundant proportion of the infrared spectrum beneficial for photobiomodulation. A unique characteristic of the Bioptron is its use of a Brewster mirror, a multilayered optical structure that produces polarized light. Some of the properties of absorption of light by living tissues are dependent on polarization, and according to several studies polarization can improve certain aspects of photobiomodulation (Ribeiro et al. 2004).

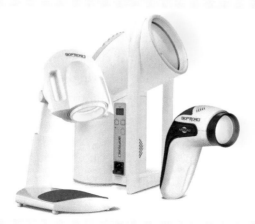

Figure 5.9. The Bioptron
(© Zepter, www.bioptron.com)

When choosing a device, one must always remember that the effectiveness of the cheaper products varies considerably and in most cases cannot compare to the effectiveness of certified medical instruments. However, they do offer us an opportunity to embark on a fascinating exploration involving no risk and can even result in some pleasant surprises!

---

*www.bioptron.com

Researchers are now interested in "sculpting" the light spectra of our artificial light sources in order to optimize their beneficial influence on our chronobiology, and also to lessen any disturbances that they inflict (see chapter 6, "Health Risks of Light"). In this case it is the lighting in our homes and workplaces that becomes a source of therapeutic light. In this we are speaking of *human-centric lighting* made possible by the new LED lighting technologies, in which one can vary the color temperature of a light and therefore its degree of influence on the circadian rhythm. Some people worry about the Orwellian danger of manipulating the productivity of workers by means of the lighting to which they are subjected—for example, by increasing the amount of blue in daytime to keep them more awake (Mills, Tomkins, and Schlangen 2007). Others, on the other hand, consider that we will bring new freedom of choice by offering each person the possibility of adapting lighting to their own preferences. In this, large interests are at stake. A recent study undertaken by a European lighting industry association evaluated at 12 billion Euros the potential gains (in terms of health and productivity) that could be realized between 2015 and 2020 if circadian-aware lighting became standard across European countries (LightingEurope 2015). The transition to this new ergonomic approach to lighting is already underway.

Lighting for Health Care

The first places where this new type of ergonomic, circadian-aware lighting is being implemented are in health-care venues like hospitals. In some countries circadian-aware lighting is being installed in patients' rooms and in postoperative units, and chromotherapy is also being used to create ambiences conducive to relaxation and stress reduction (see fig. 5.11).

One of the more promising applications is to be found in lighting for senior residences. Recent studies demonstrate that it is possible to improve the quality of life of elderly persons with dementia, such as Alzheimer's disease, wherein a person's sleep cycle is often disturbed (Hanford and Figueiro 2013). A dose of the appropriate light at the right moment of the day can resynchronize the person's circadian rhythm, leading to better sleep and thus to a reduction of symptoms such as agitation and depression.

Circadian Lighting in Space

A clear proof of how far circadian lighting has come is shown by the fact that it is now being installed 250 miles up in the sky, inside the International Space Station (ISS).

As the ISS orbits the Earth it experiences a sunrise and a sunset every ninety minutes. This unsettles astronauts' circadian rhythm to such an extent that their foremost health problem becomes one of sleep quality and the loss of sleep. Despite the use of medication, their sleep period is often reduced to barely six hours, leading to chronic partial sleep deprivation that can have life-threatening consequences in such a high-risk environment.

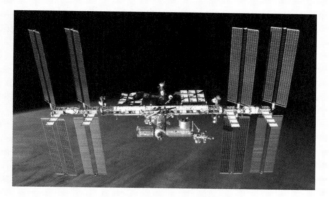

Figure 5.10. The International Space Station is a living lab
for testing the effectiveness of circadian lighting
(photo courtesy NASA)

Starting in 2016, NASA launched a research program to test and implement a circadian lighting system in the station, beginning with retrofitting astronauts' sleeping quarters. Custom LED lights were designed under the supervision of George Brainard, one of the researchers who first measured the melatonin-suppressing impact of blue light (see chapter 4), with three spectral settings adapted to normal vision (balanced), circadian shifting (blue-enriched), and sleep inducement (red-enriched). This experimental setup will enable scientists to test various hypotheses concerning the effects of lighting on sleep cycles. These enhancements to life in space will, eventually, contribute to improvements in lighting quality for all of us on the ground.

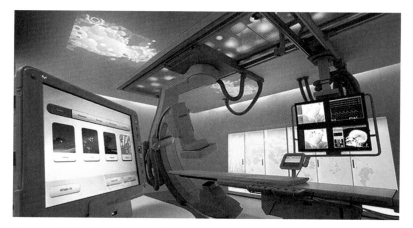

Figure 5.11. The first cardiovascular room with chromotherapeutic lighting, made by Philips AmbiScene for Catharina Hospital, Eindhoven, The Netherlands (© Philips Ambiscene)

Bright Light Therapy

In the 1980s, even before precisely understanding the mechanisms involved, health professionals began to practice bright light therapy (BLT) to treat a chronobiological disorder found mostly in northern countries—seasonal affective disorder, or SAD, a form of depression occurring during winter months. Researchers have concluded that SAD is caused by a chronic lack of sunlight beginning in the autumn, as well as habits of modern life that lead us to spend most of our days indoors under artificial lighting (Rosenthal et al. 1984). The person's internal clock no longer receives the necessary signals to properly synchronize the circadian rhythm, causing a cascade of secondary effects such as insomnia, lack of energy, and depression.

The proposed solution to SAD is simple: expose the person to a light source sufficiently bright to allow the system to resynchronize with the circadian rhythm. The prescription typically involves the use of a lamp providing 10,000 lux for thirty minutes a day, preferably upon waking. The therapy lamp must have a spectrum wide enough to include the wavelengths capable of stimulating the nonvisual optic pathway (centered on blue at 460–490 nm) because that is the best way to reach the master internal clock, the suprachiasmatic nucleus, or

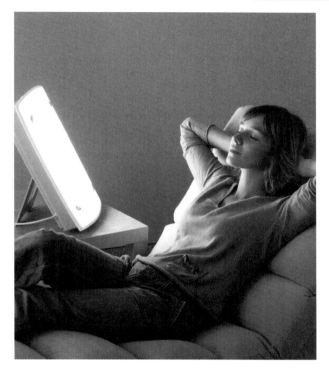

Figure 5.12. A bright light therapy session

SCN (see chapter 4). There currently are several types of these lamps (see page 99).

Numerous studies have now established that bright light therapy is at least as effective for SAD as any medication that would be prescribed (for an example, see Golden et al. 2005). Its success is such that it is commonly thought of as being synonymous with light therapy, even though, as anyone who has read this far will have realized, light therapy encompasses a much wider field than the sole bright light therapy technique.

The lack of light in wintertime affects many more people than we might think: for example, it is estimated that 10 to 15 percent of the population of France suffers from mild seasonal depression, the "winter blues," even if they do not present some of the more extreme symptoms of SAD. For those people as well, an occasional dose of bright light (using the same lamps as for SAD) can make all the difference in the world.

Today the use of bright light therapy is also being explored in the treatment of sleep disorders (Van Maanen et al. 2016), eating disorders, and Parkinson's disease. It has been observed that the technique can also be helpful for forms of depression other than SAD.

What About Jet Lag?

Jet lag is a perfect example of the desynchronization of one's internal clock, and most of us occasionally have to deal with it after lengthy air travel. Bright light therapy can be used in an attempt to minimize its impact, but studies have shown that the results do not necessarily justify the effort. That's because the resynchronization of one's internal clock follows its own natural rhythm, which is difficult to speed up, even with the aid of external light. In its reestablishment it can move forward by about an hour a day, or move backward by ninety minutes a day, which explains why it is more perturbing to travel across time zones going east (say, from New York to Paris) than going west (from Paris to New York).

In 1998, researchers proposed that the use of blue light behind the knees reduces jet lag, possibly by irradiating the blood vessels accessible at that spot. Unfortunately, subsequent studies (Wright and Czeisler 2002) failed to reproduce these results (though they were initially published in the prestigious journal *Science*), eliminating this hope. The best strategy seems to be exposure to light (either daylight or to a lamp used for bright light therapy) at judiciously chosen times, ideally starting several days before a flight. There are a few apps that can facilitate this; for example, Entrain,* which is derived from the work of biologist Daniel Forger.

Recent research at the Stanford University School of Medicine found that the circadian rhythm can be entrained efficiently by short pulses of light (typically two-millisecond flashes ten seconds apart), especially at night (Najjar and Zeitzer 2016). Since these can be applied through closed eyelids without waking up the subject, they provide a way to trick the body's biological clock into adapting to an awake cycle even when asleep. Goggles based on this principle,† worn during nights just before and after a

---

*http://entrain.math.lsa.umich.edu

†For example, the LumosTech Smart Sleep Mask (https://lumos.tech)

time-shifting flight, for example, could accelerate the jet-lag adjustment with minimal sleep disruption by generating light flashes during appropriately timed periods. Alternatively, innovative devices delivering extraocular light through the ear canals* have been shown to be effective in alleviating jet-lag symptoms. And techniques of chromotherapy such as Colorpuncture (see chapter 9) propose simple protocols for jet lag based on the activation of appropriate acupuncture reflex points with colored light.

*For example, the Valkee Humancharger extraocular light emitter (www.humancharger .com)

Which Lamp?

A brief internet search reveals a multitude of lamps for bright light therapy. They have several distinguishing characteristics:

* **Lighting technology:** As we have seen, it is the influence on the nonvisual optic pathway that is in play here, and the circadian sensitivity spectrum is centered on blue. Two technologies are capable of emitting light with a sufficient proportion of blue: fluorescent tubes and LEDs.
* **Brightness:** The majority of models are calibrated to deliver 10,000 lux of white light, the reference brightness in most studies on SAD. Recent research tends to demonstrate equivalent effects with light intensities reduced to as low as 2,500 lux (Alotaibi, Halaki, and Chow 2016).
* **Color:** Since the circadian sensitivity spectrum of the ipRGCs culminates in blue around 460 to 490 nm, some researchers prefer to use only this waveband for bright light therapy. In doing so one can work with much lower levels of light: studies have shown that 100 lux of blue light is as beneficial as 10,000 lux of white light (Meesters et al. 2016). Blue green (cyan or turquoise) light at 505 nm is almost as effective as blue (Paul et al. 2009).
* **Format:** Though most BLT devices are table lamps or "light boxes," a few others are designed as visors that can be worn like

glasses. Being portable, these have the advantage of allowing the user to go about his or her daily business. Because the light rays are aimed at the tiny area of the pupil, much less intensity is required.

* **Orientation of the light rays:** ipRGCs are more densely distributed in the lower half of the retina, onto which light from the upper visual field shines. Therefore, a light coming from above will be more efficient for bright light therapy than a light that shines on the whole visual field (Glickman et al. 2003).

The different types of bright light therapy devices each have their own proponents, and it can be difficult to choose from among them. From the point of view of conventional medicine, one can't go wrong with the most clinically validated solution, that of a 10,000-lux white fluorescent light box. However, this only takes into account the influence of light on the nonvisual optic pathway. From the perspective of this book, other factors come into play (the risks of certain forms of lighting are discussed in chapter 6). As we will see, these factors tend to discourage the use of fluorescents because of the intense lines in their light spectrum generated by the presence of toxic mercury, which is at the basis of this technology. LEDs are the preferred replacement. And even if it may be tempting to choose blue or turquoise light, the spectrum of which is optimal for this application, we will see that from a chromotherapeutic point of view each color has a profound psychophysiological influence (as discussed in chapter 8). White light, being neutral, is less likely to be disturbing than intense pure colors, which do not necessarily correspond to our immediate needs.

Another key factor is the *blue light hazard* (BLH) which determines the risk of damage to the retinal photoreceptors caused by higher-energy photons, particularly those of the deep blue wavelengths ranging from 420 to 470 nm. According to this criterion, the use of turquoise at 505 nm is preferable because the risk of BLH is reduced, while the effects on the ipRGCs are largely maintained. But even then the danger is substantial for long-term use. The overlap of the action spectra of the ipRGCs' circadian sensitivity and that of the BLH is such that one cannot be activated without the other's engagement.

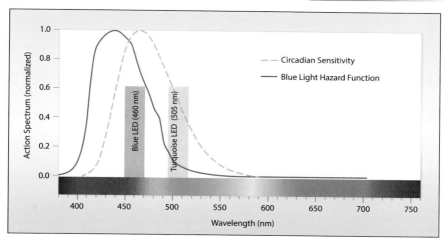

Figure 5.13. A comparison of the BLH and
the circadian sensitivity action spectra

Note: For all applications other than the mild "winter blues" it is not recommended to experiment with bright light therapy without being under the supervision of a trained specialist. Despite there being few associated side effects with bright light therapy, because it is a powerful therapeutic modality, prudence in its use is advised.

The danger of BLH (discussed in chapter 6) can be reduced by adding an infrared component to the light source. The infrared compensates for retinal degradation through the action of photobiomodulation. Unfortunately, as far as I know, no lamp on the market today has this property.

In the end there is still no device for bright light therapy that takes into account all of these factors. The ideal lamp would probably have a white spectrum of moderate intensity, including an appropriate proportion of infrared, and be oriented to shine from above. One can only hope that such a lamp will eventually come on the market. Meanwhile, my favorite solution for occasional use, such as in the case of jet lag, is a white light LED visor.* For long-term use one could consider using a white LED light box and putting a source of incandescent (or halogen) light next to it as a way of adding infrared to mitigate BLH.

---

*For example, the Luminette visor (www.myluminette.com)

SYNTHETIC PHOTOTHERAPIES

Synthetic phototherapies use light to achieve effects beyond those that occur naturally in the body. They typically involve the destructive properties of light rather than its regenerative ones and enable a range of techniques to efficiently get rid of unwanted cells.

Blue Light for Neonatal Jaundice

Even before the onset of the new light medicine beginning around 2000, one of the few phototherapy treatments that was acknowledged by conventional medicine was that used for neonatal jaundice. Its effectiveness was recognized as far back as 1958, and today maternity wards make common use of it.

Jaundice, a common condition in newborns, is caused by an excess of bilirubin in the blood, a condition called *hyperbilirubinemia*. It affects around 60 percent of babies in the first week of life. Most cases clear up naturally as the liver degrades the bilirubin, but for a few infants the condition worsens and develops into hyperbilirubinemia, which can have serious consequences. Traditional treatments involve unpleasant blood transfusions. In the phototherapy treatment, while the baby's eyes are carefully protected, its skin is exposed to blue light, the most effective range being between 460 and 490 nm. The excess bilirubin is decomposed in the skin and rendered harmless by photo-oxidation of the blood. The most recent technological innovation for this is the biliblanket, a sort of fabric made of fiber optics that shines blue light on the infant's skin.

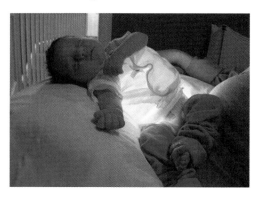

Figure 5.14. A biliblanket to treat neonatal jaundice
(photo by Chris Rugen)

Photodynamic Therapy

Photodynamic therapy (PDT) is one of the principal synthetic photo-therapies in the medical arsenal. As opposed to photobiomodulation, which uses light to stimulate natural cellular processes, PDT uses it to destroy cells. This can be very useful, for example, in the ablation of cancerous tumors that are difficult to treat by the traditional means of surgery, chemotherapy, and radiation.

PDT is based on the action of a photosensitizing agent composed of chromophore molecules that are capable, by absorbing light pho-tons, of passing from an initially neutral biological state to a toxic one. This toxicity is usually the result of the production of reactive oxy-gen species (ROS), oxygenated molecules that become highly reactive when exposed to the ionizing effect of light. Even though their action is extremely localized (spanning a few nanometers) and brief (lasting only nanoseconds), the abundance of these ROS molecules damages the neighboring cells to the point of killing them within a short period.

The success of PDT resides in the fact that once the photosensitizing agent is introduced into the body, either by injection or by application to the skin, it tends to concentrate in the cancer cells within twenty-four to seventy-two hours. At that point an appropriate dose of light is applied to the area to trigger the destructive action of the photosensitizing agent in the tumor. This is achieved by illuminating the skin, or if the tumor is in a deeper location, by the insertion of fiber optics (see fig. 5.15).

Current research in PDT focuses on the design of improved photo-sensitizing agents. The search is on to find agents that have fewer side effects, such as the excessive photosensitivity that can last for days that is commonly brought about by standard agents. Another objective is to find agents that are activated by the longest infrared wavelengths pos-sible because those are the ones capable of penetrating most deeply into the body. At first molecules in the porphyrins class were used, and now many alternatives are being tried, such as bacteriochlorins based on pig-ments found in photosynthetic bacteria. The most recent efforts use spe-cial polymer dyes* to form biodegradable organic nanoparticles featuring

---

*Notably, boron dipyrromethene molecules such as Car-BDP with a 600 to 800 nm absorption band

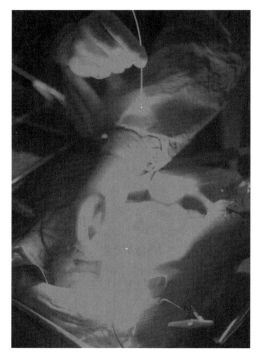

Figure 5.15. Lighting a cancerous target
by fiber optics in dynamic phototherapy

absorption in a broad near-infrared range over which tissues are most transparent, thus enabling PDT treatments with lower-power (and more cost-effective) light sources than ever before (Huang et al. 2016).

The principle of PDT has been known since antiquity, where it was used to treat skin diseases. In ancient Egypt and in India, natural photosensitizing agents were used, like the compound psoralen, which is found in many plants, notably in the bishop's-weed that grows on the banks of the Nile, as well as in the seeds of *Psoralea corylifolia* (an important plant in the ayurvedic pharmacopeia) and in the common fig, celery, parsley, and West Indian satinwood, and in all citrus fruits. An application on the skin was followed by exposure to sunlight. PDT was rediscovered accidentally at the beginning of the twentieth century by German scientists Oscar Raab, Albert Jesionek, and Hermann von Tappeiner. While performing tests on the toxicity of certain compounds on microorganisms, they noticed that samples exposed to light experienced greater harm. But it was not till the 1970s that this phenomenon was studied in a systematic way.

Even if PDT is one of the most ancient forms of phototherapy it is still not commonly practiced in the medical world today. But its use is bound to expand because in many cases it offers the least invasive and most rapid treatment, particularly for nonmetastatic cancers of the skin, the blood, and the linings of internal organs such as the esophagus, lungs, stomach, bladder, and prostate—wherever light can reach.

Ultraviolet Phototherapies

Many variations of synthetic phototherapies, called *actinotherapies,* make use of the ionizing and oxidative properties of ultraviolet light. The ultraviolet portion of the light spectrum is divided into three bands of increasing energy: UVA (315–380 nm), UVB (280–315 nm), and UVC (100–280 nm). The different ultraviolet phototherapies use the specific properties of each of these bands.

PUVA phototherapy (PUVA means "psoralen + UVA") uses a photosensitizing agent derived from psoralen that is taken orally or applied to the skin, followed by cutaneous exposure to UVA (315–380 nm). In a process similar to PDT, this combination destroys undesirable cells and is especially effective in the treatment of skin problems such as eczema, psoriasis, and vitiligo.

UVB phototherapy is used to treat the same range of skin problems but without the use of a photosensitizing agent. The more energetic photons of UVB make for a quicker treatment than is the case with PUVA and avoid the side effects associated with the photosensitizing agent—but at the risk of a possible increase in skin damage. The narrow spectrum UVB variant at 311 nm is now the preferred choice.

UVC light is essentially used for sterilization. Its photons are so energetic that they damage the DNA of cells, hence its germicidal property. Recent studies have shown that mammalian cells can better withstand UVC than microorganisms can. A judicious

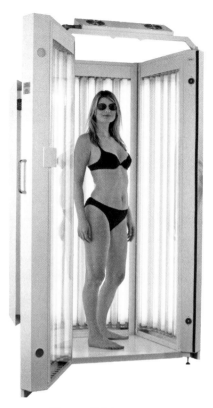

Figure 5.16. PUVA
phototherapy

dosage of irradiation (from 250 to 270 nm) is now being used in the treatment of local infections and wounds (Tianhong and Hamblin 2014).

UV Blood Irradiation (UBI) is a surprising form of phototherapy in which a small quantity of blood is taken from a patient, exposed to UV light for a few minutes, and then reintroduced into the body. Developed in the 1920s, this technique was common in the 1940s and '50s but has all but gone out of use today—another example of light therapy being eclipsed by pharmacological medicine. However, it has experienced a certain comeback of late following the results of some recent studies (Rowen 1996). UBI detoxifies the blood and has been used against viral and bacterial infections, sepsis, asthma, and hepatitis. Its operating principle has never been completely understood, but it is thought that the germicidal effect of UV acts as a type of vaccine that is transferred to the whole volume of blood. Modern practitioners of UBI* are mainly interested in its ability to stimulate the immune system and therefore to improve general health.

THE FUTURE OF LIGHT MEDICINE

Being at the frontier usually means being the first to confront obstacles. Despite light medicine's demonstrated successes, the fact remains that it has not yet found its rightful place within the medical system in terms of recognition from both health professionals and the general public. The challenges are scientific as well as financial. The medical world is largely controlled by the pharmaceutical industry, and light does not seem to lead to treatments as lucrative or patentable as those of pharmacology. Dr. Thierry Patrice, a leading pioneer of PDT, points to one of the main obstacles to its widespread acceptance:

> What makes PDT a promising medical procedure is its cost-effectiveness, which has been documented in various medical fields. However, the structure of medical expenses in our developed countries, whatever the level of analysis—for instance big-pharma companies, hospitals, doctors, or insurance companies—is not in favor of cheap treatment modalities. Each group with the exception of patients has a direct interest in using expensive methods. . . . Thanks to the debt crisis, in the future, one can expect a change in the reimbursement philosophy of health expenditures in a way that would reinforce PDT. (Hamblin and Huang 2013)

---

*I first heard about UBI from Dr. Edward Kondrot. Ed is a homeopathic ophthalmologist who has worked with several unconventional treatments based on, among other things, light and microcurrents. He offers exceptional protocols for the treatment of macular degeneration, glaucoma, cataracts, and the like at his clinic in Florida, which I have had the opportunity to visit. He has experimented with UBI and reports positive results.

Light medicine is still young, and it is evolving rapidly. Even if it is still only in its infancy, its day is definitely coming. Here are just a few examples of what is in store for us:

Bright light therapy is no longer just seasonal. Until now, bright light therapy has been known for its effectiveness in treating SAD. But an article published in the American medical journal *JAMA Psychiatry* has caused quite a stir among mental-health professionals. Lam et al. (2016) showed that bright light is more effective than one of the most common pharmacological anti-depressants (fluoxetine, better known under the brand name Prozac) in people suffering from major depressive disorders. Moreover, two important meta-analyses of the treatment of nonseasonal depression with bright light appeared at about the same time: that of Perera et al. (2016), which reviewed twenty-one studies, and that of Alotaibi, Halaki, and Chow (2016), which covered twenty-four. Both reports concluded that though the accuracy of the published studies was not perfect, a significant positive effect has been clearly established. The benefits of bright light are therefore no longer limited to seasonal disorders, and its field of application is growing. In one of the most recent examples, Valdimarsdottir et al. (2016) has been helping cancer survivors overcome their depression with the use of bright light. In another study, Sit el al. (2017) found bright light therapy effective in increasing the remission rate of patients with bipolar disorder. Intriguingly, their best results were obtained by administrating the bright light at midday rather than in the morning, as is the norm with SAD treatment, indicating that bright light therapy still holds many secrets.

New photoactive agents are coming from the ocean. The latest research into the improvement of photosensitizing agents for PDT involves more and more complex technologies, such as the use of nanoparticles. In this regard analysis of photoactive molecules already present in nature has provided inspiration. In collaboration with IFREMER (Institut Français de

Recherche pour L'exploitation de la Mer), a French institute that undertakes research and expert assessments to advance knowledge on the oceans and their resources, researchers studied 140 types of marine algae (Morlet et al. 1995). Only 2 to 5 percent of the samples were expected to be photoactive, but it turned out that photosensitivity was detected in over 50 percent, and in some by a factor of thirty times over traditional photosensitizing agents. Elucidating the mysteries of these molecules will undoubtedly enrich the field of light medicine. One of the latest trials using such new seabed-derived photosensitizing agents has shown great success in treating prostate cancer. Involving over four hundred patients, the study applied a PDT variant called vascular-targeted photodynamic therapy (VTP), in which the photosensitizing agent was injected in the bloodstream. According to lead investigator Mark Emberton, of University College London Hospital (UCLH), half of the patients treated with this new technique went into complete remission and were thus able to avoid using more invasive standard methods (Azzouzi et al. 2016).

Light is being introduced through the nose and ears. We know that light can produce effects through the visual system, the skin, and the skull (with near-infrared laser transmission). But researchers are exploring other ways to bring light into the body, illustrating what the future could hold. Intracranial low-intensity laser therapy involves the application of light in the nasal cavity. Its use is relatively common in China, where Liu et al. (2012) have been studying its effects for many years. Their studies have found it to be valuable for cardiovascular and cerebral disorders, and it is also used for many other ailments, including insomnia, migraine, and influenza, and for neuropathic and cognitive problems. With its highly vascularized mucous membranes, the nasal passages are ideal for phototherapy because they allow for direct irradiation of the blood. But Dr. Liu suspects that the effects of this light probably go beyond this. He sees a possible influence on the convergence of six meridians that according to traditional Chinese medicine pass through the nose.

Other therapists have studied the application of light in the auditory canal as an extension of research on transcranial light therapy. Since the ear canal passes through the thick bones of the skull, it is a logical pathway for irradiating the brain's neurons. This is what Jurvelin et al. (2014) tested in a study with patients suffering from SAD. Positive results comparable to those achieved with the use of a light box as in standard bright light therapy were obtained in this investigation. Furthermore, an intriguing finding is that extraocular light does not seem to influence the secretion of melatonin, a factor normally considered to be of major importance in the classical bright light therapy treatment for SAD.

Light could be an effective treatment for Parkinson's disease. In the 1980s, French neurosurgeon Alim Louis Benabid began to develop deep brain stimulation, a revolutionary treatment for Parkinson's disease and other movement disorders based on electrical stimulation of the affected neurons. Dr. Benabid is now exploring a new type of treatment based on the ability of infrared light to regenerate neurons through photobiomodulation. Transcranial irradiation cannot suffice in this case since the zones that must be reached are deeper than the few centimeters of penetration achieved with near-infrared laser transmission. Dr. Benabid proposes to bring light directly through an optic microfiber inserted into the brain. Successful trials have been performed on mice and more recently on monkeys (Darlot et al. 2016). Though this is obviously an invasive technique, it offers the extraordinary perspective of not only reducing the neuronal degradation brought on by Parkinson's, but also of preventing it and one day possibly even reversing it.

Light could be used to treat Alzheimer's disease. A remarkable result was obtained by a Massachusetts Institute of Technology team of researchers after they exposed mice suffering from

Alzheimer's disease to flickering light. They found that flickering light in the gamma brain-wave range (specifically, at 40 Hz) significantly reduced the amyloid plaque buildup in the brain that is associated with Alzheimer's (Iaccarino et al. 2016). This unexpected finding can be better understood when one considers the ability of flickering light entering through the eyes to entrain *brain waves* to resonate at the driving frequency (see chapter 9). In the progression of Alzheimer's, a reduction in gamma waves precedes the formation of harmful amyloid plaques in the brain, ultimately leading to a decline of learning and memory skills. The 40 Hz flickering light succeeded in reversing this trend, both restoring higher levels of gamma brain waves and attenuating the amyloid load. While it is too early to know how this might translate into actual treatment for humans, the potential for such a noninvasive and easily accessible light technique is enormous.

In this chapter the healing power wielded by modern light medicine has been amply demonstrated. It is now time to take a look at another aspect of the power of light, that of the detrimental effects brought about by unhealthy lighting.

6

HEALTH RISKS OF LIGHT

The Harmful Potential of Artificial Light

When trace amounts of certain wavelengths of light are missing from your "light diet," this can have a staggering effect on your health.

JOHN OTT

FOR EONS, HUMAN BEINGS have lived in harmony with the light of the sun. But only in the last hundred years or so, since its introduction, have we become rather well adapted to artificial lighting. The advent of artificial lighting liberated us from our dependence on daylight for the accomplishment of most activities, and in so doing it has fundamentally transformed human life.

The preceding chapters revealed the extraordinary healing potential of light. If this phenomenon has such powerful effects, not only on our body but also on our psyche, is it surprising that it could also have deleterious consequences if not wisely used? Present-day researchers are concerned about certain unhealthy outcomes of our relationship with light, such as the lack of vitamin D and the increase in macular degeneration, migraine, depression, and even cancer in the general population.

Why then can light sometimes be healing and other times unhealthy?

THE SUN, THE ULTIMATE REFERENCE POINT

When we consider the deleterious as well as the beneficial effects of different light sources, we must consider the ultimate reference, which is, of course, the light of the sun. The exquisite balance that our species has achieved with each one of the components of the sun's light, including not only its spectrum, but also its rhythm, is part of our evolutionary story. So first, let's review what the spectrum of the sun actually looks like as it is received on the surface of Earth. Figure 6.1 shows two important spectral curves connected to our visual system:

* **Photopic sensitivity** refers to our normal vision as generated by the cones of the retina. It is mostly centered on the maximum of the solar spectrum, which is of course not a coincidence, since the eye has adapted in such a way as to be capable of using the light of day to its best advantage.
* **Circadian sensitivity** is that to which the nonvisual optic system described in chapter 4 responds. It determines our synchronization with the natural cycle of the day, and its action spectrum culminates at 460 to 490 nm, in the blue portion of the rainbow. It is this portion that especially influences the different hormonal processes that govern our internal cycles, including the secretion of melatonin, the hormone crucially connected with sleep. The intense light of the day inhibits this secretion, which reestablishes itself spontaneously in the darkness of night. Melatonin is essential for the correct regulation of the quality of sleep.

These two sensitivity curves, *photopic* and *circadian*, direct our internal equilibrium with regard to the light that surrounds us. In all sources of artificial light we try to maximize the emission situated in the photopic sensitivity band (to obtain a light that appears more brilliant to the eye) and minimize that which is situated in the circadian sensitivity band (to avoid interfering with the circadian rhythm). Above and beyond these two elements, other factors, such as the infrared and ultraviolet portions of the spectrum, must be considered.

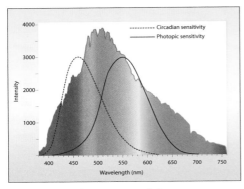

A. The spectrum of the sun
at the surface of Earth

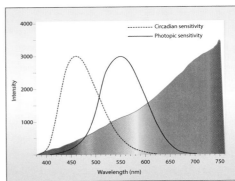

B. A typical incandescent light-bulb spectrum,
with its preponderance of infrared

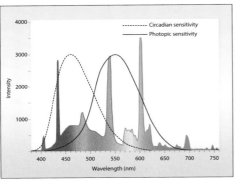

C. A typical CFL bulb spectrum,
with its uneven profile and
its bright mercury spectral lines

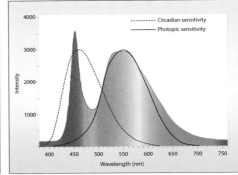

D. A typical white LED spectrum,
with the blue peak arising from
its emitter source clearly visible

Figure 6.1. Spectra of the principal sources of
modern lighting compared to that of the sun,
with superimposed photopic and circadian sensitivity curves

ARTIFICIAL LIGHTING TECHNOLOGY

Artificial sources of lighting effectively came into being in the 1870s, when Joseph Swan, a British physicist, managed to create a glass bulb with a carbonized paper filament. Shortly after this, American inventor Thomas Edison began serious research into developing a practical incandescent lamp. He filed his first patent application for "Improvement in Electric Lights" in October of 1878. His first successful test in October 1879 lasted 13.5 hours. Edison continued to improve his design and by

January 1880 he was awarded a U.S. patent for an electric lamp using "a carbon filament or strip coiled and connected . . . to platina contact wires."

Incandescents and Halogens

Let's consider the spectrum emitted by the artificial light source best known to us, Edison's incandescent light bulb (see figure 6.1b). The light of the halogen light bulb is similar to the incandescent because it is essentially an optimization of the same incandescent technology, achieved through the addition of halogen gas, which offers a gain in energy efficiency of approximately 40 percent.

It is a fortunate coincidence that these long-standing sources of artificial light rely on a principle of emission very close to that of the sun: they are sources known as thermal, which, just like the sun, emit a wide, continuous spectrum generated by their own heat. In the case of the incandescent light bulb, this heat originates from an electric current passing through a filament, resulting in a white-hot glow; in the case of the sun, heat originates in the thermonuclear reactions that activate its core. Theirs is the spectrum of the famous black body, a theoretical phenomenon well known to physicists wherein a spectrum of emission depends solely on its temperature (as described in chapter 2). Whereas the color temperature of the sun is of the order of 5,700 K, that of an incandescent light bulb is approximately 2,000 to 3,000 K. This cooler temperature of a light bulb has a spectrum noticeably shifted toward the red and infrared, perceived by our senses more as heat than light, which we can easily feel if we touch the burning surface of a light bulb.

But apart from this shift, the spectrum of these sources is actually very similar to that of the sun: it has a wide band uniformly covering the range of our photopic sensitivity, and our visual system perceives it as being whitish. Moreover, since it has a relatively small proportion of blue, its contribution to the circadian sensitivity is low. Besides introducing an artificial prolongation of the day, these incandescent light sources have never involved a fundamental difference from natural sunlight, and their universal use has afforded us a century of relatively healthy artificial lighting.

However, by its very nature a thermal luminous source such as an incandescent light bulb emits an important part of its radiation as heat, which corresponds to a waste of energy from the point of view of the specific task of producing light. For this reason, throughout the twentieth century we tried to create sources of light that were energetically more efficient than incandescent light bulbs, which exhibit rather low efficiencies of only 15 to 20 lm/W (lumens per watt), a *lumen* (abbreviated lm) being the unit of measurement of luminous flux. So at first arc lamps were developed. These are based on the discharge of electricity in an ionized gas, such as the sodium vapor lamps currently used for street lighting, which give off light at 50 to 200 lm/W, according to the different types available. Their efficiency is definitely superior to that of incandescent lamps, but their somewhat washed-out yellowish light renders them inadequate for domestic or widespread use.

The Discovery of Fluorescent Light

The exploration of arc-lamp lighting led to the fluorescent lamp, which is a more versatile solution based on the discharge of electricity in a mercury vapor.* The ionized mercury emits a strong ultraviolet light, in itself not of value for lighting purposes. The lamp has a covering of phosphorescent materials (known as *luminophores*) that convert the ultraviolet photons into photons of a visible color, most often a mixture of red, green, and blue. The final result is energetically efficient (from 50 to 100 lm/W), but its emission spectrum, with its discontinuous lines, is very different from that which comes from the light of the sun (see figure 6.1c). It is distinguished by its peaks at 436 nm and at 546 nm, the principal lines of mercury in the visible spectrum.†

---

*Mercury is a highly toxic material, and its presence in CFLs is viewed as problematic by many people, as these CFLs often end up in landfills where their content poses a long-term health threat. But since we are only considering light-related aspects in this book, we will not elaborate further on this question.

†Dr. Alexander Wunsch offers an intriguing hypothesis. He proposes that the photons of the mercury spectral lines emitted by fluorescent lighting can interact through resonance with the mercury atoms contained in our body, reactivating their toxicity, since the body stores a proportion of the mercury we absorb from the environment (from air, from food) in the epidermis, where it is exposed to ambient light.For more on this topic, see http://www.lichtbiologie.de/Downloads/PLD%2053_Alexander%20Wunsch_e.pdf.

It is here that we come across a principle that is essential to lighting: it is relatively easy to fool or trick our visual system to allow us to think that we are seeing a light as white as the sun, even if its spectrum is totally different. This will happen whenever the average of all the spectrum components (as perceived according to our photopic sensitivity) corresponds to that of sunlight. Since it can only base its perception on the total composite of the signals generated by the cone cells of the retina, which in themselves are sensitive to large bands of red, green, and blue wavelengths, our eye is unable to distinguish the precise composition of a light spectrum. It is thus that despite its obviously discontinuous spectrum, a fluorescent light appears to us as white. Adjusting the proportions of the red, green, and blue luminophores of the lamp, one can actually simulate diverse color temperatures from a range of 2,500 K to 10,000 K and higher, from the white lights with an amber hue ("warm whites") all the way to the whites with a bluish tint ("cold whites" or "daylight whites").

If you have been following until now, you will probably find it easy to understand that the biological effects of a particular light spectrum can be greater than its simple visual aspect. One of the first scientists to study the deficiencies of fluorescent light was John Nash Ott, an American who developed time-lapse photography and full-spectrum lighting (see chapter 1). Beginning in the 1950s, Ott realized that plants, animals, and even human beings could be subjected to toxic effects as a result of exposure to the unbalanced spectrum of fluorescent light.* He was the first to coin the term *malillumination* to describe this phenomenon, which he defined as a deprivation of the full spectrum of natural sunlight. His research pointed especially to the importance of reestablishing at least a minimal portion of the ultraviolet section of the spectrum, often absent in artificial light.

---

*In a classic example of conflict between independent researchers and the incumbent lighting industry, Ott's studies in the 1970s led to academic skirmishes concerning the effects of fluorescent light. For example, he found out that schoolchildren in fluorescent-lit classrooms exhibited comparatively increased agitation and reduced grades. A study sponsored by the fluorescent lighting industry leader General Electric (O'Leary et al. 1977) did not reproduce Ott's findings and instead appeared to be based on biased conditions specifically chosen to discredit Ott.

The LED Revolution

In our time, by far the most important new source of artificial light is undoubtedly the LED, which stands for "light-emitting diode." This light source has revolutionized the lighting industry, such that its use is now prevalent. Based on the photonic emission of semiconductor microstructures, it converts electricity almost directly into light by a quantum effect. It has innumerable advantages: excellent energy efficiency (from 100 to 200 lm/W in the latest versions available), great versatility in the light spectrum that it emits, and a long life span (from 10,000 to 100,000 hours). Since the size of its source is very small compared to that of previous techniques, one can also more easily shape the angular profile of its light distribution and thus create entirely new types of light fixtures. So it would seem that LED lamps will be dominating all other kinds of lighting technology for some time to come. But what is the impact of this kind of light on the body?

Because of their very nature, LEDs are emitters with a very sharp spectrum, almost monochromatic, having a typical bandwidth of 20 to 40 nm. They give off a very pure color. At present we know how to manufacture a variety of LED models covering the whole range of colors, from the infrared all the way to the ultraviolet. As a designer in electronics, I have been working with LEDs since their invention in the 1970s, though it was only around the year 2000 that they gained sufficient power to be considered a viable source of lighting. At that time the most efficient LEDs were of a yellow color, and in 2004 the team of which I was the technical director installed the very first LED tunnel lighting system in the world for a roadway project in Montreal. More than six hundred small amber-colored LEDs per fixture were then required. These very impractical constraints were eliminated by 2007 with the introduction of high-brightness white LEDs, which have been improving continuously since then. These new LEDs are based on a source emitting blue color, the most efficient technique known today. It was a discovery for which three Japanese scientists, Isamu Akasaki, Hiroshi Amano, and Shuji Nakamura, received the Nobel Prize in Physics in 2014.

As with fluorescent lamps, these high-brightness LEDs use luminophores that convert part of the blue photons into photons of a lower frequency. The resulting composite spectrum obtained, shown in figure 6.1d, is perceived as white by the eye. By adjusting the properties of phosphor blends, one can design white LEDs with a color temperature from 2,500 K to 6,500 K, ranging from warm white to daylight white.

BIOLOGICAL EFFECTS
OF ARTIFICIAL LIGHTING

The biological consequences of the lighting sources we've just considered fall into three main categories: 1) disturbance of the circadian rhythm; 2) risk of possible deterioration of the retina; and 3) impact of excessive flickering.

Disturbance of the Circadian Rhythm
The degree of influence of a light source on circadian rhythm is determined by the superposition of its spectrum on the circadian sensitivity curve. The more the two curves overlap, the higher the light source's potential for interference with the circadian rhythm. We can thus calculate a circadian stimulus coefficient representing the amount of this overlap for each light source, showing its potential for impact on circadian rhythms. It has been found that the coefficient for different light sources depends more on their color temperature than on their technology or on their detailed spectral profile. This is understandable because the preponderance of blue in a light source is directly related to its color temperature, while the circadian sensitivity profile is centered on the blue part of the spectrum: the more elevated the temperature, the greater the proportion of blue, corresponding to an increased circadian stimulus coefficient; in other words, the greater the potential for impact on circadian rhythms. For example, at a given equivalent lighting intensity, the circadian stimulus coefficient of a "daylight" LED or CFL bulb at 6,000 K is two to three times higher than that of an incandescent bulb at 2,500 K. Therefore "daylight" LEDs and CFLs have a correspondingly increased potential to disrupt the natural circadian cycle.

Our understanding of the relevance of this potential for disruption is still fragmentary, as the biological phenomena involved in the circadian rhythm are turning out to be very complex; after all, it was only in 2002 that the retinal receptors of the nonvisual optic system, the intrinsically photosensitive retinal ganglion cells, or ipRGCs (discussed in chapter 4) were identified. We are still very much in a period of discovery in the field of chronobiology, and the exact profile of the circadian sensitivity curve is evolving each year.

Our master clock, the suprachiasmatic nucleus, which regulates the circadian rhythm, is situated in the core of the brain in the hypothalamus; it controls and regulates a multitude of functions involving essentially all our internal organs—the hormonal secretion that adjusts the wake/sleep cycle, blood pressure, the release of glucose by the liver, and the production of urine in the bladder, to name just a few. Anyone who has suffered from jet lag after a long trip knows perfectly well the effects, if only temporary, of a badly adjusted internal clock: sleepiness, insomnia, digestive troubles. But when such irregularities continue over a long period of time, the consequences are more serious and can include such pathologies as obesity, diabetes, heart problems, and even cancer.

Abraham Haim, head of the Israeli Center for Interdisciplinary Research in Chronobiology at the University of Haifa, has long sounded the alarm on the significant influence of artificial light at night, a term condensed into the acronym ALAN. We now know that the level of lighting at night, even when reduced (to as little as a few lux, or the equivalent of a full moon), is sufficient to disturb circadian rhythm—and much, much higher light levels are frequently found at night in cities all over the world (Wright et al. 2001).

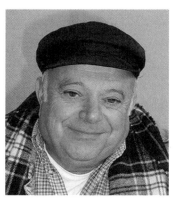

Figure 6.2.
Abraham Haim
(photo courtesy
Yoav Bachar)

Haim's team has already established the connection between the levels of ALAN and the incidence of breast and prostate cancers (Rybnikova, Haim, and Portnov 2015; Haim et al. 2010). Haim says the increased circadian stimulus generated from several types of white LEDs now in common use can be particularly problematic. A recent experiment exposed laboratory mice with existing tumors to thirty minutes of light every night for twenty-eight nights. The results showed a marked acceleration in the growth of cancerous tumors when the animal was exposed to nocturnal lighting by daylight-type LED lights, compared to being exposed to incandescent lamps with an equivalent brightness (Zubidat et al. 2015). Haim attributes this problematic effect to the increased suppression of the secretion of melatonin caused by the LEDs.

According to Haim, the conclusion is obvious: we must minimize our exposure to light before and during sleep periods. This implies the possible use of blackout curtains or a sleep mask to block out excessive sources of light from the outside, and removing things like clocks that may emit excessive light into the room in which we sleep. It is also preferable to avoid lighting that is very bright during the two or three hours preceding the time we go to bed, and to give preference to lamps of a lower color temperature (such as incandescent, halogens, or warm-white LEDs) to reduce our exposure to the blue part of the spectrum during that period.

While we are free to choose the type of lighting we want for household use, it is not so with regard to the screens on computers, televisions, and cell phones, all of which are backlit by high-color temperature LEDs necessary to offer a pleasing palette of colors. The consequences for circadian balance are inevitable, and the connection has been well established between the prolonged use of these devices in bed or before retiring and the subsequent quality of sleep (Wood et al. 2013; Chang et al. 2015). Typically, looking at the screen of an electronic device for four hours (relatively common in the West, especially among young people), even at moderate screen brightness, can retard the onset of deep sleep by ninety minutes. Over a prolonged period of time this can have a marked impact on health.

The Risk of Damage to the Retina

The photons from the blue and ultraviolet part of the spectrum (those with wavelengths under 500 nm) have the most energy and therefore have an increased potential to damage the sensitive cells of the cornea, the lens, and the retina when fully exposed to them. In practice, the lens and the vitreous humor filter the ultraviolet photons of wavelengths under 400 nm, which corresponds to the violet color at one edge of the visible spectrum. But there remains a particularly photoactive portion of the blue spectrum (peaking at 430 to 440 nm) that reaches the retina. This portion is close to the circadian sensitivity that we just examined, at 460 to 490 nm but is implicated in very different biological phenomena.

Even if the exact mechanisms involved in photoinduced retinal damage are still not completely understood, we know that large doses of blue light disturb the visual biomolecular cycle by causing the formation of toxic free radicals and oxidative species, a form of oxidant that is particularly harmful when overabundant. These factors likely play a significant role in degenerative pathologies of the eye, such as the formation of cataracts (a gradual yellowing of the lens) and age-related macular degeneration (ARMD), which is a lesion of the macula, the central part of the retina where most of our photoreceptors are located.

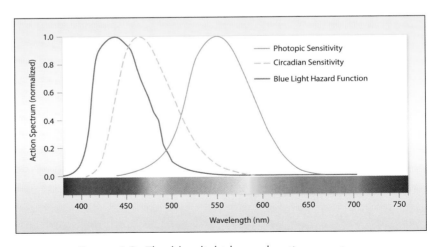

Figure 6.3. The blue light hazard action spectrum
compared to circadian and photopic sensitivity curves

Your Retina and the Risk of Blue Light

Even brief exposure to a very bright light source such as a laser can provoke immediate detrimental effects. However, what is even more pertinent to our discussion is the fact that this type of photobiological effect is cumulative, a little bit like radioactivity: even at a small dose the impact builds up gradually throughout one's life. This phenomenon has been dubbed the *blue light hazard,* or BLH. Because of it there are certain security standards in the lighting industry that govern the intensity of blue light permitted.*

The matter of age-related macular degeneration is of particular relevance. This affliction, for which there is no known treatment, is the principal cause of blindness in older people in the West. In France, for example, it affects 8 percent of the general population and 25 to 30 percent of people seventy-five years or older—and this figure continues to rise. Many causes, including genetic makeup, nutrition, obesity, hypertension, and age, are thought to contribute to this condition; the phototoxicity of the BLH has also been implicated.

Even a cursory examination of the spectra of fluorescent lamps and those of LEDs reveals a peak of blue emission that is situated precisely in the sensitive zone of the BLH, which a priori indicates an increased risk from these light sources (see figures 6.1c and 6.1d on page 114). This is confirmed if we calculate the BLH coefficient of commonly used domestic light sources, determined by the amount of overlap of the spectrum of these types of lights with that of the BLH spectrum.

We find that the risk factor of BLH is four to five times higher for fluorescent bulbs or LEDs of the daylight type (with color temperatures reaching 6,000 K) compared to incandescent bulbs, halogens, or LEDs of the warm white kind (with color temperatures of 2,700 K) (see fig. 6.4). Already in 1978 American researchers had detected photo-oxidative damage to living cells under fluorescent lighting (Parshad et al. 1978), but their warning did not have much of an impact. The French Agency for Food, Environmental, and Occupational Health and Safety (ANSES 2010) caused a much bigger commotion in the

---

*Notably, the IEC/EN 62471 standard designed to avoid lesions of the retina

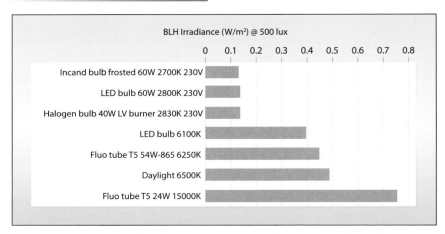

Figure 6.4. The blue light hazard (BLH) coefficients of risk for frequently used light sources (CELMA 2011)

lighting community with the publication of the report "Sanitary Effects of Lighting Systems Using LEDs," which outlined specific risks connected to LED lighting, notably the photochemical risks of BLH, while exposing the shortcomings of the accepted standards.

In recent years this report has led to a counterattack on the part of a number of government and industrial agencies favorable to the establishment of LEDs as the new universal source of lighting—and it is indeed important to note that the economic issues involved are enormous. In its report entitled *True Colors,* the United States Department of Energy (2014) pointed out that the debate on the circadian and BLH factors with respect to lighting concerns less the technology, whether it be incandescent, fluorescent, or LED, than the color temperature, as we have just been examining. Moreover, the Scientific Committee on Emerging and Newly Identified Health Risks (SCENIHR) (2012), as well as the International Energy Agency (IEA 2014) stress that the BLH coefficient of LEDs is not higher than that of sunlight, which could never be conceived as being unhealthy. Effectively, the studies on the connection between sunlight and age-related macular degeneration have never been conclusive (Winkler et al. 2007).

The case therefore seems closed, and at the time I am writing this the international lighting community appears to be satisfied that

LEDs are harmless when used within existing standards. But has this really been established? A few researchers are far from convinced.

Alexander Wunsch, mentioned earlier, is an expert on the relationship between light and health. He possesses an encyclopedic knowledge of the most pertinent aspects to be found on this subject, and he doesn't hesitate to oppose the accepted conventions when his convictions demand it. Wunsch (2016) underscores a major failing in the official argument: it does not take into consideration the essential role of the infrared part of the spectrum. To understand the importance of infrared, recall the discovery of photobiomodulation by Tiina Karu described in chapter 4. We know from her analysis that the major part of the regenerative action of light on cells is caused by the red and near-infrared portions of the spectrum, between 600 and 900 nm. Sources of light such as the sun and incandescent bulbs possess this in abundance (see figures 6.1a and 6.1b). Yet the fluorescent lamp and the LED, in the quest for greater energy efficiency, were specifically developed to eliminate the so-called wasted energy of infrared radiation, as the minimal levels of infrared in their spectra demonstrate (see figures 6.1c and 6.1d).

Infrared to the Rescue

In sunlight—and by extension, incandescent light—there exists a natural balance between the photo-oxidative properties of its blue portion and the regenerative properties of its red and near-infrared portions, which translates into a minimal risk for the retina. Many studies corroborate this. Among the most convincing are those of Janis Eells and her team (2003). I met Eells at a conference of the College of Syntonic Optometry in 2003. At that time she demonstrated how the vision of rats that had been threatened with blindness induced by a toxic injection of methanol in their retinas could be saved by brief exposure to near-infrared light (for a total time of just seven minutes at 670 nm), thus substantiating the protective power of that light. And what concerns us even more directly, in 2011 Eells found that the damage inflicted on rat retinas from a light source that was relatively bright (fluorescents of the cold white type, from 4,000 to 5,000 K) was healed by being briefly (as little as fifteen minutes at 670 nm) exposed to near-infrared light (Albarracin, Eels, and Valter 2011). Her results have been validated and even better quantified in more recent studies (Chu-Tan et al. 2016).

What should we conclude from this? It is possible that the BLH coefficient on which the lighting industry relies to confirm the supposed harmlessness of LEDs offers only a partial idea of the real risk to the retina from this light source. Solely based on a calculation of the flux in the blue part of the spectrum, the BLH coefficient does not take into account the infrared contribution of the source. For example, the BLH coefficients for a 5,500 K LED and for sunlight, both having similar color temperatures, are almost identical. This does not necessarily mean that the light from this LED would not have more long-term photo-oxidative effects (such as those resulting in age-related macular degeneration) than sunlight, because the LED does not in any way compensate for its blue radiation through the infrared protector as does sunlight—or an incandescent lamp.

A Gigantic Photobiological Experiment?

Many researchers studying the therapeutic properties of light consider the decision made by many countries to phase out incandescent light bulbs a grave error.* This decision was taken with the admirable goal of supporting greater energy efficiency and reducing greenhouse gases. Artificial lighting, for instance, uses 14 percent of the consumption of electricity in the European Union. However, this decision could result in public health problems that surpass any gains to energy efficiency. By imposing the accelerated introduction of new artificial sources of light, the spectrums of which differ fundamentally from that in which life has evolved, we are subjecting the population of the world to a gigantic photobiological experiment, the long-term consequences of which are far from being known.

---

*Brazil and Venezuela started the incandescent bulbs phaseout in 2005, and the European Union, Switzerland, and Australia started to phase them out in 2009. Other countries are implementing new energy standards or have scheduled phaseouts: Argentina and Russia in 2012, and the United States, Canada, Mexico, Malaysia, and South Korea in 2014.

The Problem of Flicker

The brain is highly sensitive to all forms of pulsation. On the positive side, this sensitivity opens the door to the whole domain of vibrational medicine (a subject we'll be looking at more closely in chapter 10). Conversely, this sensivity means we can be particularly vulnerable to a phenomenon of lighting called *flickering,* the oscillation of light, which can be found whenever a light source generates an unsteady output.

All current lighting technologies are susceptible to generating flickering that can be more or less pronounced. Our traditional light source, the incandescent bulb, when plugged into an AC power line, emits an oscillating light with a rectified frequency that is double that of the power line (50 or 60 Hz, depending on the country), that frequency being 100 or 120 Hz. But since its filament reacts slowly to changes in the current, the amplitude of this light oscillation is relatively small (about 7 percent of the total light intensity). The first fluorescent tubes also oscillated at these frequencies, but more strongly. This lighting was so badly received by the public (with reports of migraines and ocular fatigue, among other complaints) that manufacturers had to modify the ballasts powering them to elevate the pulsation frequencies to many dozens of kilohertz. Subsequently Wilkins et al. (1989) revealed a reduction of about 50 percent of the perceived symptoms from these improved fluorescent sources, but many people continued to exhibit discomfort when exposed to them for a long period of time.

For a long time it was considered that flickering could be reduced to a safe level by making sure that its frequency be higher than what is known as the *flicker fusion frequency*, the maximum flicker frequency that our visual system is capable of perceiving. Depending on the individual, flicker fusion frequency is in the order of 50 to 90 Hz. Above that frequency, the eye stops perceiving flicker. The reasoning went like this: if the light pulsation is invisible, how could it be causing problems? But already by 2010 this somewhat simplistic approach was called into question, and a number of studies have showed that even if it is invisible, flickering can lead to difficulties such as migraines, headaches, and eye stress in certain sensitive people (IEEE 2010). Newer more extensive studies in this area have begun to detect negative effects from higher and higher frequencies. In response to this, the Institute of Electrical and Electronics Engineers (IEEE, a scholarly organization that publishes and establishes standards) recommends in its latest report of 2015 that one should avoid flickering below 3,000 Hz (IEEE 2015)—a much higher limit than the 50 to 90Hz value previously recognized.

Furthermore, one can note that even these latest standards reflect only the data relevant to allopathic medicine and do not take into account the more subtle effects that are important considerations in energy medicine. According to these considerations, any vibrational information can have an effect on an organism, including at levels of stimulation well below the established threshold of normal sense perception (more on this in chapter 7). Certain people are hypersensitive to electromagnetic fields,* and it is highly likely that there exists a similar form of hypersensitivity to light. This would explain why some people become quickly affected at a flicker level that for others is inoffensive, since the latter are people who are capable of absorbing a higher level of environmental stress without experiencing any immediate symptoms. From this arises the difficulty in evaluating the criteria permitting the establishment of admissible levels of flickering, as they depend on the susceptibility of the subjects, which varies greatly. Still, whether it originates from radio waves or from light, in general such environmental stress potentially contributes in the long run to the multiple chronic pathologies that are so widespread today.†

LEDs and Flicker

Flickering is an especially acute problem when it comes to LEDs because LEDs, as semiconductor emitters, have a reaction speed beyond precedent; the fastest ones are capable of pulsating at frequencies in the terahertz range (10^{12} Hz). In an LED bulb it is the electronic drive circuit that determines the flickering effect, as the LED itself merely responds

---

*It is estimated that this phenomenon called *electrohypersensitivity* affects from 2 to 5 percent of the population.

†In addition to the problem of flickering, most CFL and LED bulbs are sources of electromagnetic interference and "dirty electricity," which refers to the electrical noise injected in the AC power line by their high-frequency power supply switching.

to the circuit's signal in a nearly instantaneous manner. Since at present there doesn't exist an applicable norm for flicker (the manufacturers do not even have to mention this factor in their specifications), we are presented with enormous differences and variability in this parameter for the commercial products now on the market. Only a small number of bulbs have almost no flickering, whereas others have extreme flickering, and the rest run the gamut.

The following figure 6.5 shows the flickering profile of some typical LED bulbs from 2013, illustrating the modulation depths and frequencies to be found. While the average LED bulbs have improved since then, they still exhibit a similarly wide variety of flickering profiles.

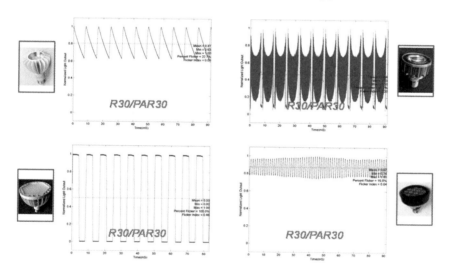

Figure 6.5. The luminous flickering of some typical LED bulbs
(© CIE 2013, International Commission on Illumination,
courtesy of Pacific Northwest National Laboratory, as shown in
Poplawski and Miller 2013)

Luminous Cacophony

Laxity of standards around flickering is unfortunate because most of the time flickering is not discernible to the naked eye. Its effect is perceivable only in the long term, as it contributes to the overall environmental stress load. To measure it one has to use a type of meter that converts light to an electric signal or to sound.* Most people are quite shocked when they hear the audio version of the intense *light noise* given off by certain LED fixtures—a veritable cacophony of a very disturbing quality, one that would not be bearable for any length of time in our sensorial environment.

Even though such measurements are available, they still do not enable us to make a list of LED bulbs that we can recommend, because the technology as well as the market is so fluid that models change every month. Bulbs made by the large international manufacturers have a better chance of having a more reasonable flicker level than those that are fabricated by anonymous companies or offered at bargain prices.

Another point to consider with regard to LED flickering is to avoid the use of dimmers, even with bulbs that are supposedly compatible. Even if an LED bulb has a low flicker level when it is fully lit, it will most likely emit a higher flicker when its brightness is reduced by a dimmer. This is due to a feature of dimming known as *pulse width modulation,* which is based on rapid switching on and off of the LED power supply to vary the light bulb brightness. The majority of LED devices use this process unless it is explicitly specified that they dim through a nonswitching (direct current) control.

PROBLEMS WITH COLOR RENDERING

Light sources can appear to our visual system as having the same shade of white, so long as the combination of the various wavelengths comprising their spectrum result in a similar stimulation of the cones of the retina. But this does not guarantee that when these apparently similar light sources are used to illuminate a colored object they will render its hue in the same way. This is because the object can have a precise color that is lacking in the spectrum of the light source, and therefore the color cannot be highlighted by that source.

---

*For example, the LightBee light-to-sound converter, a simple and inexpensive light noise detector which I designed (www.sensora.com\lightbee)

In Defense of LEDs

After reading the preceding one might tend to think that LED is a lighting technology that is fundamentally incompatible with the principles of healthy lighting. But that is not the message I am trying to convey. Instead, my intent is to point out that the current versions of LED lights have design flaws originating from an incomplete knowledge of the relevant photobiological factors.

As a lighting technology, the LED possesses extraordinary versatility. We can adjust its spectrum at will, as well as its power and optical properties. Its light is very pure, stable, efficient, and highly adapted to general use. It is even suitable for therapeutic use. By applying the appropriate photobiological knowledge, with a clear intention of producing LEDs without economic compromise, it is quite possible to create new versions of LEDs for domestic use that would be much safer in terms of health impact. Among the improvements that can be implemented: the elimination of the blue peak of their spectrum, the inclusion of some near-infrared radiation to ensure a photobiomodulation-induced balance in the retina, the suppression of all flickering in their power supplies, and an increase of their color rendering index to at least 95.

It is probable that these modifications would lead to slightly lower energy efficiency and could result in a price tag that is slightly higher. But from the point of view of one's health, these considerations would far outweigh the cost.

The capacity of a lighting source to accurately illuminate colors is quantifiable: it is known as the *color rendering index,* or CRI, and it varies substantially according to the lighting source. By definition, the sun, which is the ultimate reference point, has a CRI equal to 100, and so do incandescent sources of light. In comparison, fluorescent bulbs have a CRI of around 80, and those of ordinary LED bulbs vary from 70 to 85. Regarding these latter two technologies, a number of special models exist where the CRI is at least 95, the minimal level recommended for a true rendering of color, but these kinds of bulbs are not common.

At present the lighting industry regards the accuracy of colors to be only of relative importance, less important than energy efficiency or cost. After all, the reasoning goes, the eye can adapt to various colors. From the point of view of a holistic approach to light, their reasoning is less persuasive, especially if you take into consideration the perception of skin tone, a variable to which we interact with daily. Evolution has equipped us with a very fine perception of the color of the skin, which permits us to evaluate at a glance the health of those with whom we interact. Illness (for example, jaundice or anemia) produces changes, even if subtle, which we pick up or sense, even unconsciously—like the pallor that precedes death (known as *pallor mortis*). As it happens, changes of the same magnitude can routinely be produced by a deficient color rendering index.

The decision is yours. Would you prefer a light source offering a natural perception of the environment, or one that gives even a healthy person the pallor of sickness or even the appearance of being at death's door?

THE ULTRAVIOLET QUESTION

For a number of years now we have been warned about the dangers of ultraviolet rays from sunlight. UV has been implicated with certain problems ranging from wrinkles and accelerated aging of the skin and damage to the retina, to cancers such as melanoma, which is almost always fatal. The medical establishment consequently recommends that we avoid the sun, and if we don't have a choice, then to protect ourselves with a thick application of sunscreen, sunglasses, and clothing that blocks the sun's rays.

This concern is relatively recent. The human species has been evolving for millions of years without the use of sunscreen under the full light of the sun, including its ultraviolet radiation. And as recounted in chapter 1, it's been barely a hundred years since heliotherapy (exposure to the sun) was considered the treatment of choice for a number of different illnesses. Pioneers in this field, like the "Sun Doctor" Auguste Rollier, established their many clinics at high altitudes in the Alps precisely to maximize patients' exposure to ultraviolet light. So what has happened since that time to make us run for cover?

The thinning of the ozone layer of Earth's atmosphere has often been blamed for these changes. For the last fifty years this natural filter and UV radiation protector has been steadily depleted due to the massive production of industrial compounds such as chlorofluoro-carbons. This has produced a global increase in the level of the average UV, which by 1995 in the United States alone rose 10 percent over levels established in 1970. Fortunately, the worldwide mobilization that occurred as a result of the 1987 Montreal Protocol on Substances that Deplete the Ozone Layer has succeeded in stemming this terrible progression, to the extent that the levels of UV have returned to an increase of just 5 percent at this time, and they continue to decline. These values are far from being negligible and surely merit sustained vigilance, but in themselves they do not justify such radical measures as those recommended to us by the medical establishment.

What is alarming medical authorities is a disturbing increase in the number of cancers of the skin. According to the Canadian Skin Cancer Foundation, one in every three cancers now diagnosed worldwide is a type of skin cancer. Deep tanning, which had been popular not so long ago, is discouraged because exaggerated exposure to the sun and sun-burn are among the principal risk factors for skin cancer. However, as is often the case, this has been a one-size-fits-all solution. So let's examine more closely the factors that are responsible for the rise in skin cancer.

Radiation from UV is divided into three bands, illustrated in figure 6.6: near UV (UVA), middle UV (UVB), and far UV (UVC).

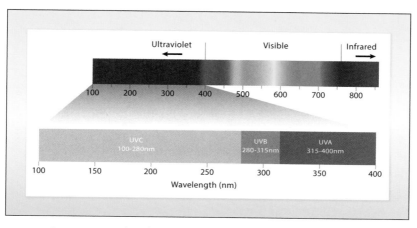

Figure 6.6. The three bands of the ultraviolet spectrum

Getting Sufficient Vitamin D

Vitamin D is indispensable for good health: an insufficiency of this vitamin can cause rickets in children, and in adults it can increase susceptibility to osteoporosis, fractures, diabetes, cancer, hypertension, infections, and autoimmune diseases. Depending on the country, up to 70 percent of us are deficient. The recommended daily dose is from 800 to 1,000 IU (certain researchers suggest up to 4,000 IU per day), which we cannot obtain from food sources alone. Our principal source of vitamin D is sunlight; specifically, the UVB portion of the solar spectrum. And this mechanism is remarkably efficient: when the body is fully exposed to bright sunlight it can generate between 10,000 and 20,000 IU in less than twenty minutes. Furthermore, there exists in our skin an autoregulatory mechanism by which the UVB produces vitamin D and the UVA disintegrates it, reducing the chance of an overdose in natural conditions.

The conclusion is simple: we need to be balanced with regard to our daily exposure to the sun. The difficulty lies in the fact that the UVB is so well diffused by the atmosphere (unlike the UVA, which even pierces through the clouds) that it does not come to us in sufficient quantity except when the sun is high in the sky, at fifty degrees or more above the horizon. For those of us who live in high latitudes, this restrictive condition implies that we cannot synthesize vitamin D adequately except in the middle of the day—and not at all in wintertime. Our bodies adapt to the seasons; consequently, it is important to take in as much light as possible during the summer months.

The optimum strategy to maximize the biosynthesis of vitamin D and at the same time minimize the risk of damage to the skin could appear surprising, even going directly against those ideas that are in now in vogue:

Expose yourself to the sun when it is at its zenith, because at that time the highest proportion of UVB is being emitted, which is necessary for the production of vitamin D.

Expose the largest possible surface of your body, but for only a relatively brief period of time. This allows you to maximize the production of vitamin D (proportional to the surface of exposed skin) while reducing the risks of sunburn (proportional to the highest UVA exposure on any skin area).

Make your exposure gradual, not exceeding more than a few minutes a day at first, and never get to the point of sunburn according to the sensitivity of your skin (fair-haired people tend to burn more easily). This is of great importance, as statistically it is estimated that the risk of developing a melanoma is twice as high in someone who has had more than five sunburns in the course of a lifetime.

Protect your face and the eyes, as they are the most vulnerable. This is especially true for children in whom the transmission of UV through the eyes can be ten times higher than it is for adults, and also for people who have had a lens replacement, as happens after an operation for the removal of a cataract, since the lens is our principal filter of UV for the eye.

In this instance it is counterproductive to use sunscreen, since it blocks especially the UVB rays and as a result radically diminishes the synthesis of vitamin D (Webb 2006).

When it is not possible to have proper exposure to the sun, especially in wintertime, a vitamin D supplement in capsule form is recommended, preferably of the D3 type, especially if one has brown or black skin because its capacity to absorb UV is even further reduced.

The UVC, which is farthest from the visible light spectrum, is also the most energetic and dangerous, having both sterilizing and germicidal properties; luckily, it is for the most part filtered by Earth's atmosphere. The UVB, and even more so the UVA, reach us more easily, and in larger proportions. Both UVB and UVA provoke cutaneous reactions that promote tanning. In strong doses they generate free radicals, which burn the skin and accelerate its aging. Eventually, damage is done to the DNA, which can lead to cancer. The most dangerous and fatal form of skin cancer is melanoma, which is mainly caused by overexposure to UVA. Contrary to popular belief, however, melanoma occurs mostly in people who work indoors rather than outside in the sun. In fact, one of the contributing factors currently being investigated is the effect of long-term exposure to light that is filtered through a glass pane, which in most cases blocks the UVB but allows the UVA to pass, resulting in an unbalanced UV spectrum (Godar 2011).

Photobiologist John Ott (1985) had already observed that minimal but balanced doses of UV are indispensable for the optimal growth of plants and animal cells. These results have been reproduced in subsequent experiments. Jacob Liberman (1990) enumerates many beneficial effects coming from UV radiation: a reduction in blood pressure, the strengthening of the cardiac system, a reduction in cholesterol, weight regulation, an increase in the production of sex hormones, and most important of all, the production of vitamin D.

THE IMPORTANCE OF NATURAL LIGHT

One of the most efficient ways of cultivating a healthy relationship to light is to maximize lighting by the natural full spectrum of the sun at home, in schools, and in the workplace. Many architects are now more aware of this, and the tendency is to optimize the use of daylight in new buildings, not only from the point of view of energy efficiency, but also for the health of occupants.

Rosemann, Mossman, and Whitehead (2008) are exploring techniques that permit the efficient transmission of daylight up to fifty meters deep into the interior of large buildings, even in spaces without windows. In the near future we will see more of such new technologies as automated mirrors that follow the path of the sun, and optical guiding systems that regulate light delivery like the way ventilation conduits manage air flow.

IMPROVING YOUR RELATIONSHIP TO LIGHT

How can we improve the quality of our daily relationship to light? The following are some practical recommendations you can apply in the home. Note that some of these suggestions do not necessarily correspond to the official line of the medical establishment or the lighting industry, but they do reflect a wider perspective about light stemming from the accumulated knowledge that has been compiled over the years by my colleagues of the ILA.

Prefer halogen or incandescent bulbs, because of their significant infrared content as well as because their light spectrum is closest to that of sunlight's broad continuous spectrum. A side benefit

Sunlight Combats Myopia

As we explore the incomparable qualities of natural light I am reminded of a recent article by British engineer Richard Hobday, an authority on sunlight and health in the built environment. Hobday (2015) has established a connection between the rapid increase of nearsightedness in schoolchildren over past decades and the quality of light they are exposed to on a daily basis. This question is significant because in China, for instance, it is estimated that now as many as 80 percent of students are nearsighted by the end of high school.

This worldwide development seems to have begun in the 1960s, at a time when the accepted norm for the interior of schools went through a transition, moving from the natural light of day, with large windows, to artificial, usually fluorescent lighting. Obviously, there were probably many other factors involved, but recent studies have confirmed that myopia can be countered by increasing the number of hours that children spend outdoors, no matter what physical activity they are involved in.* Many researchers conclude that being exposed on a regular basis to very bright daylight (generally of the order of 100,000 lux, as opposed to 1,000 lux under artificial lighting) is essential to the visual health of children.

*Hobday (2015) quotes a 2013 Taiwan study that found a 50 percent reduction in myopia in children who go outdoors during class recesses.

to using incandescent and halogen bulbs during a good part of the year in Nordic countries is that the energy "wasted" through heat is not lost because it contributes to the heating of the house.

Avoid, as much as possible, fluorescent and compact fluorescent bulbs because of the strong, discontinuous lines in their light spectrum as well as the toxicity factor from the presence of mercury.

If you use LEDs, choose the "warm white" type (2,500 to 3,000 K) to minimize the effect of blue within their spectrum, which can interfere with the circadian rhythm, especially in the evening.

Avoid fluorescent and LED bulbs with excessive flickering, to minimize exposure to unnecessary environmental stress caused by "noisy" light. Since flicker levels are not readily visible to the naked eye a light noise detector (such as a light-to-sound converter) may be useful to select better light bulbs. Avoid the use of dimmers with LED bulbs, as dimming commonly leads to increased flickering.

Avoid all light sources in your bedroom at night, including alarm clocks, night lights, and the like. Use curtains or shades to shield all excess light from the outside, which is to say anything that is brighter than the light of a full moon. If you need to use an illuminated alarm clock, choose a red or orange color to minimize any interference with the circadian rhythm.

Spend as much time as possible outdoors in daylight to maintain a properly synchronized circadian rhythm.

Try to expose your body (without using sunscreen) at least occasionally to the full light of the sun. While carefully respecting the sensitivity of your skin, allow it to benefit from the effects of heliotherapy and natural ultraviolet light. Expose the largest possible surface of your body, at the same time giving proper protection to the eyes and head. A few minutes will suffice. Aim for those periods when the sun is high in the sky to optimize the biosynthesis of vitamin D. At other times of day you risk being sunburned without receiving the benefit of increased vitamin D.

Expose yourself at least occasionally to daylight without your glasses or contact lenses (including sunglasses) on. While carefully respecting the sensitivity of your eyes, allow them to receive the natural total light spectrum. Of course, never look directly at the sun, which could damage your retina.

In this second part of the book we learned about the scientific discoveries that led to the rise of modern light medicine, which has been gradually embraced by the medical community as it becomes more aware of the paramount influence of light on health. We are now ready to explore new applications of light concerned with energy medicine and chromotherapy—the intriguing world of alternative light medicine is ahead.

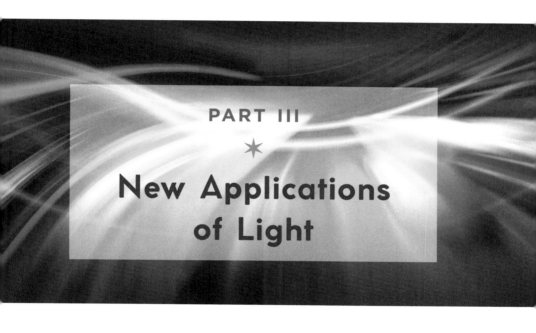

PART III

✳

New Applications of Light

7

THE DAWN
OF ENERGY MEDICINE

Integrating Vitalism and Science

Scientists are trained doubters, but the traditional bias against energy medicine has gone deeper than skepticism. . . . Some approaches to the body are rarely able to tap into the continuum methodology and consciousness because their philosophical base is advertised as rational and unemotional science, while the energy continuum is repeatedly rejected on irrational and emotional grounds. The history, psychology, and biopolitics of this rejection is a fascinating subject. The point is that a medicine that fails to look at, and function from, life's most fundamental attributes is destined to become irrelevant and obsolete.

JAMES OSCHMAN

THE MEDICINE OF LIGHT has already demonstrated remarkable applications of its use, and it continues to deliver major new discoveries, a few of which are highlighted in chapter 5. There exists, however, a whole other category of applications for therapeutic light, those that are related to energy medicine (also called *subtle-energy medicine* and *vibrational medicine*) (Rosch 2015). These are the healing modalities that have been labeled "alternative" because they have not been recognized by the official medical establishment.

In a certain way, all biochemical and genetic processes at the core of any form of medicine are processes of energy exchange at the molecular level. We could therefore say that all medicine is energetic. But we are giving a more specific sense here to subtle energy, which is quite different from the conventional understanding of modern medicine.

VITALISM, THE ULTIMATE CRIME

In this chapter I offer an overview of the extraordinary work accomplished up till now by a whole generation of courageous and creative researchers who have devoted themselves to understanding this energy that has been called *chi, prana, bioplasma, vital force,* and the like. The point of view held by these scientists is sometimes called *vitalism,* in contrast to the conventional mechanistic or materialistic viewpoint. My goal is to underscore the scientific basis of current research on vital energy, which is now substantial enough to justify a serious scientific evaluation of the role of energy in living matter. By extension this will contribute to the validation of the different approaches that involve light in so-called alternative medicine.

One of the pioneers of this type of research, Nobel Prize winner Albert Szent-Györgyi, once remarked that in a scientific circle to be a vitalist is far worse than to be a Communist—and this statement was made during the Cold War! This state of affairs has improved a little since then, but there is still a long road ahead.

The Official Paradigm
The only medical science officially sanctioned as a result of scientific reductionism is based on the following principles:

* All phenomena, whether biological or not, can ultimately be explained through the action of fundamental physical forces (electromagnetism, gravity, etc.) on inanimate elementary particles.
* All biology, including all those processes that have to do with life itself, result from biochemical interactions between molecular structures of various complexity.

∗ The organization and the functioning of living beings can be completely explained by the functioning of their DNA. Once its code has been properly deciphered, it is then possible to understand and heal the majority of illnesses.

∗ Memory and consciousness reside in the physical brain and result from the bioelectric activity within the massive network of neurons. All information circulating in a living being is transmitted either by electrochemical signals that move through the central nervous system, or through the diffusion of messenger molecules (such as hormones) carried by the circulatory system of the blood.

This view was summarized by James Watson and Francis Crick, codiscoverers of the double helix structure of DNA. Watson once said, "These successes . . . have created a firm belief that the current extension of our understanding of biological phenomena to the molecular level will soon enable us to understand all the basic features of the living state" (1970). Crick ironically added, "No longer need one spend time attempting . . . to endure the tedium of philosophers perpetually disagreeing with each other. Consciousness is now largely a scientific problem" (1996).

The extraordinary successes in molecular biology and the genetic sciences that we are witnessing today reinforce the dominant paradigm. These two fields absorb almost all of the gigantic resources expended for medical research and development in the world today. Any deviation from this point of view is generally ignored, dismissed, or denigrated by the scientific community, the media, and government authorities.

Some Cracks in the Model?

Regardless of the dominant paradigm, a steady stream of research is emerging that shows that this mechanical, materialist model is incomplete. Biologist James Oschman (2003, 2015) is one of the most articulate spokespersons of the new trend, and this chapter, which is based in large part on his work, demonstrates the multiple facets of an evolving vision of living beings that is held by energy medicine.

Oschman points to a number of issues that are still unresolved in the classical model of medicine. To name just a few:

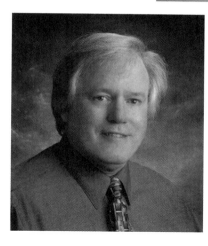

Figure 7.1.
James Oschman

* The essential function of DNA consists of managing the synthesis of proteins, those complex molecules of which we are composed. There exists an enormous discontinuity, entirely unexplained, between this basic function and the perfect organization of the trillions of cells that make up a living being. No one can explain where in the DNA a "master plan" can be found that directs the growth and interconnectedness of the organic structures of our body.

* Life can function perfectly well without the central nervous system. It suffices to look at a paramecium, a single-cell protozoan, an organism that moves about, avoids predators, finds its nourishment, and reproduces without the slightest trace of a nerve or synapse. It follows that different systems for the transmission of information must be at work.

* A careful examination of the speed of muscular action occurring in athletes at the highest level, or even the simple visceral reactions happening within ourselves or in animals, indicates delays of less than a millisecond. When one looks at the speed of transmission of signals in neurons (about 100 meters per second, plus 0.5 milliseconds for each synaptic crossing), these delays are too short to be explained by a normal neuromuscular process, even when taking into account the accelerated circuits of reflex arcs. Another, more rapid communication system has to be operating.

WE ARE CRYSTALLINE

Oschman offers us a model that has gradually established itself and constitutes one of the best we now have in energy medicine. According to his model, living beings are equipped with a hitherto unrecognized communication system: the whole assemblage of connective tissues that compose the major part of the body. It has now been confirmed that these tissues have crystalline properties that enable them to transmit energy signals. Oschman (2015) expresses it in this way: "We do not usually consider our bodies to be crystalline, because when we think of crystals we usually think of hard materials, like diamond or agate. Living crystals are composed of long, thin, pliable molecules, and are soft and flexible. To be more precise, these are liquid crystals. . . . materials that are intermediate between solids and liquids and display properties of both." Such quasicrystalline tissues are to be found everywhere in our anatomical structure: in cellular membranes, in the contractile part of muscles, and in the connective tissue of bones, fascia, tendons, ligaments, and cartilage—as well as in the DNA itself.

Meetings with Dr. James Oschman

Jim, as his friends call him, possesses a very affable personality and a delightful sense of humor that masks a formidable erudition and a complete mastery of his subject. This turns each of his presentations into a gratifying experience, where in between two slides addressing particularly arduous scientific points the unexpected image of an adorable kitten can suddenly appear. We have invited him to ILA conferences many times because his message is of utmost importance to all those looking to establish a junction between conventional and alternative medicine, as the ILA seeks to do in the field of light. The association named him an honorary member in 2013 in recognition of his important contributions in the field.

Jim has met most of the scientists and researchers working to establish energy medicine, starting with his mentor, the great biologist Szent-Györgyi, whose lab was just across the hall from his own at the Marine Biological Laboratory in Woods Hole, Massachusetts, in the 1980s. Jim is an inexhaustible source of facts and anecdotes about these pioneers, their work, and the challenges that they face while pushing the envelope of conventional science.

He likes to recount how he and Szent-Györgyi became fascinated with the "blind-spot" in modern biomedicine regarding the role of energy and why modern medical researchers gave no consideration to successful medical traditions of the past. "Eventually we learned that one reason for this is that physicians are not taught basic physics in medical school, and are therefore bewildered when we try to talk to them about energy fields" (Oschman and Oschman 2015).

In recent years Jim has become more and more convinced of the primary role played by light in the energy processes driving life within organisms. At the 2017 ILA meeting he shared with us: "During the evolution of life, organisms had millions of years and a host of physical phenomena to 'choose from.' We can ask, 'given a choice of physical processes, why would evolutionary selection choose random diffusion of signal molecules—probably the slowest and least specific mechanism available?' Light has played many roles in the evolutionary process. Why would nature not utilize light for its vital regulations? Light has a great advantage over random diffusion because it travels at the speed of light and is precisely specific, i.e. from molecule to molecule."

Jim's message, that a scientific point of no return has been reached and that it is just a question of time before a new energetic vision of life transforms the present reductionist view, is particularly heartening for the therapists and practitioners who must endure the intellectual and legal restrictions imposed by the dominant model of institutionalized medicine.

BIOLOGICAL COHERENCE

Szent-Györgyi was ridiculed by the scientific community in 1941 when he suggested that the organic proteins of connective tissues such as collagen were perhaps semiconductors, which permitted them to transmit electronic signals at much higher speeds than that of the nervous system itself. It was necessary to wait until the 1960s (Rosenberg and Postow 1969) for the validity of this hypothesis to become accepted.*

---

*These studies led to the discovery of conductive polymers, for which the discoverers, Alan J. Heeger, Alan G. MacDiarmid, and Hideki Shirakawa, were jointly awarded the 2000 Nobel Prize in Chemistry.

Around this time, German-born British physicist Herbert Frölich, who had been studying the properties of the crystalline molecular structures of connective tissue, concluded that they allowed for the existence of "coherent excitations in active biological systems" (1988). These structures are "excitable," which is to say they respond to external stimuli with great sensitivity, far below the level of ambient energetic noise, and can project their signals in the form of coherent waves throughout the whole matrix (Adey 1990). His calculations predicted resonances at frequencies in the microwave band, in the order of 10^{11} Hz, which were in fact detected years earlier by Webb and Stoneham (1977). Such waves are global: they interconnect with all the elements of the body, the "continuum," and even the interior of each cell. They are guided by the connective tissue that surrounds the cell, then transmitted through its envelope, the cytoskeleton, as far as the DNA (Scott 1984; Pienta and Coffey 1991). It is these waves that maintain the integrity of an organism and permit it to function in perfect synchronicity, with simultaneity far too rapid to be explained by the random diffusion of chemical messengers, a theory postulated by classical medicine (Adolph 1982).

In the 1970s, Ukranian physicist Alexander Davydov discovered that these waves could take on a particular form, called a *soliton,* possessing remarkable properties (Davydov 1987). Differing from normal waves, these "solitary waves" are not dispersive and can transmit energy at great distances without structurally degrading (a tsunami, or tidal wave, is a classic example of the soliton propagating on the surface of the ocean). This quality would give an extraordinary efficiency to energy communication in the body.

Becker (1991) confirmed that the connective tissue that surrounds each one of our neurons in the continuity of the connective matrix possesses semiconductive properties and is sensitive to magnetic fields, therefore concluding that this is a perineural system; basically, a parallel nervous system synergetically connected to the neuronal system, but which from the point of view of evolution is older and is ideally placed to send the energy signals of the organism all the way to the brain.

The Emergent Order of Nature

From the 1940s on the development of *general systems theory* by Austrian biologist Ludwig von Bertalanffy in concert with his Viennese colleague Paul Weiss provided support for the holistic viewpoint espousedd by subtle-energy medicine, as it taught how the synchronized action of independent elements can lead to an "emergent order" at a level of superior organization (von Bertalanffy 1976). This emergent order, characteristic of all living beings, is nowhere to be found when looking at each separate element and is therefore beyond the reach of reductionist analysis as practiced by conventional science.

Subsequently, Belgian chemist Ilya Prigogine, who received the Nobel Prize in Chemistry in 1977, developed *dissipative structures theory* and offered a new view on how a living organism sets in motion the spontaneous organization of its components, a biological concept known as *self-organization*. Such self-organization may appear to contradict the second law of thermodynamics, which states that all isolated physical systems tend to move into a state of total equilibrium, with maximal entropy—the very opposite of organisation. To Prigogine this contradiction is resolved with the understanding that a living organism is not isolated, but rather exists in a state of perpetual nonequilibrium maintained by an ongoing influx of external energy through food, light, and other sources (Prigogine and Nicolis 1977).

This Mysterious Coherence

The late Chinese geneticist Mae-Wan Ho (2008) showed how maintaining that state of nonequilibrium implies a continuous cooperation of its components, at all levels of organization. And these levels are multiple: living processes occur in a vast spectrum ranging on a time scale of 10^{-14} seconds (at the scale of atomic resonances) to 10^7 seconds (the duration of annual cycles); and across spatial extensions from 10^{-10} meters (the dimension of intermolecular interactions) to the meter (the size of the body). The fact that life manages to operate with perfect cooperation across such enormous time and space scales cannot occur without a profound state of coherence, the determining factor in all living beings.

And what could this coherence actually be? For a living organism it manifests visibly in the regular, crystal-like assembly of vast quantities of molecules, such as those to be found in the connective tissue. These structures are capable of initiating patterns of collective vibrations, for example, in the form of electric or light waves. When such vibrations reach a certain level of coherence, a global wave is generated that can only be described in quantum terminology. Ho uses the metaphor of the laser, which at the start consists of an emission of disorganized photons that then synchronize to form a coherent ray of great force when it goes beyond a certain threshold of energy.

The existence in a living organism of such a state of quantum coherence, the nature of which is still unknown, would have significant consequences with regard to our understanding of homeostasis and health. It opens the door to a whole series of phenomena that are difficult to explain in terms of isolated biochemical reactions, the latter being the only category worthy of consideration by conventional medicine. It implies, for example, that an intervention of energy applied to any point on the body could instantaneously be transmitted through the living matrix and have an effect on the whole organism—an occurrence frequently observed by practitioners working with therapeutic light in the field of alternative medicine.

This macroscopic coherence is illustrated by the images of living organisms obtained by Mae-Wan Ho thanks to a technique derived from the polarized microscope, normally used to photograph the structures of crystalline minerals (see fig. 7.2). Here one finds shimmering interferometric waves with pure colors of the kind usually only seen in the perfectly aligned molecular arrays of crystals, the revealing sign of quantum coherence in all its dynamic aspect. Ho (2008) explains: "The reason living organisms could appear like a dynamic liquid crystal display is because all of the molecules in the tissues and cells . . . are not only globally aligned as liquid crystals, but also moving coherently together as a whole."

ENERGY AS THE BASIS OF ACUPUNCTURE

Acupuncture (and its sister therapy, acupressure) is one of the most ancient techniques of energy medicine still being used today all over the world. It

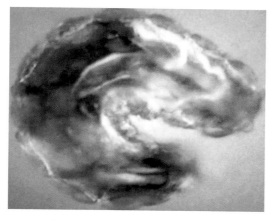

Figure 7.2. Coherence revealed: drosophila larva as seen under a polarizing microscope, from Mae-Wan Ho.
(photo courtesy www.i-sis.org.uk)

is based on the application of pressure or a needle to specific cutaneous reflex points or acupuncture points, which are all interconnected along energetic passageways called *meridians*. In the original model of traditional Chinese medicine (TCM), these meridians are a sort of highway along which vital energy, or chi, circulates. Although the clinical validity of acupuncture has been amply demonstrated, it has proved nearly impossible to detect these hypothetical meridians at the anatomical level. It could be because they are none other than circuits embedded within the matrix of connective tissue, indistinguishable from this matrix.

Whatever the case may be, many researchers have been able to locate acupuncture points using measurement instruments that detect variations in the flow of tiny electrical currents applied at various points on the body. Some have come across differences in the electric impedance at the level of the acupuncture points, while others have succeeded in tracing the meridians through impedance or electrical capacitance measurements. Ahn et al. (2008) completed a meta-analysis of eighteen studies of this type that offered a partial proof of the physical existence of meridians. Using a different approach, Cho et al. (1998) stimulated some acupuncture points on the foot and observed through functional magnetic resonance imaging (fMRI) the corresponding cerebral reaction, which closely matched the type of vital function associated in traditional Chinese medicine with the meridian being stimulated.

Other researchers have developed sophisticated systems based on the bioelectric measurement of acupuncture points. Among the most notable is that of Dr. Reinhard Voll, a German medical doctor who, starting in the 1950s, dedicated more than forty years to elaborating his theory of electro-acupuncture. His method was documented and proven in over a decade of hospital studies in Germany and is today widely used throughout Europe. In the United States it is growing in acceptance, particularly by medical practitioners who specialize in a holistic approach.

Are Meridians Energetic Rather than Physiological?

It seems possible that the meridians are not physical at all but purely energetic. Chinese biophysicist Chang Lin Zhang (2008) says that acupuncture points might correspond to the nodes of resonance of internal electromagnetic waves. These waves hypothetically issue from a coherence network in the body and form relatively stable standing wave patterns.

One can visualize patterns of this type through a method invented in 1787 by German physicist Ernst Chladni, which enables us to see the standing waves that naturally occur in many vibrational phenomena. Several modern

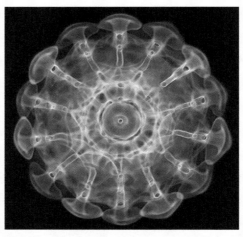

Figure 7.3. Cymatics standing wave pattern within a small disc of water having a diameter of roughly 1 cm, formed by a sound composed of five pure tones (© 2008 Cosolargy International)

versions of this technique exist, notably in *cymatics,* a term coined by Swiss physician Hans Jenny to refer to the visualization of multimodal vibrational patterns in various media. The surprising complexity of the shapes obtained when, for example, sound vibrates water droplets on a flat surface beautifully illustrates the organizational power of resonance and coherence (a subject discussed further in chapter 10).

Professor Zhang's theory has the advantage of explaining certain puzzling bioelectrical observations, such as the fact that the position and electrical conductivity of acupuncture points fluctuate according to one's health, and these fluctuations affect all points simultaneously. If the points are nodes of resonance on an internal wave, one would expect that any change in the conditions sustaining that wave would affect the whole internal interference pattern. According to this concept, wherein the meridians are a reflection of vibrational phenomena, it would be useless to try to establish their physiological traces in the body.

As we will see in the following chapter, many systems of therapeutic light used in alternative medicine today are based on a variation of acupuncture and consist of applying colored light rather than acupuncture needles to the points. These different approaches accept that the meridians are capable of transporting luminous energy, which is entirely plausible when one considers the crystalline, semiconductive nature of the connective tissue. This viewpoint received support in 1991 when Russian physician Vlail Kasnacheyev projected light on acupuncture points and observed their reemergence from other points located along the same meridian (Pankratov 1991). Similar findings were documented in a 1992 study by Yan et al. in which channels with high luminescence properties were observed in places where meridians are expected. This was confirmed by a study by Schlebusch, Maric-Oehler, and Popp (2005), in which infrared thermography revealed meridians during light stimulation performed with moxibustion (a technique in which a burning herbal stick is brought near acupuncture points).

In recent years, Korean biophysicist Kwang-Sup Soh has revived results claimed by a North Korean researcher in the 1960s, Bong-Han

Kim. The latter had reported the discovery of a system of previously unknown microscopic threadlike structures running throughout the body, in the skin as well as on the surface of organs and inside blood vessels. No one could reproduce his findings until 2004, when Soh and his team developed special staining techniques enabling the observation of these transparent, nearly invisible structures (known as *Bonghan ducts*) barely 50 micrometers across, which are now considered to be meridians (Soh 2004; Soh, Kang, and Ryu 2013).

BIOPHOTONS, LIVING LIGHT

One of the most remarkable energetic manifestations of life is the biophoton. Coined by a pioneer in this field, German biophysicist Fritz-Albert Popp, this term refers to light photons emitted by biological organisms. It was in the 1970s, when Popp served on the faculty of the University of Marburg, Germany, that he began to study the interaction between life and light. At that time, several other researchers were independently studying the phenomenon called *ultraweak photon emission,* or UPE, in which living organisms emit light.

If UPE was previously very little known, it was because this form of light really is *ultra* weak. It can be compared to the light of a candle shining twenty kilometers away and is one million times weaker than a star in the night sky. These levels (in the order of 1 to 100 photons per cm^2 per second) are completely invisible to the naked eye and can only be detected with the most powerful photomultiplying instruments. It is a very different manifestation from bioluminescence, which is photochemical in nature and is easily observable without magnifying help. Bioluminescence only concerns a few species, such as fireflies, glowworms, and certain phosphorescent mushrooms, whereas UPE seems to occur in most life forms.

Despite its extreme faintness, this light had been observed as early as 1922 by Soviet biologist Alexander Gurwitsch (1923). Since the technology of that time could not measure such low light levels, Gurwitsch had to establish its existence indirectly by studying interactions between organisms. In one of his now-famous experiments, he placed two onion roots in close proximity and observed that their

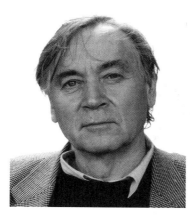

Figure 7.4.
Fritz-Albert Popp

growth was amplified on the side where they were closest. The effect disappeared when he placed an object between them, unless that object was transparent to ultraviolet light (for this he used a piece of quartz). He deduced that the two plants were exchanging invisible rays that he named *mitogenetic radiation*. The continuation of Gurwitsch's work elicited such interest that he was nearly awarded the Nobel Prize (missing only one vote) in 1930. But the effect was so difficult to quantify that the conflicting results obtained by other researchers, as well as the rise of molecular biology, led to his theories being largely forgotten.

When UPE was rediscovered in the 1970s, most researchers attributed it to the occasional leaks of energy occurring during normal chemical oxidation, and thus it was considered to be devoid of any particular biological significance. But when Popp first made his observations he suspected that it concerned something far deeper, and he named this light emitted by living tissue *biophotons*. He began an intensive investigation that lasted forty years, during which time he published hundreds of articles. In 1992 he founded the International Institute of Biophysics and subsequently became an inspiring figure for many researchers around the world. What Popp and his colleagues have discovered together has opened up new horizons in our understanding of life.

A Biological Laser

One of the main voices in this field is that of German scientist Marco Bischof, a long-time president of the International Institute of

Biophysics and the author of important works on biophotons (2003, 2005, 2008). I have had many occasions to meet Marco, and his presentations on the latest aspects of energy medicine are always fascinating.

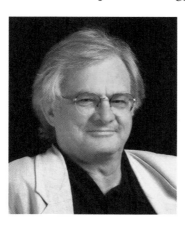

Figure 7.5. Marco Bischof

Early on in the research on biophotons it became clear that their emissions are correlated with various internal processes of living organisms. Bischof (2005) expresses it thus:

Unlike chemical bioluminescence, before the death of an organism its (biophoton emission) intensity increases steeply, more than a 100- or a 1,000-fold, and then decreases down to zero at the moment of death. The radiation also increases during mitosis (cell division) and undergoes very characteristic changes during all phases of the cell cycle. It reacts very sensitively to all disturbances, external influences, and inner changes in the organism. For this reason, its measurement can be used as a reliable and sensitive indicator for such influences and changes.

The wavelengths of biophotons are more or less evenly distributed from 260 to 800 nanometers, which covers the entire visible light spectrum. There is every indication that they do not originate from random thermal emission but are rather highly ordered, somewhat like a biological laser. Years of systematic measurements of cell cultures, microorganisms, plants, animals, and humans have confirmed that

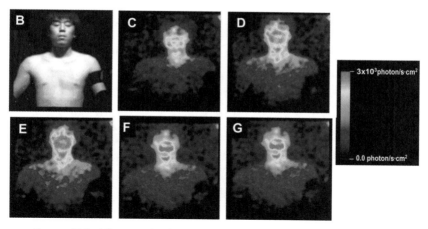

Figure 7.6. Ultraweak photon emission of a human subject (B) on the same day, showing variations at hour 10 (C), hour 13 (D), hour 16 (E), hour 19 (F), and hour 22 (G) (from Kobayashi, Kikuchi, and Okamura 2009)

biophotonic activity is universal. In humans, the emission is highest around the hands and the head. There are cyclical variations of ultraweak photon emissions during the day, the week, and the year, as though it is adapted to the biorhythm of the individual as well as to the outside world. An increase in stress leads to an increase in the UPE. Lateral asymmetries between the left and right side of the body are correlated with health problems, and treatments such as acupuncture have been observed to rebalance them. A treatment on one part of the body can restore the UPE elsewhere, indicating the global nature of the biophotonic field.

More and more sensitive instruments have been developed, and some are now capable of imaging the UPE of the whole body. The teams of Dr. Roeland van Wijk in the Netherlands and of Dr. Masaki Kobayashi in Japan are actively pursuing this research today.

The Light of the DNA

From his measurements, Popp (and Li 1993, and Yan 2002) deduced that biophotons have a high degree of coherence that grants them remarkable properties. They can easily propagate in opaque environments such as biological tissue. They can establish coherent electromagnetic fields over great distances, potentially over the whole organism, as Frölich had envisioned. And their interference patterns could constitute a veritable language adapted to intra- and intercellular communication (Popp 1999). This language also allows living organisms to communicate with one another, as Gurwitsch observed in plants. Physicist Sergey Mayburov (2011) has studied the biophotonic exchanges within populations of eggs from fish and frogs. He found that this exchange occurs in short, quasiperiodic bursts, with characteristics similar to those developed in network communication technology to optimize the transmission of signals in noisy environments. The eggs use this exchange to synchronize their growth.

For Popp, biophotons are more than mere random biological emissions. They are a means of information exchange playing a crucial role in living processes in which cells continuously emit and receive biophotons, using them to direct and regulate metabolism.

Even more extraordinary, Popp and Nagl (et al. 1984) concluded that the principal source of biophotons in the cell is none other than its DNA. They theorize that the DNA emits and stores biophotons within its molecular helix. This would enable it to act like a master tuning fork, entraining the molecules of the body to resonate with the "tone" of its biophotons.

While some of Popp's most audacious interpretations are still too controversial for the scientific community,* he has undeniably given us a revolutionary vision of biology in which living processes are guided by the interplay of coherent fields extending far beyond the reach of biochemistry.

Biophotons, Put into Service

The science of biophotons is still in its infancy, but we can already speculate on some practical applications. One of the most promising is related to the diagnosis of certain pathologies that perturb the UPE in ways that can be analyzed. For example, a cancer cell emits more

---

*See, for example, Cifra et al. 2015. The authors conclude that biophoton coherence, a central component of Popp's theories, is still not proven beyond all doubt. According to them the method used to infer this coherence, based on the statistical count of the number of photons emitted during UPE, does not exclude interpretations not relying on coherence.

biophotons than a healthy cell, and its degree of coherence is reduced. In a healthy organism biophotons are mostly emitted and recaptured internally, and relatively few escape to the outside world. Cancer leads to a loss of organization in the organism, which manifests as an increased leakage of biophotons (Takeda et al. 2004).

UPE measurement is already being used in the food industry to evaluate the freshness of food. As with the cancer example, the healthiest foods emit fewer biophotons, and those that they do emit are more coherent. The technique can even differentiate between the eggs of free-range chickens and those of chickens raised in cages; the light emitted by the former is more coherent (Grashorn and Egerer 2007).

If allopathic medicine is not yet ready to make use of the information provided by biophotons, some proponents of energy medicine have already developed experimental treatment techniques that do. One of these is Johan Boswinkel, a Dutch biophysicist who coengineered a device called Chiren,* which uses fiber-optic technology combined with biofeedback to conduct biophotons to and from the body. Boswinkel reports that the Chiren combines diagnosis (performed by Electroacupuncture according to Voll) with a treatment based on the detection of biophotons to retransmit an inverted corrective signal by means of fibre optics.

Another practitioner of light medicine is Dr. Dietrich Klinghardt, who integrates modalities of light therapy into a range of energetic techniques that are taught at his academy.† One of them uses polarized filters for diagnosis and is based on polarization properties specific to biophotons.

Biophotons and Consciousness

It seems that the more evolved the organism, the lower the density of its ultraweak photon emission. The UPE of a human is ten times less than that of morphologically more primitive animals or plants. For all organisms this emission is lowest when health is optimal. These factors

---

*See www.biontology.com
†See www.klinghardtacademy.com.

indicate that the higher the order within an organism, the more its biophoton emission remains internalized. Remarkably, this is not only true for physical health but for mental health as well.

Roeland van Wijk, a Dutch biochemist who authored the reference book *Light in Shaping Life: Biophotons in Biology and Medicine* (2014), shared some fascinating studies with us at the 2012 ILA conference. By comparing the UPE of subjects trained in meditation with that of subjects who were not (all being in good health), van Wijk and his team observed that the biophotonic emission was significantly reduced in the first group (et al. 2006). He concluded—not surprisingly—that long-term practice of meditation seems to contribute to internal order. But what he observed in a subsequent study is even more intriguing (van Wijk et al. 2008). By looking not only at the quantity but also the quality of the UPE, he and his team established a correlation between meditation and the degree of coherence of the biophotons emitted by the subjects.* This means that perhaps for the first time we can surmise that the light emanating from a person reflects an aspect of his or her state of consciousness. In the future we may be able to use light not only for its energetic properties, but also as a carrier of information about an organism's subtle internal condition.

THE ASTONISHING ROLE OF WATER

An essential concept in energy medicine is the role played by water in living organisms. Although it may be the most ordinary of the elements, water is, in fact, one of the most mysterious. This matters, as 99 percent of the molecules of our body are molecules of water.

The molecule H_2O has exceptional properties, with consequences that we are only beginning to uncover. It is dipolar, which is to say that it can easily undergo an internal displacement of its electrical charges

---

*This type of real-time measurement of the optical quantum coherence is still at the limit of our technological capabilities. In this study it was extrapolated from an analysis of the quantum squeezed states of the biophotons (see Van Wijk, Van Wijk, and Bajpai 2008). Squeezed states of light belong to the class of nonclassical states of light and occur when photons achieve exceptionally high coherence, as biophotons are thought to do.

between the pole of its oxygen atom and those of its two hydrogen protons. In so doing, it creates an electrical force called the hydrogen bond that attracts it to neighboring molecules. This very special property enables it to create vast electrical assemblies through which it can associate with other organic molecules. The whole structure of our organism is surrounded by such lattices, which are made up of 15,000 water molecules on average surrounding each of our proteins. Each molecule of water generates but a minuscule force field. But this force is multiplied by an astronomical number of water molecules, so many that together they literally maintain our body's structure (Corongiu and Clementi 1981). Remarkable simulations have shown that the DNA double helix of amino acids is electrically unstable without the presence of a large number of water molecules embedded within its matrix (up to fifty per amino acid), forming a highly resonant crystalline structure.

It is also thought that the network of water molecules intimately attached to those of the connective matrix could play a significant role in the transmission of energy waves. For example, a study demonstrated that a variation of barely 10 percent of the water content in proteins is capable of multiplying the transmission of electrical charges by a factor of one million (Gascoyne, Pethig, and Szent-Györgyi 1981).

In vibrational medicine, it has already been long considered that water is capable of adjusting the organization of its molecules to conform to external signals, and as a result it takes in or absorbs information. A new science about the energy properties of water is emerging* that purports to explain this and other properties of water.

I mention the role of water because it is intimately connected to light. Several traditions in chromotherapy are based on methods where water is exposed to colored light in order to "charge" it with specific properties related to the different colors.

University of Washington professor of bioengineering Gerald Pollack, who has elaborated the theory of structured water, describes the intimate relationship between water and light. A large portion of the water

---

*As demonstrated by the annual Conference on the Physics, Chemistry and Biology of Water (see www.waterconf.org)

contained in the human body exists in a state that until only recently we had never heard of. Pollack (2013) calls this state the *fourth phase* (beyond the three familiar states, solid, liquid, and vapor). This fourth phase is characterized by properties that most likely play a key role in its interaction with a living organism. In the intermediate phase between liquid and solid water has a higher viscosity and density and is more alkaline. In this state it possesses a negative electrical charge, and its molecules are more ordered. In fact, this fourth phase is activated by light—more precisely, the infrared light that is generated by the heat of our body.

A Connection between
Water and Photobiomodulation?

An intriguing link between water and photobiomodulation has recently been proposed (Sommer, Haddad, and Fecht 2015). To understand it we must recall the cellular respiration taking place in the mitochondria (discussed in chapter 4). This process generates ATP molecules, the power units essential to innumerable metabolic processes in living cells. In her discovery of photobiomodulation, Tiina Karu identified one particular enzyme (cytochrome c oxidase) within the respiratory chain as being susceptible to stimulation by light, thus explaining the capacity of light to accelerate cell metabolism. It turns out that another component of cellular respiration may be influenced by light as well: it is the very last link of the chain, a large enzyme complex called *ATP synthase*.

ATP synthase is a truly remarkable miracle of biology. It is a veritable molecular rotary motor, a nanoscale machine barely 10 nanometers across (see fig. 7.7). Each enzyme is composed of a motor head embedded within the mitochondria inner membrane (the FO motor) that entrains a second module (the F1 motor) through a central rotor shaft. This rotor has an asymmetrical "bump" and works like a camshaft, exerting a pressure in the F1 module with each rotation. It is this pressure that transfers the energy necessary to generate the precious ATP molecules.

How would light intervene here? Surprisingly, through its influence on the water surrounding this whole molecular machinery. Biologists now know that nearly all water within cells is in the fourth state due to its prox-

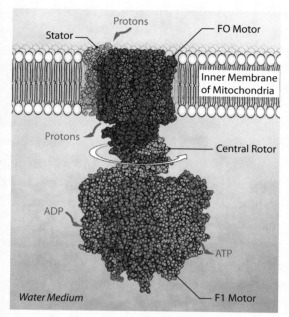

Figure 7.7. Molecular model of ATP synthase
(constructed from x-ray crystallography)

imity to cellular membranes. In this state, water has an increased viscosity, exerting substantial friction on the ATP synthase rotor. But Sommer, Caron, and Fecht (2008) have demonstrated that light in the near-infrared range (they tested 633 nm and 670 nm) significantly increased the lubricating properties of water inserted between the moving molecular parts. When one considers that the mitochondrial nanomotor turns at up to 9,000 revolutions per minute, it's easy to appreciate how this viscosity change may be a significant factor in reducing friction and thereby increasing ATP production.

Together with Karu's original finding, we now have a second photobiomodulation mechanism within cellular respiration, enabling light to stimulate cell metabolism through the acceleration of ATP synthesis—both mechanisms operating at similar near-infrared wavelengths. Any such influence is bound to be vital, given the astounding effectiveness of the process: our body's mitochondria generate on average 60 kg of ATP every single day!

THE LIVING MATRIX

In 1993, James Oschman gave the name *living matrix* to designate the collective assembly of matter, energy, and spontaneous organization that is the source of all living organisms (Oschman and Oschman 1993). A living matrix is a network that is simultaneously mechanical, vibrational (capable of oscillation), energetic, electronic, and informational. This explains the transmission of energy signals throughout the whole of our body in a multitude of forms, which we are only now beginning to identify: electrons, protons, solitons, phonons (electromechanical waves) and, of course, photons of light—and perhaps others as yet unknown.

This enigmatic and hidden vital energy so long sought after may be none other than a form of energy that we already know very well, whether it be electric or luminous. But it could also be that its nature is more in the order of information rather than something material, as in, for example, a wave of coherence that organizes an assembly of inanimate particles into which it breathes life during a fleeting moment.

The scientific study of subtle energy is only beginning. It has not yet gained the necessary attention (in terms of assembling a quantity of accepted scientific facts) to satisfy the criteria established by conventional medicine. This isn't surprising, if only for the simple reason that subtle energy is a new frontier that covers a vast array of entirely unknown phenomena. We await the coming generation of scientists daring enough to venture into nonconventional avenues to cement the proofs that grant this field unassailable acceptance by the scientific community.

While science has not yet given us a complete model of the living matrix, it has already offered us extremely promising indications for what will unfold in the future. Meanwhile, we are witnessing the discovery and application of a multitude of alternative therapeutic techniques involving subtle energy based on electromagnetic and photonic methods, as well as a variety of other modalities. Nothing should stop us, therefore, from benefiting from the best that *both* the conventional medical approach as well as the energetic approach can offer. This is the vision of a new, genuine integrative medicine.

8

COLOR MEDICINE

The History and
Uses of Chromotherapy

Color possesses me. I don't have to pursue it. It will possess me always, I know it. That is the meaning of this happy hour: Color and I are one.

PAUL KLEE

COLOR MEDICINE—CHROMOTHERAPY—UTILIZES the distinct properties of the colors of the visible light spectrum. It is a so-called alternative medicine capable of intervening in all aspects of our being. At the physical level it can ease chronic issues that sometimes stump conventional medicine. At the emotional level it can provide precious support to psychotherapy. At the mental level it can bring harmony and expansion.

Chromotherapy is a complement to the medical approach. It in no way replaces medicine or, for that matter, the light medicine that we explored earlier in this book. Chromotherapy is an energetic modality rather than a biochemical one, and it is meant for subtle fields of application that are generally ignored or overlooked by conventional medicine.

THE PATHWAYS THROUGH WHICH
COLOR INFLUENCES US

After all the successes of the new light medicine, one would think that the mystery of color would have been elucidated by now. In reality, the medical world is still perplexed when it comes to the therapeutic effects of color. At present, light medicine evaluates the healing properties of color through two mechanisms: the nonvisual optic pathway and photobiomodulation (refer to the discussion of the biological pathways of light in chapter 4). However, these two mechanisms work essentially in black and white and thus do not perceive color. Of course, the receptors involved in these mechanisms do have their own action spectra and react more or less to each color, but in a way that only influences the magnitude of the activation and not the quality. These two mechanisms depend on only one type of receptor: the ganglion cells (ipRGC) in the case of the nonvisual pathway, and the cytochrome c oxidase enzyme of the mitochondrial respiratory chain in the case of photobiomodulation. These receptors encode only a single variable, light intensity—similar to an old-fashioned black-and-white TV. So this makes these forms of light medicine intrinsically achromatic—without color.

Nevertheless, some studies have attempted to explain the effects of color through one or the other of the two mechanisms of light medicine, the nonvisual optic pathway and photobiomodulation. For example, they consider only the proportion of blue within each color and the consequential level of activation of ipRGCs of the nonvisual optic system, and thus its influence on our internal clock. Or else they consider only the biochemical effect of photobiomodulation, triggered by photons of various wavelengths inside the cell. Though these effects are real and important, this approach can only provide fragmentary insights into the profound influence of the different colors. In contrast, chromotherapy embraces this deep influence by recognizing that each color has distinct qualities. Our visual system allows us to perceive the quality of each color because it transmits specific chromatic information to the brain. It does this by means of the three types of cones in the retina that generate a signal with multiple variables capable of encoding color—again, to use the TV metaphor, just like the RGB (red-green-blue) signal of color TV.

To understand and appreciate the value of chromotherapy, one must take into account the whole optical system, including the visual optic pathway, that which is the most capable of perceiving color. And one must recognize that the perception of color is not purely a physiological phenomenon; it is also cognitive, and consequently it affects the mind as well as the body. Furthermore, chromotherapy cannot be fully understood without allowing for the phenomenon of resonance (mentioned earlier and discussed at greater length in chapter 10). Understanding resonance will perhaps one day explain how certain wavelengths of light can interact with various aspects of our internal energy field, as in the concept of the living matrix, discussed in the previous chapter.

Since chromotherapy is related to holistic concepts like consciousness and energy fields, notions that are still foreign to the present medical system, it is not surprising that it lies at the fringes of conventional medicine. Yet in truth no one can say for certain exactly how color affects us. As we mentioned at the beginning of this book, its influence is multidimensional; it acts simultaneously at the biophysical, energetic, and mental levels. So let's take a closer look at how this occurs.

Color through the Visual System

The primary way that light, and thus color, influences us is through the visual system. In chapter 4 we looked at the two main optic pathways: the visual optic pathway (or retinocortical pathway) that gives us sight, and the nonvisual optic pathway that links the retina to the hypothalamus and synchronizes our internal clock. Beyond these two main pathways are other neuronal connections, the retinotectal pathway and the accessory optic tract, which issue from the optic nerve and show the extent to which light reaches into most of the brain's centers. The four optical pathways stimulated by color are thus far-reaching, influencing every level of the cerebral processes: physiological, emotional, and cognitive, both conscious and unconscious.

As if this brief exploration of visual brain function is not already complex, I will add this last note: multiple feedback loops crisscross the various optic pathways, rendering the separate study of each one rather complicated, since they are interrelated. Ultimately, brain function is wonderfully unified. Indeed, Vanderwalle, Maquet, and Dijk (2009) have described how, using functional magnetic resonance imaging (fMRI), they were able to see the effects of a blue light stimulus targeting the hypothalamus through the nonvisual optic pathway gradually diffuse to other zones until it reached the whole cerebral cortex—and this entire process took place in about twenty minutes.

The Four Chromatic Pathways of the Visual System

Vision, the "royal road" of color: From the visual cortex where the visual optic pathway ends, the neuronal signals initiated by color are transmitted to a multitude of brain areas involved in cognition that are in the cortex, as well as in the regulation of emotions in the midbrain (see fig. 8.1). This optic pathway of color has a conscious as well as an unconscious influence. Color information from the visual pathway is thus brought all the way to the limbic system, where the amygdala controls our most instinctive emotional reactions. This opens the way for the psychotherapeutic use of chromotherapy as well as its use in treating physical ailments through psychosomatic processes.

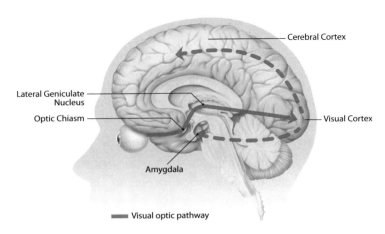

Figure 8.1. The visual optic pathway

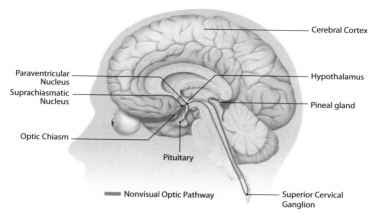

Figure 8.2. The nonvisual optic pathway

The blue pathway: The nonvisual optic pathway (fig. 8.2), for its part, is mostly influenced by the color blue, to which the ipRGC ganglion cells driving it are most sensitive. It is clearly involved in the physiological reactions to color, especially in the blue to green part of the spectrum. Because of the relatively slow reaction time of the ipRGCs, chromotherapeutic effects on this system will usually require several minutes of exposure at comparatively high intensities. However, these generalities are increasingly qualified as our knowledge of neurology improves (Vanderwalle et al. 2007).

The retinotectal pathway: A third network is the retinotectal (subcortical) pathway that connects the retina directly with the

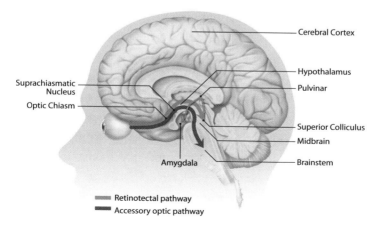

Figure 8.3. The retinotectal and accessory optic pathways

superior colliculus (SC), the small midbrain structures that play a role in the sensory motor control of the eyes, somewhat like an internal gyroscope. The SC is also involved in unconsciously perceived emotional stimuli and is linked to other structures of the brain implicated in this function, such as the pulvinar and even the amygdala, which is connected to the eyes by more than one pathway (Tamietto and de Gelder 2010). The retinotectal pathway originates in the ganglion cells, which are joined to the cones of the retina and are therefore sensitive to color.

The accessory optic tract: This fourth network connects the retina directly with the brainstem. Light is thus involved in the multiple physiological functions of the brain stem, including regulation of the heart rate and breathing, and managing our level of alertness and the quality of sleep. We have known since the 1960s that this optic pathway is color sensitive, each color activating distinct sets of neurons (Hill and Marg 1963).

Color through the Skin

Several types of chromotherapy are not directed to the visual system, but instead depend on the effect of light on the whole body. We have already seen how light, especially red and infrared, has an effect on the skin through the process of photobiomodulation. There are probably many other biochemical reactions that are catalyzed by other wavelengths of light. For example, blue green photons, at 460 to 490 nm, have a photochemical effect on the blood of newborns by decomposing bilirubin (recall chapter 5).

Since Dinshah Ghadiali, several other chromotherapists have established a link between the elements of the periodic table and colors as revealed by their spectroscopic properties. The spectra show which wavelengths are absorbed and emitted by the electronic orbitals of the atoms and therefore indicate which colors are likely to interact with it through resonance. Neuropsychiatrist Christian Agrapart (2016, with Delmas 2011) identifies the main color that appears in the spectrum of each trace element and associates its therapeutic properties to that color. For example, we know that zinc has immunostimulating properties. Since its main spectroscopic lines are violet, we can therefore deduce that shining light in this color range on the skin will have analogous immune-stimulating effects.

We know that light projected on the skin penetrates several layers of epidermal cells and irradiates blood though the capillaries. Any resulting biochemical reaction would be distributed throughout the organism by the circulatory system.

Color's Interactions with the Subtle-Energy System

The effect of color on the subtle-energy system is more speculative but potentially more far-reaching. Several different types of chromotherapeutic modalities act on acupuncture points to establish a link between the meridians and colored light. This is possible because as energy medicine asserts, the meridians are most likely electromagnetic in nature.

Along the same lines, if the whole body is animated by a field of coherence, this means that an application of colored light, whether localized or general, can produce a resonance that will be felt throughout the entire organism.

COLOR SYSTEMS
USED IN CHROMOTHERAPY

There are many approaches in chromotherapy, each following different color systems that have been developed, some of which we will present here. Most of these systems can be best visualized in the form of a chromatic wheel, a technique first used in the seventeenth century by English physicist Sir Isaac Newton. Newton took the seven colors that he observed in the linear spectrum projected by his prism and arranged them in a circle by joining the red and violet edges (see fig. 8.4). In doing so he was mainly interested in studying the mathematical and harmonic interrelationship between the colors.

A century later, Goethe, whose literary efforts addressed a wide range of subjects, including treatises on botany, anatomy, and color, became interested in the "allegorical, symbolic and mystical" properties

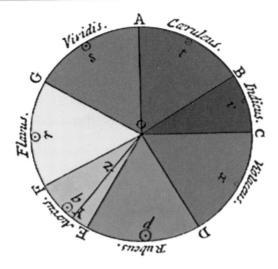

Figure 8.4. Newton's original chromatic wheel, with its seven colors.

of color as he called them. He identified three main colors: red, yellow, and blue. These colors are said to be primary because they form the basis of this color system. All other colors can, in principle, be obtained by mixing the primary colors, and for this reason they are called *secondary* colors, or even *tertiary* in the case of more nuanced hues.

By inserting three secondary colors (orange, green, and the synthetic color magenta*) between his primary colors, Goethe obtained a wheel with six colors (see fig. 8.5). His method had the advantage of bringing out colors that are diametrically opposed around the circle: red against green, yellow against magenta, blue against orange. These pairs of colors are considered complementary and are very important in chromotherapy, as they are often seen to have opposite effects. If one color has a certain effect, its complementary color will have the opposite effect. They can therefore be used conjointly to amplify or reduce their associated qualities.

It's important to realize that in chromotherapy the choice of primary

---

*Magenta is called "synthetic" because it is not found in the rainbow spectrum of visible light. Rather, it is physiologically and psychologically perceived as the mixture of red and violet/blue light, with the absence of green.

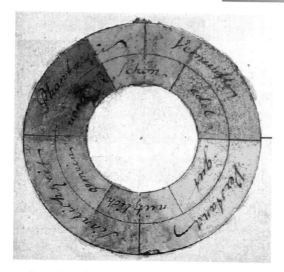

Figure 8.5. Goethe's chromatic wheel, with six colors

colors (and hence secondary colors) is not absolute since it depends on subjective considerations related to our appreciation of color. Thus different theorists have arrived at different interpretations, although this has not prevented them from developing perfectly coherent systems. For example, at the beginning of the twentieth century Dinshah Ghadiali based his Spectro-Chrome system on a more complex wheel. He selected three primary colors (red, green, and violet), between which he inserted three secondary colors (yellow, blue, and magenta). In between these six colors he added an additional six tertiary colors (see fig. 8.6). According to Dinshah, certain opposite colors are obtained by diagonal symmetry (red/blue, orange/indigo, yellow/violet) and others by mirroring along the green axis (lemon/turquoise, scarlet/purple). In his system green has a central role, being the physical balancing color.

In the 1930s, American physician Carl Loeb developed his own method, called Spectroband therapy. The mentor of Harry Riley Spitler (who earlier had developed his method of *syntonic phototherapy,* as recounted in chapter 1), Loeb was a contemporary of Dinshah, whose color model he adopted for his color velocity diagram (see fig. 8.7). This diagram clearly underscores the polarity of complementary colors.

A modern pioneer of chromotherapy is Theo Gimbel. Considered

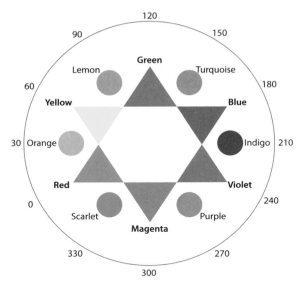

Figure 8.6. Dinshah Ghadiali's chromatic wheel
with twelve colors

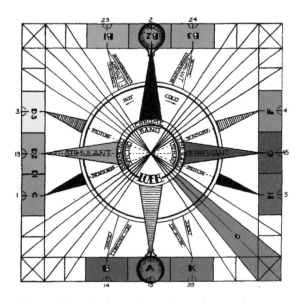

Figure 8.7. Carl Loeb's color velocity diagram
with twelve colors

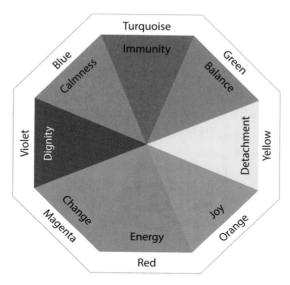

Figure 8.8. Theo Gimbel's chromatic
octagon

one of Britain's most experienced color researchers and practitioners, he focuses on the deeper spiritual aspects of color. Gimbel prefers an eight-colored wheel (see fig. 8.8). Here we can see how his chromatic octagon led to new pairs of complementary colors, such as orange/ blue and red/turquoise.

Belgian color researcher Pierre Van Obberghen created a twelve-colored wheel (see fig. 8.9 on page 176). His method resembles that of Dinshah but is based on a triad of primary colors better adapted to the physiology of our eyes, with their three types of cones: red, green, and blue. He has added three secondary colors: yellow, cyan (which he renames "sky blue"), and magenta. Six tertiary colors are inserted between these.

I have personally found Van Obberghen's wheel to be the most rational, and I use it to define complementary colors in my own Sensora system (red/turquoise, green/magenta, blue/yellow). Visually, the light patterns based on these combinations are remarkably powerful.

The Color Industry

Color is at the heart of the activity of numerous painters, graphic artists, lighting designers, and other artists who know how to use it to influence us, to enchant us, and to make us dream. Since color is so important in our lives it's not surprising that a whole industry has sprung up around it that is primarily concerned with the means of reproducing color: inks and machines for paper printing, tints and dyes for textiles and architecture, light control for video displays and colored illumination.

The study of color has led to a psychology of color that attempts to understand the influence of color on our tastes, desires, and preferences. Investigated by people such as American color theorist Faber Birren, color psychology is now used by designers, architects, and of course experts in marketing and advertising. One of its most noteworthy tools is the color test that Swiss psychotherapist Max Lüscher created in 1947, which uses color preferences as a means of assessing a person's psychophysical profile (Lüscher and Scott 1969).

The whole domain of color is much vaster than that of chromotherapy. How is the latter different? The color industry wants to master the utilitarian use of color in our daily lives, while chromotherapy aims to relieve physical and psychological ills by the case-specific application of color. Of course, there is some overlap between these aims, color being universal. For example, the lighting designer will want to avoid inadvertently triggering the kind of intense emotional reaction that the chromotherapist may wish to elicit in a controlled therapeutic setting.

Then there is the new field of "mood lighting" that seeks to create a beneficial living environment through illumination. Among the lighting industry's mood-lighting products, few are truly chromotherapeutic. Those that are, like my own spherical mood-lighting device, the SensoSphere,* have been conceived with the knowledge of the therapeutic properties of color and are generally more subtle and nuanced. But the majority of gadgets that inundate the market today are rather garish and do not respect the health implications of lighting (see chapter 6), as they typically have high levels of

*www.sensora.com/sensosphere_e.html

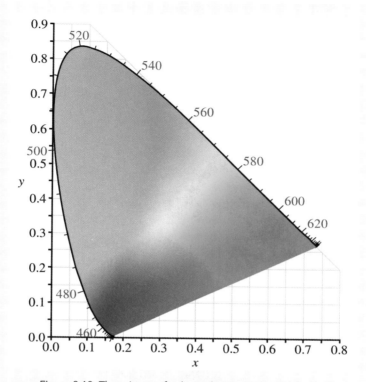

Figure 8.10. The science of color, *colorimetry*, is regulated by organizations like the Vienna, Austria–based International Commission on Illumination (or CIE, for its French name, Commission Internationale de l'Éclairage). This science analyzes and quantifies all aspects of the perception of color according to the properties of our visual system. This is the 1931 CIE color space diagram defining the gamut of all reproducible colors as a function of two standardized colorimetric parameters, *x* and *y*. The pure colors of the rainbow are distributed along the periphery of the diagram, shown with their wavelengths in nanometers (nm).

flickering and display excessive blue light. Given the explosion of hyper-colored light in our environment, a recent phenomenon made possible by the extensive availability of LED technology, one wonders if human beings will become desensitized to the influence of color in the coming years. Accordingly, many forms of chromotherapy use as dark an environment as possible in order to amplify the effects of the pure colors that are presented.

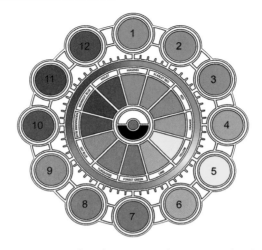

Figure 8.9. The "harmonic chromatic wheel"
of Van Obberghen, with twelve colors.
Reproduced with permission from *Treatise on Color Therapy Practice,*
Guy Trédaniel Publisher, 2014.

THE PRACTICE
OF CHROMOTHERAPY

The Properties of Color

We now come to the heart of this discussion; namely, what are the particular properties of each color? When I began my own exploration of light therapy in the 1980s I naively expected to find the answers in any good reference library. I quickly became disillusioned; it turns out that there are many different interpretations of the properties of color. It is by no means an established or exact science. When one considers that light has an effect on multiple levels, it's understandable that there is no simple and absolute answer to this question. A color can have a certain effect on one level and act quite differently on another. Its effect can depend on the state of the organism or on the interactions with other chromatic influences within the organism.

Fortunately, since the first experiments in chromotherapy in the nineteenth century there is some consensus regarding its general principles. It is by and large accepted that there are two main categories of colors: colors that are said to be warm and colors that are regarded as cool. Warm colors are stimulating, fortifying, and energizing. Cool colors are calming, sedative, and analgesic. The specific colors associated with these two categories vary somewhat, but in general the warm colors in the spectrum range from red to yellow, and the cool colors span from turquoise (or sometimes green) to deep blue or indigo.

Early on, researchers like Harry Riley Spitler established a link between the two categories of color and the autonomous nervous system (ANS), the part of the nervous system that is not under conscious control and functions in an autonomous way to maintain vital functions. It is divided into two complementary and antagonistic systems: the sympathetic nervous system (associated with action under stress, as in the fight-or-flight response) and the parasympathetic nervous system (associated with rest, relaxation, and regeneration). Warm colors naturally correspond to the sympathetic nervous system and cool colors to the parasympathetic nervous system. The equilibrium of the ANS is fundamental to our health, and the possibility of influencing it is a driving force in chromotherapy.

Observing colors on a chromatic wheel, we see that at the junction of the warm and cool halves are two intermediate areas: on the one hand is the band between yellow and turquoise (lime green, green), and on the other the band between deep blue and red (violet, magenta). The colors in these two areas are generally considered to have a balancing effect that makes them particularly valuable in facilitating transitions; for example, in breaking a pattern of chronic illness (see fig. 8.11 on page 179).

Beyond these general principles, a more extensive analysis of the properties of colors depends on the system, and the reader wishing to learn more can study the specific type of chromotherapy that he or she is interested in.

Table 8.1 of the general properties of colors contains information gathered from Van Obberghen (2014) and Deppe (2013), both of whom have compiled the interpretations of several other authors. These properties are not absolute and are mostly of an empirical and analogical nature. They are included here because they offer a good representation of contemporary chromotherapy color interpretation.

TABLE 8.1. GENERAL PROPERTIES ASSOCIATED WITH COLORS, ACCORDING TO VAN OBBERGHEN (2007) AND DEPPE (2013)

COLOR	WAVELENGTH	PHYSICAL PROPERTIES	PSYCHOLOGICAL PROPERTIES	ASSOCIATED BODY PARTS
Red	760–635 nm	Tonifying Warming Antianemia Antimigraine	Extroversion Passion	Reproductive system Urogenital system Increases blood pressure
Orange	635–590 nm	Invigorating Adrenal stimulant	Antidepressant Joy Sociability	Adrenal glands Vasomotricity Musculoskeletal system
Yellow	590–570 nm	Digestive stimulant Lymphatic stimulant	Intellectual strength Optimism Detachment	Digestive system Intestine Spleen Pancreas
Lemon	570–550 nm	Antiallergy Detoxifying Addresses chronic conditions	Flexibility Peace Opening	Joints Gallbladder Diaphragm Vision, visual field
Green	550–520 nm	General balancing Neutralizing Anti-infection	Love Abundance Adaptability	Liver Lungs Thymus Immune system
Turquoise, Cyan	520–490 nm	Cleansing Refreshing Addresses acute conditions	Wholeness Autonomy Fulcrum of emotion vs. thought	Arms and hands Parathyroid glands Skin
Sky Blue	490–460 nm	Calming Anti-inflammation Antipyretic	Antistress Introversion Endorphins stimulant	Nose, throat, neck Thyroid gland Breathing Ears and hearing
Deep Blue, Indigo	460–430 nm	Sleep-inducing Muscle relaxant	Intuition Imagination Anxiolytic	Sinuses Pituitary Forehead and occiput Limbic system
Violet	430–380 nm	Immunostimulant	Spirituality Trust Dignity	Cerebral cortex Pineal gland Memory
Magenta	Synthetic color (red-blue mix)	Cardiovascular normalizer Aphrodisiac	Mood enhancer Capacity of letting go Intimacy	Heart Cardiovascular system Lips and mucous membranes

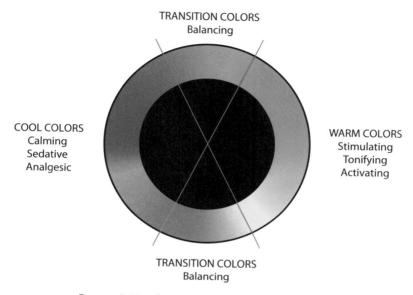

Figure 8.11. The warm colors, the cool colors,
and the transitional colors of chromotherapy

The Tools of Chromotherapy

Certain types of chromotherapy are practiced with tools as simple as cards, filters, or other colored objects. But most systems are based on the application of colored light and consequently require instruments capable of producing and delivering light with precision. These instruments come in a variety of forms depending on the intended use. Some are specifically designed to shine light in the eye, as in syntonic phototherapy. Others are designed to illuminate specific body areas, like the Spectro-Chrome projector. Some work on specific points, as in *Colorpuncture*. And yet others illuminate the whole body, as in Samassati. Finally, some are aimed at the visual field indirectly by projection on a screen, as with the Sensora.

Nearly all these instruments rely on one of two main technologies for producing colored light:

* **A wide-spectrum white source** paired with a filter that will produce the desired color. The source may be incandescent,

halogen, or in the more sophisticated instruments requiring the widest spectra, xenon. The filters can be of different types. Gels can be used to obtain colors of moderate saturation. Dichroic-type filters, obtained by vapor deposition of optical microlayers on glass, provide purer colors. And filters made with holographic structures or optical gratings result in quasimonochromatic colors.

∗ **An LED source** with a narrow spectrum (20 to 50 nm wide according to the LED color), which in itself produces a pure color. This technique has the drawback of being limited by the range of commercially available colors on the LED market, which prioritizes the primary colors, red (630 nm), green (530 nm) and blue (460 nm), along with a few others such as amber (590 nm) and turquoise (505 nm).

These two technologies are perfectly suitable for chromotherapy, and the choice depends on the type of intervention required.

With LED technology it is possible to produce a vast range of colors by combining the three primary colors, red, green, and blue (RGB). That is precisely the technology used, for example, in our video screens and TVs. I am often asked if this is appropriate for chromotherapy.

The Blue Paradox

That the nature of blue is relaxing and sedative is one of the most universally acknowledged particulars of chromotherapy. Blue is a characteristically cool color, and yet hundreds of recent clinical studies on the properties of the nonvisual optic pathway have established blue as the color that suppresses melatonin, the sleep hormone, and keeps us awake and vigilant even against our wishes. How can we resolve the paradox of these seemingly opposing influences? Till now I have not found a convincing answer to this question, whether from chromotherapists or biologists. This paradox illustrates the limits of our present knowledge of color.

A comparison of scientific articles inexorably leads to mixed and contradictory results. For example, research on the effects of blue and red (two chromatic polarities) on the autonomous nervous system (ANS) does not reveal any clear and simple effect, despite the conviction of chromotherapists since the time of Spitler. As well, studies on the comparative impact of blue and red on cognitive performance (Mehta and Zhu 2009) or cardiorespiratory synchronization (Edelhäuser et al. 2013) often reach opposite conclusions. Coherent results are hard to obtain because the effects depend on too many variables that are difficult to control in a clinical setting, including wavelength, intensity, and the context in which the colors are presented (Meier et al. 2012). Most biologists and psychologists keen on the study of color agree on the difficulty of this endeavor.

As for the opposite effects of blue, my own impression is that they are related to the intensity of the light. The intensities for which melatonin suppression has been observed are generally above 100 lux with long durations (over 30 minutes), whereas the intensities commonly used in chromotherapy are relatively low, often less than 100 lux and of a rather short duration (a few minutes). In the first case, light interacts with the hypothalamus; in the second it probably interacts with the visual cortex. Given the complexity of the brain, should we be surprised that the same color can interact dissimilarly with different cerebral areas?

Currently the scientific literature can neither confirm nor refute the foundations of chromotherapy. So as long as this is the case, it's not unreasonable to rely on the clinical observations of generations of chromotherapists.

It is heartening to see that a few scientists are at last beginning to venture into the field of chromotherapy. In a recent article anesthesiologist Mohab Ibrahim (et al. 2017) and his team at the University of Arizona found that shining soft green light (525 nm) into the eyes of lab rats reduced their neuropathic pain. Intigued by this result, he is now testing the same treatment in small-scale human trials, with most test subjects reporting a significant reduction of pain from migraines, fibromyalgia, and arthritis. While the exact mechanism that makes green light so helpful is still unknown to the investigators (they suspect it acts on the brain's central opioid circuits), Ibrahim says his initial inspiration came after realizing that sitting among trees helped to mitigate his own headaches—a balancing effect of the green color that chromotherapists have known about from age-old experience.

The simple answer is that it depends on the modality. It is particularly efficient in approaches aimed at the visual field because it is well adapted to the three types of cones in the retina. A wide variety of colors can be obtained by mixing the red, green, and blue sources, and these colors will appear to the eye just like those in the rainbow spectrum. Only visual applications requiring monochromatic light (such as Karl Ryberg's Monocrom) cannot use RGB.

RGB has some drawbacks, one being the poor quality of the yellow color normally obtained by the combination of red and green; this can be remedied by adding a fourth primary color, amber, as I have been doing in my Sensora system. RGB performance is also limited at the extremities of the visible spectrum, where violet and deep red cannot be adequately simulated by the combination of blue and red, which instead produces magenta.

For nonvisual approaches in which the aim is to illuminate areas of the skin or to interact with the energy field of the body, the RGB technique is not recommended. This is because the spectrum that is simulated by the combination of the RGB frequencies may fool the visual system but will in no way have the vibrational signature of the specific bandwidth of a pure color—especially when the color sought after is not one of the three primary colors.

Treating Color "Allergies"

For some therapists who work with color, an overly strict interpretation of their properties does not take into account one important reality: each of us reacts differently to color. Some colors we naturally gravitate toward, while with others we might feel an aversion. The mental processes triggered by color inevitably depend on our past experiences, our conditioning, and our personality. Nobody expresses this more clearly than Jacob Liberman, who in the 1980s developed his system of Spectral Receptivity Training, thereby initiating a new understanding of chromotherapy:

> Having used color therapeutically since 1971, I empirically discovered that color is inseparably linked to our emotions. Different

people react to the same color in different ways and the effect of a specific color is not based on its supposed attributes (as claimed by most methods), but rather on how an individual relates to that color.

Each person is comfortable with some colors, and uncomfortable with others. When a person is exposed to colors they dislike, it can evoke agitation, releasing feelings and memories that trace back to unsettled experiences. Some colors elicit joy, a sense of safety and comfort. Others can trigger sadness, fear, and a variety of other emotions. It's as if we recoil from certain colors because they awaken painful memories and the feelings that accompany them. . . . Just as some life experiences are easy for us to accept and others are difficult, the energetic frequencies underlying these experiences are either comfortable or uncomfortable for us to embrace. Light and life are inseparable, which is why colors affect us so deeply and so differently. In essence, we respond to specific colors in the same way we respond to specific life experiences. Whether the color is viewed or visualized, the impact is obvious and often immediate, offering deep insight into one's psyche.

The colors we withdraw from represent the portions of the visible spectrum we are allergic to. And when we are allergic to a certain color, like red, we will do our best to avoid the spectrum of light that we perceive as red, as well as the spectrum of life that corresponds to red. . . .

By systematically viewing colors that feel uncomfortable, you can gradually desensitize to the habitual triggers that catalyze stress in your lives, embracing that which you previously avoided. Based on my observation and clinical experience, colored light—the energetic foundation of our life's experiences—circumvents our conscious defences before the intellect can dilute its potency. You can overcome allergies to color—and therefore to life—by gently visualizing specific colors at your own pace. And as you become more comfortable with those colors, you may experience greater physical vitality and wellness, as well as an increased ease and receptivity to all aspects of life.

184 New Applications of Light

For the experienced therapist, this understanding of chromatic "allergies" is a great advantage. Exposing a person to his favorite colors can bring about harmony and regeneration. Conversely, exposing someone to colors he dislikes, within the safe setting of a chromotherapy session, can help him overcome the associated negative experiences.

It is inherent in the nature of noninvasive interventions such as chromotherapy that only memories or traumas that a person is ready to integrate will be brought to consciousness. During chromotherapy sessions with the Sensora, we have observed again and again the spontaneous emergence of past traumas happening in a nonthreatening and effortless manner; for example, during treatment for post-traumatic stress disorder. Color radiates an essential beauty, pure and impersonal, that facilitates new realizations and the dissolution of blockages.

Meetings with Dr. Jacob Liberman

I have had many occasions to hear Jacob Liberman speak at various syntonics and ILA conferences, and each time I have appreciated the pragmatism and clarity of his talks. Jacob is undeniably one of the most influential pioneers in the development of light therapy in the course of the last thirty years. His book *Light: Medicine of the Future* is today the most read book on the subject and has inspired a whole generation of researchers, myself included. Jacob has always been closely involved with the light community and has generously supported many causes, such as that of the College of Syntonic Optometry (CSO), the International Society for the Study of Subtle Energies and Energy Medicine (ISSSEEM), and the international conference LIGHT'98* that was the forerunner of the ILA, which was founded a few years later, as well as the ILA itself.

I've met with Jacob many times, but it was on a trip to his adopted place of residence in Maui, Hawaii, that I benefited the most from his kindness.

---

*LIGHT'98 took place in 1998 at the University of Reading in the UK and brought together researchers and therapists from the four corners of the world who had been working with light. This historical meeting was organized by the late Primrose Cooper, a woman of shining wisdom who was also a founding member of the ILA (see Cooper 2000).

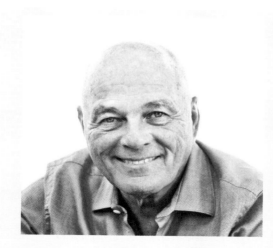

Figure 8.12.
Jacob Liberman
(© Cansu Bulgu,
www.cansuart.com)

I was there on vacation with my companion, Deva. Jacob organized a wonderful stay for us on the island, complete with lodging and car, and received us in his home on the slopes of the Haleakala volcano. He and I embarked on a local tour, lecturing on light, and our presentations complemented each other's very nicely.

In the 1980s and '90s, Jacob developed the chromotherapeutic projectors known as the *Color Receptivity Trainer*, as well as the *Spectral Receptivity System*. He also designed a visual trainer, the *Eyeport*. Notably, after having contributed so much to the technical dimension of light therapy by producing clinical studies, books and articles, and other innovative instruments, Jacob has gradually turned his attention toward the spiritual dimensions of light, as attested by his latest book *Luminous Life: How the Science of Light Unlocks the Art of Living*. But that has not prevented us from imagining a few new instruments that we could design by combining our respective expertise. Time will tell if we manage to realize one or another of these ideas.

Determining the Right Color

How does one determine what the appropriate colors are for a particular person? Pierre Van Obberghen, a specialist in the field, likes to say that for the chromotherapist, the answer to that question is a veritable "quest for the Holy Grail" since there are as many answers to the question as there are types of chromotherapy, each one having its own approach.

In most approaches that apply to the body, such as *Chromatothérapie* or Spectro-Chrome, a medical diagnosis is first established and a precise, systematic protocol then applied. For example, syntonic phototherapy, another form of chromotherapy that falls into this category, relies on an optometric evaluation to determine the sequence of colors of treatment.

When chromotherapy is used at a psychological or energetic level it relies on tools capable of evaluating more subtle parameters. For example, Esogetic Colorpuncture, a technique combining acupuncture and colored light developed by Peter Mandel, uses a variation on Kirlian photography that he calls *Kirlian energy emission analysis* to complete an energetic diagnosis.

One technique used in alternative medicine involves the vascular autonomic signal (VAS), which analyzes the radial arterial pressure of the pulse of a person to reach a clinical evaluation. An experienced practitioner, by holding the wrist of a patient or client, can instantly detect the response to various energetic interventions such as color. This technique is used by Pierre Magnin, MD, one of the pioneers of chromotherapy in France who developed Photonomedicine (Magnin and Vidal 2017).

Other practitioners rely on verbal evaluations to determine the psychotherapeutic needs of a client, as is done with my Sensora system. This kind of evaluation facilitates the selection of the most appropriate program from a whole library of color combinations.

Therapists using other techniques expose the client to certain colors and observe their verbal or emotional responses in order to direct the course of treatment. This is the case in *Emotional Transformation Therapy* (ETT). Others use color testing methods such as the Lüscher test, which measures a person's psychophysical profile based on his or her color preferences. Color therapist Pierre Van Obberghen has developed his own color test, which is based on the client's chromatic preferences and aversions. Yet another approach is to have the client choose the colors, trusting in the ability of each person to perceive which colors he or she needs. This is what happens in the Monocrom and Aura-Soma systems. Last but not least, some practitioners simply rely on their own intuition when it comes to selecting colors, as in Samassati Colortherapy, a form of psychotherapy based in meditation practice developed by Nishant Matthews.

If this enumeration of some of the many methods of chromotherapy arouses your curiosity, the next chapter will go into detail on how some of these systems work. Each method relies on the different aspects of how color influences us, whether at the physiological, the psychological, or the spiritual level. The extraordinary variety offered within the field of chromotherapy demonstrates the richness of our interaction with color.

9

ALTERNATIVE
LIGHT MEDICINE

Modern Chromotherapy Technologies

In every culture and in every medical tradition before ours, healing was accomplished by moving energy. Treating humans without the concept of energy is treating dead matter.

ALBERT SZENT-GYÖRGYI

FORTUNATELY FOR THEM, ancient civilizations never had to wait for scientific confirmation to enjoy the benefits of light. Certainly many modern innovators have developed healing systems in advance of any blessing by establishment medicine. Many of these systems are considered "alternative" because they rely on an energetic aspect of healing that is simply not understood by allopathic medicine today. Though many light-medicine practitioners are scientists, some are not; yet all of them are moved by a passion for light, and most have intuitively discovered new ways to use its healing powers.

The overview of alternative light medicine presented in this chapter offers a sampling of what's available in the field, but by no means does it include all approaches, since it would be impossible to thoroughly chronicle the profusion of ideas emerging today. My sole criterion for selecting the systems mentioned in these pages is that I have either experienced them myself or I have met their creators and heard them speak of their vision—often in the context of one or another of the international conferences on light that I regularly attend and organize. Though I am not necessarily able to quantify their effectiveness, I know at least that they have touched and helped many people in a positive way. In the individual descriptions and case studies included in the chapter, the creators have granted me the privilege of quoting directly from their responses to my request to summarize the essence of their system for the purpose of this book.

Very few of the alternative methodologies mentioned here have been clinically validated yet, either due to lack of funding or because the very nature of the interaction does not readily lend itself to such study. Technological means of measuring subtle energy are rare, and even those few methods that are available are generally not recognized by the medical establishment and are therefore unsuitable for clinical studies. Furthermore, traditional or natural methods are not usually patentable and therefore cannot attract the financial investment necessary for rigorous clinical investigations. Still, several of these methods are taught and practiced by thousands of therapists throughout the world, which gives a good indication of their value.

Even those alternative systems that have been developed by legitimate scientists have often been firmly opposed by the more conservative elements within established medicine, while the creators of these systems have been accused of practicing pseudoscience. Such was the case of optometrist Harry Riley Spitler and his syntonic phototherapy system in the middle of the last century, and more recently of neuropsychiatrist Christian Agrapart, the originator of Chromatothérapie, and neuropsychiatrist Anatoly P. Chuprikov, who conceived *lateral light therapy*.

Some general principles apply to nearly all these diverse modalities of chromotherapy. The influence of color on the autonomic nervous system (ANS) is used in several systems, and so is the application of colored light to specific points: the reflex points and meridians of acupuncture as defined by traditional Chinese medicine. One thing common to all methods is the use of color, the influence of which is too intangible and thus poorly understood to be quantified by the methods of conventional medicine.

Some chromotherapeutic systems work by interacting with the body while others are oriented to work with consciousness, a subtler but no less powerful approach. Still others make use of both dimensions.

Note: The use of any alternative or parallel modality should never replace medical treatment. All persons who are under medical supervision should check with their physician that the use of a chromo-therapeutic method will not conflict with their treatment.

• • •

Spectro-Chrome

The Spectro-Chrome method was developed in the United States between 1920 and 1940 by Dinshah Ghadiali (see chapter 1). It has since acquired the questionable honor of becoming one of the most denigrated methods of chromotherapy, showcased in museums dedicated to quackery and cited as an example of delusion about the supposed magical powers of color.

Dinshah was unfortunate to live during the time of the rising power of Big Pharma and the associated medical establishment. He was brought to trial in 1931 and again in 1947 for inaccurately describing his product, at which time he lost his case and received a three-year prison sentence. In 1952 the FBI destroyed all his instruments and documents. Then, from 1958 on, the U.S. Food and Drug Administration banned his work permanently, a ban still in effect today. However, Dinshah Ghadiali's son, Darius Dinshah, today strives to keep alive the method invented by his father. As it is still under FDA injunction he must limit his efforts to education. To that effect, in 1975 he founded the Dinshah Health Society and later published the manual *Let There Be Light,* which describes the core of his father's method.

As a result of its suppression, the original Spectro-Chrome method

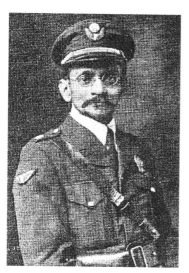

Figure 9.1. Dinshah Ghadiali (photo taken in 1920 when he was a colonel in the New York Police Reserve)

has not evolved very much since Dinshah Ghadiali's day and has become a sort of relic of chromotherapy from the last century. So what is the truth about its validity? Surprisingly, the general properties of color as established by Dinshah (1933) for the Spectro-Chrome method are still the foundation of most modern chromotherapy methods. Dinshah (as he preferred to be known, since he considered his family name too difficult to pronounce for most Americans) seems to have come to an understanding that is still pertinent today. Several modern researchers have taken his work and adapted it by making use of the new possibilities offered by the advance of technology.

One of these is Alexander Wunsch, a holistic physician who describes the Spectro-Chrome method as follows.

It is a color system which arranges nine spectral and three extra-spectral colors of light in an equidistant distribution pattern within a circle. The Spectro-Chrome color wheel provides the same clear orientation as we know it from a classical clock face, each hour representing another color. Equidistant arrangement allows a clear definition of the relationships between the colors, such as infra-green, ultra-green or opposite colors. It also allows the classification of primary, secondary, and tertiary colors. Equidistance also enables the therapist to extrapolate the expected effects of colors based on the observed effects of another color. The Spectro-Chrome color wheel is like a precise compass for optimal orientation in the color world.

It is a chromotherapy system using the Spectro-Chrome colors for the treatment of large skin areas. This systemic treatment modality represents the classic Spectro-Chrome method, in which the color perception via the eyes plays only a secondary role. The main targets are the cellular structures of the skin and the molecules and cells in the bloodstream, which are located not more than 1/10th of a millimetre beyond the body surface. Dinshah's attuned color waves, in fact the specific wavelengths of the photons, resonate with the different biomolecules. Each "colored" photon carries a typical amount of quantum energy, which (in case of absorption) modifies the structure and/or behaviour of the absorbing molecule. In contrast to the retinal photoreceptors, which can only discriminate between three different colors, the biomolecules in human skin and blood provide a much broader absorption bandwidth. This makes the systemic application of colored light so interesting for a light therapist, since it addresses the body structures and functions in a primordial manner. . . . If skin, blood and eyes are addressed simultaneously, the best efficacy can be expected—for this reason the eyes should also look into the colored light during a systemic application.

The classical systemic Spectro-Chrome treatment requires a (ideally small) room which can be heated in order to provide an environment which allows the patient to undress without feeling cold. Room ventilation between two sessions is crucial. The light in the treatment room should be blacked out during the session, because white light "dilutes" the therapeutic colors and reduces or even eliminates the desired effects.

Note that the three *extra-spectral colors* of the Spectro-Chrome system are the synthetic colors magenta, scarlet red, and purple, obtained by mixing various proportions of red and blue (see fig. 9.2).

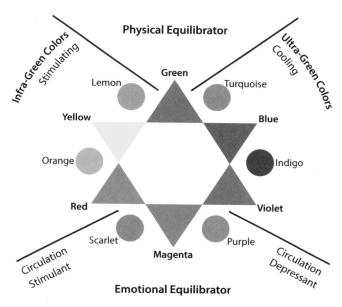

9.2. The Spectro-Chrome color wheel

The Spectro-Chrome method involves projecting colored light on various parts of the body during sessions lasting up to an hour, a process that Dinshah called *tonation*. He had established chromatic protocols adapted to over three hundred pathologies—a therapeutic intention that only increased the antagonism of the established medical system, the only authority legally permitted to heal. Dinshah perfected several generations of light projectors in which colored filters were carefully selected. He used a set of five basic filters (colored glass plates) that could be combined to make up the twelve colors of his chromatic wheel. Modern versions of these filters are now available, and one can reproduce the Spectro-Chrome colors with a set of nine gel filters commercially manufactured by Roscolene. It is easy and inexpensive to combine these filters with a white-light projector in order to experiment with this method at home. Spectro-Chrome is thus still accessible to all who wish to use it to improve their well-being.

Dr. Wunsch developed a professional version of a Spectro-Chrome projector that uses a light source with an optimized spectrum as well as a direct-current power supply to eliminate any parasitic flickering. Having added Spectro-Chrome to the multiple methods by which he practices light therapy, he continues to study its applications, proving that interest in this system is still valid today and that it should not be reduced to a mere historical curiosity.

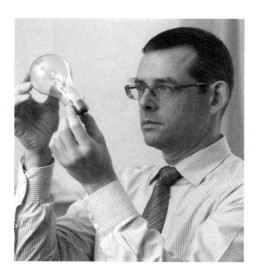

Figure 9.3.
Dr. Alexander Wunsch

In collaboration with the German company Innovative Eyewear, Dr. Wunsch has also developed a series of twelve colored glasses reproducing the twelve colors of Spectro-Chrome. These glasses provide an ideal way to explore for oneself the psychophysiological effects of each color. One simply has to wear them for a few minutes or a few hours.

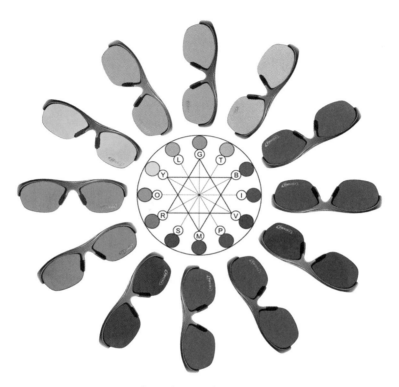

Figure 9.4. A set of twelve SpektroChrom PRiSMA glasses
(© Innovative Eyewear)

Resources

www.dinshahhealth.org

www.innovative-eyewear.shop (SpektroChrom glasses)

Darius Dinshah, *Let There Be Light,* 11th edition. Dinshah Health Society, 2012.

Spectro-Chrome Case Study

(from Dr. Alexander Wunsch)

Presenting problem: Second- and third-degree burn

Case details: The subject's lower arm was burned due to contact with boiling water.

Treatment: The treatment began with tonations (projecting colored light on different parts of the body for up to an hour) in indigo to reduce inflammation. After one week the indigo color was replaced with turquoise in order to promote skin cell regeneration. After two weeks, a period of orange was incorporated into the tonation to stimulate the production of ATP by photobiomodulation (see fig. 9.5).

Outcome: The healing of this type of burn usually requires several months and leaves permanent scars. Here we can observe that the application of colored light significantly accelerates the natural healing process, and six years later no sign of the wound is visible.

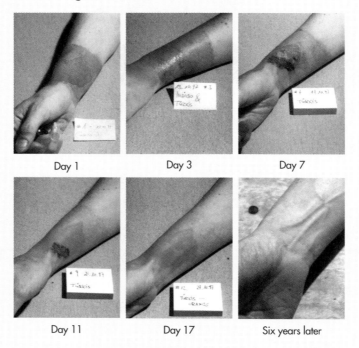

Figure 9.5. Spectro-Chrome treatment of a second- and third-degree burn: condition at days 1, 3, 7, 11, and 17, with control six years later

Colorpuncture

Colorpuncture is a remarkable union of light and acupuncture and one of the most evolved and complex forms of modern chromotherapy. It was created by Peter Mandel, a pioneer in the development of new technologies for healing, whose expertise in naturopathy, homeopathy, acupuncture, and chiropractic informs his research into new diagnostic systems and therapies.

His technique has inspired many practitioners to apply the principles he discovered in their own way.

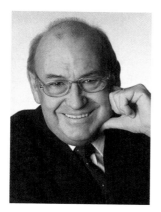

Figure 9.6.
Dr. Peter Mandel

Mandel originally studied the relationship between vital energy and the meridians of acupuncture as revealed by the form of high-voltage discharge photography known as Kirlian photography.* Specifically, Kirlian photography captures the phenomenon of electrical coronal discharges. Mandel was the first to use Kirlian photography as a medical and energetic diagnostic tool, analyzing over three million Kirlian photos to arrive at a technique he called Energy Emission Analysis (EEA). In 1985 he published his book *Energy Emission Analysis,* and this work was the foundation for the development of Colorpuncture.

In his 1986 book, *Practical Compendium of Colorpuncture,* Mandel writes about how he developed Colorpuncture:

---

*This form of photography was invented in 1939 by the Russian Semjon Davidovitch Kirlian. It has since led to the development of several modern digitalized versions of Kirlian discharge analysis, notably the gas discharge visualization (GDV) system for bio-electrography developed in Russia by Dr. Konstantin Korotkov.

It was the general fascination with color, a fascination expressed by Goethe and in numerous publications since then, which gave me the impulse to search for correlations between energy emission phenomena and color vibrations. . . . Assuming that human bio-energy is a carrier of information, it can be expected that a normal, harmonious flow of energy will result in normal and harmonious functioning of the cells. However, since information never flows in one direction only, it can be assumed that the relationship between cell and energy is a two-way one. If the information involved should undergo change for any reason, it will no longer pulsate in a balanced rhythm, meaning that the functioning of the cells will also be affected. . . . Since this energetic principle calls for correspondingly energetic methods of treatment which make use of the resonance behaviour of the cells, it seemed obvious to make use of color to restore a lost state of harmony. Emission Energy Analysis provided me with decisive theoretical information concerning the energy-oriented use of color as a means of treatment.

This intuition led Mandel to create a sophisticated system based on the stimulation or sedation of acupuncture points when applying complementary colors. Using Goethe's chromatic system described in chapter 8, he chose three primary colors and their complementary colors: red/green, yellow/violet, blue/orange. For each pair he identified one "cool," yin, or sedating color (green, violet, blue), and one "warm," yang, or stimulating color (red, yellow, orange). As in acupuncture he established protocols that are appropriate for many treatments, both on the physical and energetic levels. Whereas acupuncture is limited to specifying the location of points to be treated, Mandel's system introduces an additional parameter, that of the color to be applied on these points, thus adding many more treatment possibilities. In this way, deeper layers of the organism can be reached through the transmission of information in the form of light (see fig. 9.7). Mandel perfected instruments that can carry light with great precision without generating unwanted heat, even on tiny reflex points in the pinna of the ear, as used in his Colorpuncture version of auriculotherapy (a form of acupuncture for the ear developed by French medical doctor Paul Nogier).

Echoing the discoveries of Fritz-Albert Popp, with whom he has collaborated, Mandel (1986) says,

> Light is life. This is not a belief system but something that is confirmed by science. Specifically, light is present in the communication between cells in the body, and illness occurs when the cells can no longer speak the same language. Giving light to the body has a resonance effect, bringing cells into the same language again, and thus supporting the body's natural healing process.

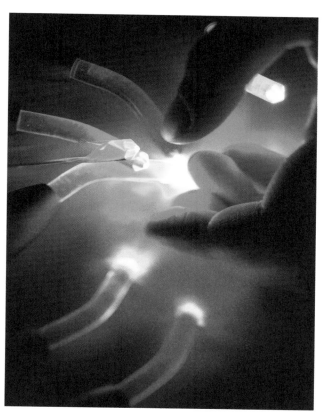

Figure 9.7. Colorpuncture tools
(© Esogetics GmbH, Int.)

I first encountered Colorpuncture early in the 1980s. My spiritual master, Osho, with his customary foresight, had instantly recognized its merit and asked Peter Mandel to come and teach it at his ashram in Pune, India. But it was not until 2006 that I met its inventor in person at an ILA conference. A tireless innovator, Mandel had by then expanded his system into what he now calls "esogetic medicine," a term that derives from the union of esoteric wisdom, energetic medicine, and recent scientific discoveries in neurology and noetics.

Colorpuncture is taught throughout the world in various Mandel institutes; practitioners of this healing technique number about 2,500 worldwide. The Mandel International Institute is now directed by Mandel's son Markus Wunderlich.

Colorpuncture Case Study
(from Markus Wunderlich, Managing Director at Esogetics GmbH)

Presenting problem: Long-term headaches and stress

Case details: A female patient, Sabine M., age thirty-eight, suffering headaches ascending from the neck, experienced regularly over a period of many years; heart palpitations (tachycardia); difficulty falling asleep because of restlessness and occasional anxiety; wakes several times during the night. The patient feels permanently stressed out and has recurring stomach pain and gastric reflux. Underwent a tonsillectomy at age nine and an appendectomy at age twelve. She reports that even as a child she was anxious and restless. The parents were good, and she felt loved. During the sixth month of her pregnancy her mother had a car accident resulting in a concussion and a hospital stay. As an adult, the patient had a hysterectomy due to a myoma at age thirty-six and no other significant illnesses. She has three children; the family is, she says, functioning well. All clinical exams have been without findings so far. She received some prescription drugs for her headaches and the recurring heart palpitations, as well as some tranquilizers. As she did not notice any changes with these drugs she discontinued their use. A psychiatric evaluation was proposed.

Treatment: During Sabine's first visit to our clinic she seemed hurried and tense. The energetic emission analysis (EEA) indicated an endocrine insufficiency. She had edema around her eyes, especially in the lower lids. We discerned swellings at the sacrum (pelvic organs) and tension in the area of the left shoulder that radiated to the left side of the neck (heart segment). Overall, this diagnosis pointed toward endocrine dysregulation. Esogetic medicine has some systems that treat the entire axis of endocrine regulation, from the pituitary and hypothalamus to the thyroid, pancreas, genital organs, and the adrenal cortex. These sequences are distributed across the entire body and were treated with Colorpuncture as well as Peter Mandel's induction therapy, an additional technique which is part of Esogetics medicine. In this case we decided to use the stress hormone program. This program is a sequence of frequency oscillations that resonate with brain rhythms. It is particularly well suited for the balancing of endocrine disorders. We also prescribed the color sound "psychosomatic balance" based on a laterality disturbance that was visible in the Kirlian picture, plus we recommended the application of herbal oil to the zones that stimulate dream activity. Included as well was a program of self-treatment that acted as a support in helping the patient become responsible once again for her own health.

Outcome: Sabine M. received treatments over a period of four months. The control examination half a year later showed that all complaints had disappeared.

Resources

www.esogetics.com

www.colorpuncture.org

Peter Mandel. *Energy Emission Analysis: New Application of Kirlian Photography for Holistic Health*. Synthesis Publishing, 1985.

———. *Practical Compendium of Colorpuncture*. Edition Energetik, 1986.

———. *Esogetics: The Sense and Nonsense of Sickness and Pain*. Medicina Biologica, 2006.

Chromatothérapie

Chromatothérapie is a highly refined system of colored light therapy that is the invention of French neuropsychiatrist Christian Agrapart, one of the first western physicians to have studied acupuncture in China.

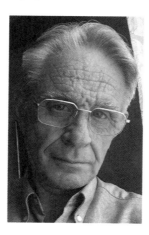

Figure 9.8.
Christian Agrapart

Dr. Agrapart describes how he created his system:

In 1983 I attended the first Franco-Chinese symposium on acupuncture. During this trip to China I met scientists and lectured at conferences. Upon my return I began my own research on the energetic effects of the use of acupuncture needles, both in the university lab and with hundreds of clinical cases. Based on the most recent discoveries concerning the electromagnetic emissions of visible light and the results of my own experimentation, it became possible for me to decode the influence of each color as defined by a precise wavelength for living beings. A living being always actively reacts to any stimulation. This observation helps to understand how an organism adapts to the environment with which it is in symbiosis. This work led to the understanding that applications to an area of just a few millimetres can have an effect on the whole body. The next step was to find the corresponding properties between acupuncture and color.

Not satisfied with the traditional Chinese understanding of the function of color, which Agrapart considered to be uninterpretable in scientific terms, he formulated his own theory based on hypotheses that he considered to be generally in accord with most of the ancient texts. This led him to a system based on the properties of the trigrams of the I Ching* and on the four Chinese climactic factors: cold, heat, humidity, and dryness (see fig. 9.9). These climatic factors correspond to energies that exist not only in the environment but in the human body as well, and they can be influenced by colored light according to the following description:

* Red has an anticold effect by calling up heat
* Orange has an antiheat effect by calling up cold
* Green has an antihumid effect by calling up dryness
* Blue has an antidryness effect by calling up humidity

Agrapart further describes his system:

Chromatothérapie is the therapeutic use of colored rays according to a strict protocol based on a diagnosis that is both medical and energetic. The bases of this therapy are both scientific and mathematical. The projection of colored light rays can be done in three different ways:

♦ Through the eyes, when the pathology is global (fever, heat stroke, nervousness, aggression, fear, anxiety, depression, sleep disorders)

♦ On the affected zone (trauma, burns, frostbite, rheumatism in a joint)

♦ On an acupuncture point (this is an elaborate medical method practised by acupuncturist physicians having been trained in Chromatothérapie)

It is therefore a complete medical system that has its own applications. It is not in conflict with established medicine but rather complements it.

---

*The eight trigrams of the I Ching, the ancient Chinese classical text dating from approximately 1000 BCE, are binary archetypes.

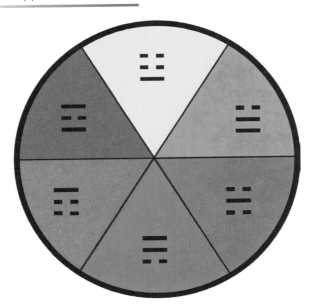

Figure 9.9. The six colors of Chromatothérapie
(© CEREC)

Agrapart founded the *Centre Européen de Recherche sur l'Énergétique et la Couleur* (European Center for Research on Energetics and Color), which has been offering training since the 1980s. Instruction in Chromatothérapie requires several years and is intended mainly for health professionals. Today there are certified practitioners in many countries.

The best argument for the validity of this system is doubtless its therapeutic successes. Agrapart and his wife, psychologist Michèle Delmas, who incorporates Chromatothérapie in her psychotherapy practice, shared some impressive case studies with us in their presentations at ILA conferences. These included healings at speeds well beyond that of classical treatment in cases of severe burns, joint inflammation, and the aftereffects of brain trauma. Chromatothérapie has been shown to be very effective in cases of stroke as well as phlebitis of the lower limbs, with a particularly fast treatment response.

Chromatothérapie Case Study
(from Dr. Christian Agrapart)

Presenting problem: Immediate stroke relief

Case details: Cerebrovascular accident during a lavish meal at a physician's home. A sixty-year-old man was suddenly afflicted by paralysis of the right arm.

Treatment: After examination, the physician diagnosed a stroke. Naturally, the family of the afflicted man plan for an emergency hospitalization in order to eliminate the embolism responsible for the cerebrovascular accident as soon as possible. While waiting for an ambulance to arrive, the physician host proposed applying Chromatothérapie. He chose the left side of the man's head, specifically the area of the sylvian segment of the middle cerebral artery that is situated just above the ear, which is the area that corresponds to the right arm. On this area he projected two Chromatothérapie colors: red for four minutes followed by green for five seconds. The treatment was given in total darkness to ensure that only the wavelengths of the Chromatothérapie filters were present without being diluted by other light. Once the treatment was complete, the subject remained lying down in darkness for twenty minutes, after which time the paralysis completely disappeared. The man was hospitalized afterward in order to have a complete medical examination to understand the cause of the stroke and to establish preventive measures.

Resources

www.chromatotherapie.com

Christian Agrapart. *Se soigner par les couleurs: Guide pratique de la chromato-thérapie.* (Healing with colors: practical guide to chromatothérapie). Sully, 2016.

———— and Michèle Demals. *Guide thérapeutique des couleurs: Manuel pratique de chromothérapie, médecine énergétique, principes, techniques et indications* (Therapeutic guide to colors: handbook of chromatothérapie and energy medicine, principles and applications) Dangles, 2011.

Michèle Delmas. *Quand la couleur guérit: Psychologie et chromothératie* (When color heals: psychology and chromatothérapie). Paris: Guy Trédaniel éditeur, 2010.

Polychromatic MIL
(Magneto-Infrared-Laser) Therapy

MIL-therapy, described in chapter 5, was developed in Russia in the 1970s. It relies on the use of a magnetic field in order to boost the effectiveness of light. In recent years a number of devices have been developed that are derived from this principle, but with the addition of colored light.

coMra Therapy

The coMra (Coherent Multi-Radiances) system is one of the more recent developments of MIL-therapy. In 2009, following their intuition and based on lengthy therapeutic experience, the creators of coMra added two new components to classic MIL-therapy: colored light and ultrasound. The company Radiant Life Technologies was founded to manufacture and teach the use of these new multiradiant therapy devices, and it was at the 2012 ILA conference in Berlin that I met Dr. Arzhan Surazakov, director of research and development at the company. Surazakov firmly believes in the importance of noninvasive, gentle energetic modalities in the therapeutic process. For him, the cellular intelligence inherent in a living being will bring about healing as long as one supplies it with extra energy and necessary stimulation in cases of trauma or chronic deregulation. He considers the combination of the four stimulants within coMra to be ideal for supporting the neuronal and biochemical cascades characteristic of the natural resolution of pathology (see fig. 9.10).

The colored light component of coMra is supplied by tricolored LEDs (red at 650 nm, yellow-green at 570 nm, indigo-violet at 420 nm) that have been sequenced in an innovative way according to two specific patterns:

* The first pattern is the regenerative type and uses a sequence that corresponds to the natural progression of the healing of wounds: red (inflammation) to indigo-violet (cell proliferation growth) to yellow-green (structural remodeling).
* The second pattern is the rejuvenation type based on the

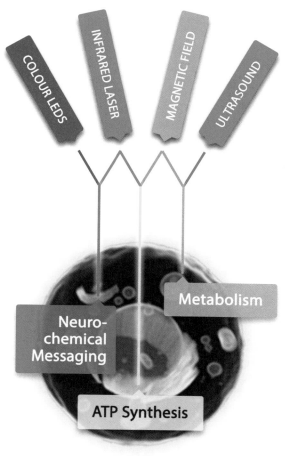

Cell

Figure 9.10. The roles and synergy of the four radiances of coMra
Therapy in supporting three aspects of healing
(© Radiant Life Technologies)

sequence red-yellow to green-indigo to violet and is used to
benefit healthy tissue; for example, in cosmetology.

In addition, the ultrasound component uses 40 KHz emitters to
stimulate enzymatic metabolism, while a near-infrared laser diode (at
905 nm or 980 nm) and permanent magnets supply the classic components of MIL-therapy.

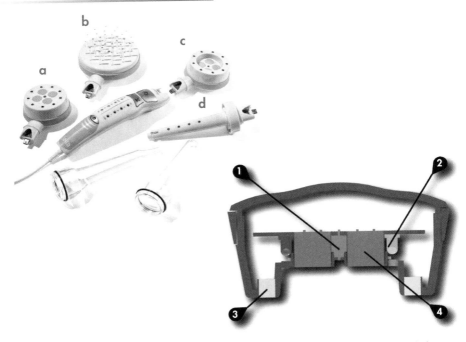

Figure 9.11. Delta Series coMra instrument and terminals. Above left, four attachments: (a) aesthetic, (b) meridian, (c) medical, and (d) probe. Right, a cross-section of a typical terminal showing 1) near-infrared laser, 2) color LEDs, 3) permanent magnets, and 4) ultrasound emitters.
(© Radiant Life Technologies)

The creators of coMra have designed a variety of protocols based on the instrument's built-in programs to treat over two hundred pathologies. These are suitable for personal use (for home use, to alleviate backache, chronic pain, allergies, etc.) as well as for more refined medical application by specialists.

Classic MIL-therapy has been validated in many studies. Its coMra variation, currently used by several thousand people around the world, has been accumulating an increasing number of convincing case studies.

Resources

www.radiant-life-technologies.com

Milta Therapy

Milta therapy, developed in France by the company PhysioQuanta, is another variation of MIL-therapy. In addition to the standard MIL components (laser diode and infrared LED for photobiomodulation and magnets to create a magnetic field), it has a polychromatic component implemented through a red-green-blue LED. A distinctive aspect of Milta is its use of what its creators call a *photonic accelerator*, which shapes the magnetic field into a tunnel, with the intention of increasing the penetration of light rays.

The Milta is available as a handheld device for personal use and as a panel version for professional application. The latter has multiple MIL emitting sources to increase both the speed and the surface area of the treatment (see fig. 9.12).

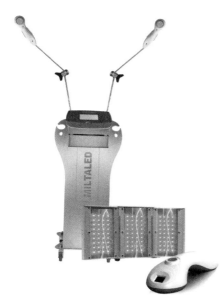

Figure 9.12. Milta instruments: the control station (left), photonic panel (center), and handheld emitter (right)
(© PhysioQuanta)

The Milta is recommended for treatment of pain and reduction of inflammation, for healing and regeneration of scarring, as well as for bone repair.

Resources

www.physioquanta.com

Syntonic Phototherapy

Syntonic phototherapy is among the methods of light medicine having the longest history. It was in 1933 that its originator, Dr. Harry Riley Spitler, founded the College of Syntonic Optometry in Ohio, to promote the study of the light therapy method that he had been developing since the 1920s. In 1941, Spitler published *The Syntonic Principle,* still considered the preferred reference book in this field. Spitler died in 1966; however, the college, now based in Pueblo, Colorado, carries on his work and has hosted an annual conference every year for the past eighty-five years.

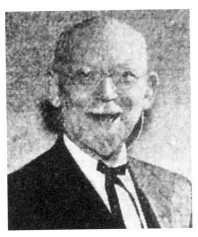

Figure 9.13. Harry Riley Spitler, founder of syntonic phototherapy, here seen in a rare and badly damaged original photograph

Spitler, an optometrist, was one of the first to systematically explore the therapeutic application of colored light via the eyes, and his technique essentially works through the visual system. Spitler called his approach the *syntonic principle,* where the term *syntonic* refers to "equilibrium" or "balance." His undeniable clinical successes quickly attracted many practitioners among optometrists of his time. Used mainly by certified health professionals, this form of chromotherapy has always had a more solid reputation than many more marginal methods. The extraordinary clinical experience and many case studies that have accumulated over the past eighty years have helped ignite renewed interest in chromotherapy. It is therefore not surprising that some of its principal players were involved in founding the International Light

Association (ILA) in 2003, and that is where I met Dr. Larry Wallace, president of the College of Syntonic Optometry at the time, as well as Dr. Ray Gottlieb, its dean, and Sarah Cobb, editor of the *Journal of Optometric Phototherapy* (a publication of the College of Syntonic Optometry). I was immediately attracted to their open-mindedness and their immense enthusiasm for light. Dr. Larry Wallace went on to become president of the ILA from 2009 to 2011.

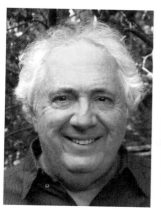

Figure 9.14.
Larry Wallace

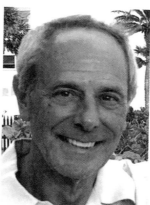

Figure 9.15.
Ray Gottlieb

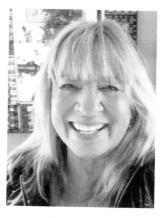

Figure 9.16.
Sarah Cobb

Ray and Larry are among syntonics' best teachers today. For the *Journal of the International Light Association,* they described syntonic phototherapy in these words:

> Spitler concluded that many bodily, mental/emotional and visual ailments were caused primarily by imbalances in the autonomic nervous and endocrine systems. He was the first to elaborate on this function of the retinal-hypothalamic pathways. Spitler proposed that applying certain frequencies of light through the eyes could restore balance within the body's regulatory centers, thereby directly correcting visual dysfunctions at their source. His model suggests that red (low energy, long wavelength) at one end of the visible spectrum stimulates the sympathetic nervous system related to action and stress, green (middle frequencies) yields physiological

balance, and indigo (high energy, fast frequencies) activates the parasympathetic nervous system related to the relaxation response (Gottlieb and Wallace 2011) (see fig. 9.17).

Spitler developed the Syntonizer, a light projector that uses a white-light incandescent source positioned behind a support in which one places a colored filter or, if needed, a combination of two or three filters. A set of thirteen standardized filters is commonly used with the equipment. To avoid the imprecision of the common names of colors and to make their work less vulnerable to American medical authorities who persecuted them till the end of the twentieth century, practitioners of syntonic phototherapy gave coded names to these thirteen colored filters, such as Alpha, Delta, Pi, Omega, and so forth. Today, several modern variations of this instrument are in use.

A syntonics session consists of looking at a light source for twenty minutes. Generally, a course of treatment takes about twenty sessions, with an average of three sessions per week.

Syntonic phototherapy is mostly employed in the alleviation of ophthalmological and visual problems, but it is also helpful for a wide range of applications, such as improving memory and learning, reducing ADHD, and relieving migraine headaches. It is especially effective in accelerating recovery from head injuries and stroke. An estimated

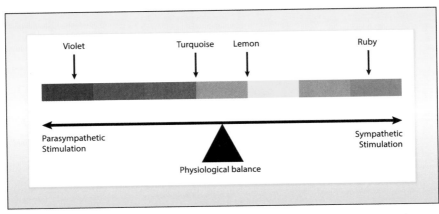

Figure 9.17. The syntonic physiological balance according to Spitler

1,300 optometrists all over the world practice this form of therapy today.

Syntonic optometrists use a variety of techniques to diagnose and assess a person's progress; notably, the measurement of the functional visual field, how far one's visual field extends in each radial direction for each of the three primary colors of the retinal cones (red, green, and blue). Originally done with an instrument called a *campimeter,* this measurement is now done with computerized instruments. Whereas in conventional medicine the functional visual field is used to detect certain physical ailments (such as toxemia, or cardiovascular or endocrine disorders), it is of even greater importance to Syntonists, who see it as an indicator of the overall physical and emotional health of a person. While a normal visual field extends quite evenly over a radius of 20 to 40 degrees in all directions, it can sometimes happen that the visual field is reduced to 1 or 2 degrees; for example, in children who have learning or behavioral difficulties. During the course of a syntonic treatment it is frequently observed that the visual field gradually expands back to normal, which is an excellent objective indicator of progress.

Some researchers in syntonics have brought the interpretation of functional visual fields to a high degree of refinement. In 2010, Denise Hadden, a South African optometrist, published her book *New Light on Fields,* in which she explains how the analysis of what she calls *subtle visual fields* can be a real tool for inner exploration and personal growth.

Resources

www.collegeofsyntonicoptometry.com

www.denisehadden.com

Harry Riley Spitler. *The Syntonic Principle.* Eugene, Ore. Resource Publications, 2011.

Denise Hadden. *New Light on Fields.* 2010. Available at http://www.bernell.com/category/s?keyword=denise+hadden

Syntonic Phototherapy Case Study
(from Dr. Larry Wallace, OD, PhD)

Presenting problem: Neonatal toxemia

Case details: A six-year-old girl was experiencing difficulties in school, including a seeming inability to learn to read; she also suffered from severe hyperactivity and exhibited aggression toward classmates and family members. She had a medical history of prenatal exposure to toxins (neonatal toxemia) and a difficult birth. Her history also included continual head-banging on a daily basis. A diagnostic exam revealed a host of visual dysfunctions, with constricted visual fields being the most significant.

Treatment: She was treated through the eyes with ruby light for ten minutes, followed by yellow-green for ten minutes, and underwent these treatments three times a week for a total of twenty sessions. Ruby is an emotional stabilizer, while yellow-green is a detoxifier and physiological stabilizer.

Outcome: The girl's visual fields expanded and her visual anomalies normalized (see fig. 9.18). Her hyperactivity disappeared, and she started to read, with performance approaching her grade level. She began gymnastics with great enthusiasm. The parents were thrilled to have their daughter become a cooperative, loving, gentle child. The fast-acting changes could only be explained by the power of color to restore her disrupted nervous system and her emotional health. These changes were dramatically demonstrated by the expanded visual field.

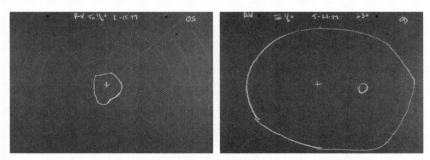

Figure 9.18. Functional visual field of the patient: highly contracted prior to treatment (left); *expanded and normalized post-treatment, four months later* (right)

The PhotonWave

Having developed his Syntonizer in the 1930s, Spitler confirmed the impressive therapeutic power of ocular stimulation by colored light. Several generations of phototherapists, particularly in the United States, have subsequently worked to improve the original Spitler model. John Downing, OD, PhD, developed the Lumatron in 1986, and a smaller portable version, the Photron, followed in 1993. In a parallel development, Jacob Liberman created the Color Receptivity Trainer, and then in 1990 developed the Spectral Receptivity System. These inventions make use of technological advances in optics, light sources, and colored filters. The devices didn't reach Europe until 1986, when Belgian light therapist Leona Vermeire-Van Raemdonck brought the first Lumatron to Belgium and began a long career dedicated to the spread of light therapy in Europe. When the Photron ceased to be available after the death of its manufacturer in 2000, Vermeire-Van Raemdonck took it upon herself to ensure the continuity of the work of both Downing and the manufacturer for the European medical community. In the same year, she formed a partnership with Dr. John Searfoss, a syntonic optometrist who had developed a new device for ocular stimulation. But only three months after partnering with Searfoss, just as they had finished their prototype, he died. Leona and her team persevered nevertheless and completed the PhotonWave, probably the most advanced ocular stimulator currently available (see fig. 9.20).

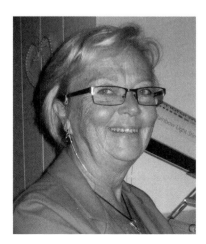

Figure 9.19.
Leona Vermeire-Van Raemdonck

What makes the PhotonWave stand out is the quality of its filters and the very sharp bandwidth that produces colors of near mono-chromatic purity. It is equipped with two filter wheels that can be superimposed on each other to produce a wide variety of colors. It generates pulsed light between 1 and 35 Hz for *photic brain wave entrainment*, a process useful to bring patients toward mental states associated with various brain wave frequencies (see also chapter 10).

The most recent version of the PhotonWave features an automated system for color selection. Years of experience using this technology along with input from specialists such as Dr. Dietrich Klinghardt have led to a design of chromatic protocols adapted to the most common ills, which have been programmed into the device.

As is often the case with chromotherapy, the PhotonWave is mainly used by various types of therapists, for whom it is a complement to their main practice, whether that be psychology, medicine, or naturopathy.

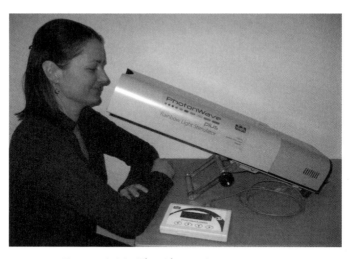

Figure 9.20. The PhotonWave in action
(© Rainbow Flash)

Resources

www.photonwave.be

Emotional Transformation Therapy (ETT)

Emotional Transformation Therapy (ETT) is a form of psychotherapy based on brain stimulation through the visual pathway. The name refers to its capacity to resolve emotional distress within minutes or even seconds. Its creator, American psychologist Steven Vazquez, is a Texas-based professional in family therapy and counseling who has studied epigenetics, optometry, neurobiology, and quantum physics and incorporated aspects of these into ETT.

In the early 1980s Vazquez discovered the psychotherapeutic technique Spectral Receptivity, created by Dr. Jacob Liberman. Inspired, he went on to develop his ETT technique and the various light-therapy methodologies used in its practice. These include a spectral resonance technique that utilizes highly saturated colors with a visual impact that rarely occurs in typical visual environments; this results in an improved connection with one's emotions. The light sources can be dialed to any one of hundreds of colors and are capable of pulsing light for brain-wave entrainment (more on this in chapter 10). Special light-blocking goggles are available that are particularly useful for people who are hypersensitive to light, such as those who suffer from migraine.

ETT is used to treat acute stress, PTSD, addiction, depression, bipolar disorder, anxiety conditions, ADHD, schizophrenia and other psychotic states, insomnia, and chronic pain. Vazquez considers that the use of this form of light medicine brings about a remarkable acceleration in the psychotherapeutic process. He explains:

> ETT uses the principles of memory reconsolidation and neuroplas-
> ticity (the brain's ability to reorganize itself by forming new neural

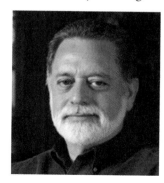

Figure 9.21.
Steven Vazquez

connections). Underlying most distressing symptoms that are a part of conditions like depression, anxiety, and addictions are unresolved core emotional memories. These memories normally continue to exist life-long if they are not treated. Since ETT possesses strategies to access and resolve these core emotional memories, it results in permanent change of psychological conditions. . . .

A chief mechanism of action in ETT involves the application of precise visual stimulation at the exact time emotional distress is active. How could visual stimulation affect the brain? When light enters the retina of the eyes, photosensitive cells convert incoming light into neural impulses that travel throughout almost all of the brain's neural circuits. These light-initiated neural pathways extend far beyond those circuits that simply allow vision to occur. They extend into brain mechanisms that control thoughts, behavior, physiology, and states of extreme well-being. These brain mechanisms produce the transmission of neurotransmitters like serotonin and dopamine. By the use of precise external visual brain stimulation, specific brain mechanisms responsible for a symptom, such as sadness, can be directly and immediately targeted, resulting in rapid change.

Vazquez's team organizes training seminars in ETT in several countries, and the technique is enjoying renewed interest since publication of his books. It is estimated that there are currently about two thousand therapists employing ETT.

Resources

www.ettcenter.com

Steven Vazquez. *Emotional Transformation Therapy: An Interactive Ecological Psychotherapy.* Lanham, Md.: Rowman & Littlefield, 2014.

———. *Accelerated Ecological Psychotherapy: ETT Applications for Sleep Disorders, Pain, and Addiction.* Lanham, Md.: Rowman & Littlefield, 2015.

———. *Spiritually Transformative Psychotherapy: Repairing Spiritual Damage and Facilitating Extreme Wellbeing.* Lanham, Md.: Rowman & Littlefield, 2016.

Lateral Light Therapy

Lateral light therapy is one of those rare instances of a chromotherapy modality that has been validated in multiple clinical studies. Though this modality arguably belongs more to conventional medicine than to alternative medicine, it nevertheless is considered marginal by the medical establishment. This lack of recognition is likely due to the fact that most of the studies have been done in the Ukraine and published in Russian.

I heard about Lateral Light Therapy for the first time at the 2005 ILA conference, when biologist Frances McManemin* and psychologist Mary Ross spoke to us about some interesting reports coming out of Russia about research done by neuropsychiatrist Anatoly P. Chuprikov, which were translated by one of their Russian-speaking students and circulated privately. In the 1990s, after studying the relationship between mental health and cerebral lateralization (the tendency for some neural functions or cognitive processes to be more dominant in one hemisphere than the other), Chuprikov developed a technique based on applications of complementary colors to each of the two sides of the visual field. The working principle is based on three premises.

First, Chuprikov identified the distinct functions of the two brain hemispheres. The left hemisphere is associated with verbal thinking and with anxiety-provoking aspects of the emotional range; its activation is associated with an increase in the sympathetic tonic activity of the autonomous nervous system (ANS), which is related to increased activity and stress. The right hemisphere is in charge of internal figurative cognition of the external world and with aspects of the emotional range relating to sadness and relaxation. Its activation is associated with an increase in the parasympathetic ANS activity and is related to energy conservation.

---

*Frances McManemin, PhD, was president of the International Light Association in 2004–2005. After her untimely death in 2011, the association established the Frances McManemin Prize that is awarded each year to the person who has played a determining role in the advancement of therapeutic applications of light.

Next, Chuprikov took into account the fact that our visual system is organized in such a way that the left and right sides of the visual field of each eye connect to the opposite hemisphere of the brain; the optic nerves coming from the left and right portions of the retina cross at the optic chiasm, located at the bottom of the brain immediately below the hypothalamus (see fig. 9.22). Hence, the laterality of the stereoscopic visual field is transposed in the cerebral hemispheres. We can therefore stimulate each cerebral hemisphere separately by illuminating its corresponding visual field.

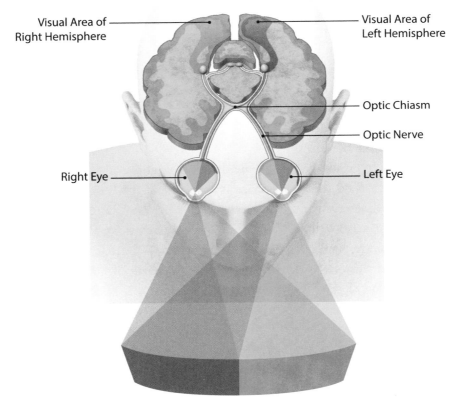

Figure 9.22. The visual field is lateral, with separate left and right halves. Each half of the visual field is connected to the visual cortex of the opposite cerebral hemisphere.

Third, Chuprikov adopted fairly classical chromotherapeutic interpretations of the properties of the different colors. Colors with a longer wavelength (red, orange, and yellow) he considered stimulating; colors with a shorter wavelength (green, blue, and violet) he regarded as calming.

The logic of his system is clear: to influence one hemisphere into being dominant over the other, one stimulates that hemisphere while calming the other by applying appropriate complementary colors to each half of the visual field. Chuprikov defined two types of lateral light projections, a direct type and a reverse type, the properties of which are listed in the chart below. By varying the chromatic interval between the complementary colors, Chuprikov regulated the intensity of the desired effect of each type of projection: the farther away on the scale of the rainbow the color on the left is from that on the right, the more the lateralization effect was amplified. Hence a projection using yellow and green would have a moderate effect since the two colors are very close, but a projection using red and violet would have the maximum effect because these colors are at the opposite ends of the rainbow. An intermediate combination such as orange and blue would be of a medium intensity.

TABLE 9.1. THE TWO TYPES OF LATERAL LIGHT PROJECTIONS ACCORDING TO CHUPRIKOV

DIRECT TYPE	REVERSE TYPE
stimulating color (red, orange, yellow), over **right** visual field, **sedative** color (green, blue, violet), over **left** visual field	**stimulating** color (red, orange or yellow), over **left** visual field, **sedative** color (green, blue, violet), over **right** visual field
stimulation of the left hemisphere, sedation of the right hemisphere	stimulation of the right hemisphere, sedation of the left hemisphere
Psychostimulant Effect: • Elevation in mood, emotional tonus • Increase in speed of thinking • Decrease in length and depth of night sleep and ease of morning awakening • Extroversion	**Psycholeptic Effect:** • Decrease in emotional tonus and motivation • Decrease in speed of thinking • Ease of falling asleep, increase in length of sleep • Introversion

Chuprikov (1994) says,

The main principle of lateral therapy is the directed transformation of an individual's profile of inter-hemispheric interactions by
suppressing the hemisphere with the pathological determinant and
activating the opposite hemisphere.

Based on these principles, he established protocols appropriate
to the treatment of a range of psychiatric disorders by adjusting the
type of projection (direct or reverse), the intensity (determined by the
choice of colors), the number of treatments (five to twenty-five), and
the duration of each treatment (five to thirty minutes). The treatments are given with special goggles into which one inserts colored
filters in such a way as to illuminate separately the two halves of the
visual field.

A number of clinical studies have been conducted on lateral
light therapy, especially in the 2000s by Dr. Igor A. Palienko of the
University of Kiev in the Ukraine. It was found that the usefulness
of this technique goes beyond psychiatry—not surprising when one
considers its impact on the autonomic nervous system. Palienko (2000,
2001a, 2001b, 2001c) published studies on chronic illnesses as diverse
as hypertension, arrhythmia, and rheumatoid arthritis, all conditions
that come under the influence of the ANS.

It is difficult to estimate the number of lateral light therapy practitioners there are out there, but clearly this healing modality has not
had the attention that it deserves in the West.* Personally, I have been
sufficiently impressed by the effectiveness of this method of light medicine that I have integrated certain aspects of it into my own system, the
Sensora, described later in this chapter.

---

*Eventually I found out that Dr. Chuprikov has a dubious reputation in certain academic
circles because he was in charge of psychiatric research associated with a coercive form of
mental-health practices in post-Soviet Ukraine. However, this concerns other aspects of his
work and not what is described here, which unfortunately (and perhaps unjustly) has been
condemned by association.

Resources

Anatoly P. Chuprikov et al. *Lateral Therapy—Guide for Therapists*. Kiev: Zdorovja, 1994.

A. P. Chuprikov, V. N. Linev, and I. A. Martsenkovskii. "Lateral Phototherapy in somatoform mental disorders" (in Russian). *Lik Sprava* 10–12 (1993): 56–59.

A. Palienko. "Hemodynamic effects of lateralized colored-light stimulation of the brain hemispheres in patients with essential hypertension" (in Russian). *Ukr. Kardiol. Zh.* Nos. 5/6 Issue II (2000): 46–48.

———. "Effect of different light and color stimulation of the cerebral hemispheres on cardiac rhythm self-regulation in healthy individuals" (in Russian). *Fiziol Zh* 47 (1) (2001a): 73–75.

———. "Modifications of the EEG activity upon lateralized stimulation of the visual inputs to the right and to the left brain hemispheres by light with different wavelengths." *Neurophysiology* 33, no. 3 (2001b): 169–74.

———. "Spectral analysis of heart rate responses to light and color stimulation of the cerebral hemispheres" (in Russian). *Fiziol Zh* 47 (2) (2001c): 70–73.

The Monocrom Method

The Monocrom method relies on the aesthetic and psychological properties of monochromatic light, the light that makes colors so highly saturated that their spectra are reduced to a single frequency or to a very narrow bandwidth of frequencies (as described in chapter 3). It was developed by Swedish architect and psychologist Karl Ryberg. His affinity for light is perhaps innate—his great-uncle was none other than Neils Ryberg Finsen, the Danish doctor dubbed the "Father of Phototherapy" (see chapter 1). Karl Ryberg's interest in monochromatic light took root during his studies in laser biology with Tiina Karu at her laboratory in Moscow (see chapter 4). There, Karu's experiments demonstrated that the effect of light on biology is increased the closer the light is to being monochromatic; in other words, the purer and more saturated a color, the greater its potential to interact with a cell, in particular if its bandwidth is below the 5 to 10 nm range.

Ryberg had the extraordinary idea of making what he calls a "super light" available by developing projectors capable of generating light

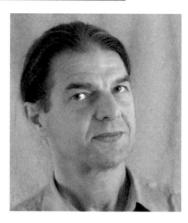

Figure 9.23.
Karl Ryberg

sufficiently monochromatic to satisfy Karu's criteria. To do this he worked with xenon lamps, intense thermal sources of wide-band spectrum light sources, which he combined with holographic gratings, a type of optical component capable of filtering a tiny frequency band.

When I first met Karl in 2003 he had been involved in developing his Monocrom Dome since 1996. This is an impressive dome more than two meters in diameter in which he uniformly diffuses the purest monochromatic light. To enter this dome is to be transported into a *ganzfeld* (total field in German)—a uniform field in which the eye cannot focus and in which all external references disappear. I immediately recognized a close connection to the immersive concept in my own invention, the Sensora. Karl has since become a friend and collaborator, as we faced similar practical difficulties in developing our systems. Such large-scale installations, even if they are very effective, are too heavy and expensive to be accessible to most therapists. Karl has since developed a portable version of the Monocrom, which consists of a helmet worn over the head. His most recent creation is a fiber optic mask. Both smaller versions operate under the same ganzfeld principle as the original dome (see fig. 9.24).

Karl describes the experience of immersion in a total field of monochromatic light:

> The subjective experiences are quite intense. The brilliance of spectrally pure light quickly alleviates depression and stress. Higher brain functions readily respond to the light stimulation as precise

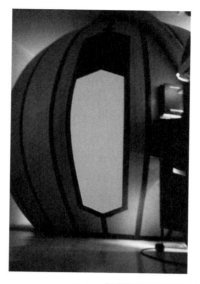

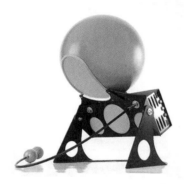
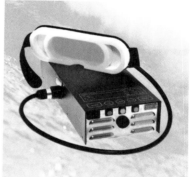

Figure 9.24 The three versions of the Monocrom projector: top, the dome (1996); bottom left, the helmet (2006); and bottom right, the mask (2011)
(© Monocrom)

optical software to upgrade the cognitive functions. The concentrated information content of the monochromatic light enables short treatments acting long-term, much like an optical vaccination.

It is recommended that Monocrom exposure be limited to five to ten minutes per month. During a session the user is free to choose the colors that he or she wishes to "drink in"—the control handle is very simple and intuitive to use, allowing one to go through the whole visible spectrum in a continuous manner, somewhat like the glissando of a violin. Karl is a free thinker who considers it presumptuous that a therapist should choose the colors that a client needs. According to him, it is for each person to follow his or her own intuition while exposed to this full range of colors of surreal purity. It is a way of seeing things that I have always shared and appreciated. To date, several thousand people have benefited from the various Monocrom projectors, and hundreds of therapists currently use this method in a clinical setting.

An inveterate inventor, Karl has also designed powerful and versatile sources of infrared for the treatment by photobiomodulation of tinnitus and other physical ailments. Recently he developed a reading lamp of nonhomogeneous radiation to treat persons suffering from dyslexia; he has found that following such treatment they can triple their reading speed. And he now offers a set of colored filters for people to experience the benefits of chromotherapy in their own homes.

Resources

www.monocrom.se

Karl Ryberg. *Living Light: On the Origin of Colors.* Self-published in Göteborg, Sweden: Typografia. 2010.

Audiovisual Entrainment (AVE)

Audiovisual entrainment (AVE) is a phenomenon that makes use of the natural tendency of the brain to enter into resonance with a vibrating sensorial stimulus that is within its frequency range. We will explore this in more detail in the next chapter, but here we will introduce the chromotherapeutic instruments based on this principle.

The therapeutic interest in brain-wave entrainment lies in the relationship between the mental state of the brain and the electroencephalographic (EEG) waves that it generates. In the same way that each mental state generates specific EEG waves, one can inversely produce the same mental state by exposing the brain to the corresponding frequencies. Brain-wave entrainment can be achieved either by visual stimulation (with pulsing light) or by auditory stimulation (with pulsed sounds) and is most effective when both modalities are combined in AVE.

Many different devices using this principle have been manufactured beginning in the 1970s. For a long time these consisted of a set of goggles equipped with light bulbs and earphones and driven by a processor generating the desired frequencies. With the advent of LED technology new versions have appeared that use polychromatic red, green, and blue (RGB) LEDs. These offer the possibility of combining AVE and chromotherapy. In this chapter I present three such devices that I consider state of the art. They've been designed by people whom I know personally. These inventors have the tenacity and the dynamism essential for this type of creative innovation.

Note: Stroboscopic pulsations such as those produced by AVE devices must be avoided by persons subject to epileptic seizures; the reason will be explained in the next chapter.

The DAVID

The Digital Audiovisual Integration Device—shortened to DAVID—is the work of Canadian design technologist Dave Siever, a pioneer in AVE. Since the 1980s he has been designing many generations of these instruments, and his latest polychromatic models are very versatile (see fig. 9.26).

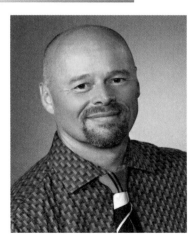

Figure 9.25.
Dave Siever

An essential aspect of this type of instrument is the quality of the programs controlling the sequences of audiovisual pulsations. Siever has extensive experience in this area, and since 2000 he has implemented an excellent series of studies demonstrating the effectiveness of AVE in applications for the treatment of various affective disorders (mood disorders such as depression, bipolar disorder, and anxiety disorder), post-traumatic stress disorder, and seasonal affective disorder (SAD), and also as an aid to learning.

I was particularly impressed by the models in his Delight series because they include two separate light sources for each eye, each illuminating one half (left or right) of the visual field. This makes it possible to program them for the lateral light therapy, discussed earlier in this chapter. Aside from the Sensora, I don't know of any other AVE instrument having this capability.

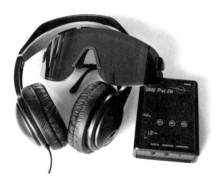

Figure 9.26.
The DAVID
(© Mind Alive Inc.)

Resources

www.mindalive.com

www.mindalive.com/index.cfm/research/research-articles-by-dave-siever

The PSiO

Created by Belgian Stéphane Krsmanovic, a specialist in relaxation and mental preparation for athletes, the PSiO is one of the most technologically advanced polychromatic AVE instruments. The quality of the light diffusers in its visor provides a beautifully uniform visual field that comes close to that of a ganzfeld, a total field (see fig. 9.28).

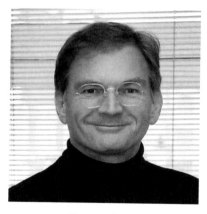

Figure 9.27.
Stéphane Krsmanovic

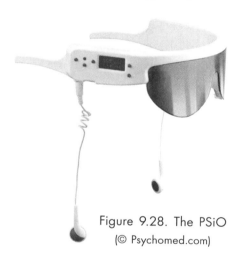

Figure 9.28. The PSiO
(© Psychomed.com)

The PSiO's audiovisual programs are designed for applications such as stress management, depression, insomnia, weight loss, and drug and tobacco withdrawal. Because these programs often include voice guidance or music, the PSiO is presented as a combination of light and relaxation therapy rather than as a simple AVE instrument.

Resources

www.psio.com

The Lucia N°03

The Lucia N°03 is one of the most unusual light-therapy instruments I have had the opportunity to try. Though it does not have an audio component, it still is grouped with these other AVE devices because of its brain-wave entrainment function. Created by psychologist Englebert Winkler and neurologist Dirk Proeckl, both from Austria, the Lucia N°03 is a highly sophisticated stroboscope intended to induce hypnagogic experiences (see fig. 9.30).

Here is how Winkler and Proeckl describe the techniques:

> This light system combines a stroboscope (flickering light) with variable speeds and intensity and a constant light. Lucia N°03 provides us with a powerful stimulator that generates EEG wave patterns that normally only occur after several years of meditation practice.
>
> A hypnagogic trance is a state of consciousness between being awake and alert and being asleep. Most people experience this state when they fall asleep and when they wake up. Throughout history this state of consciousness has been sought after by many people, with the aid of various techniques, simply because it feels wonderful, and to find inspiration and answers to the deeper questions about life.

The stroboscopic technology of the Lucia N°03 produces intense hallucinogenic effects. Ever since the invention of the Dream Machine by British artist Brion Gysin (see the next chapter), many have tried to exploit the psychedelic potential of visual stimulation. It took specialists like Winkler and Proeckl to finally develop—and present as such—an instrument specifically designed for the exploration of altered states of consciousness to be used in the context of personal development.

Resources

www.gesund-im-licht.at

www.lucialightexperience.com

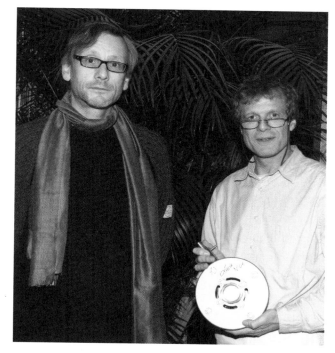

Figure 9.29. Englebert Winkler (left) and Dirk Proeckl (right)

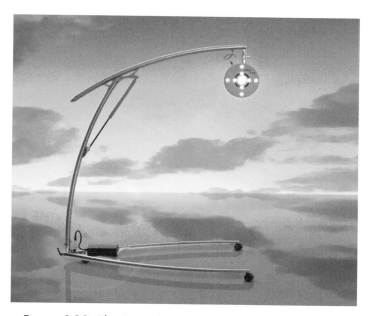

Figure 9.30. The Lucia N°03 (© Light Attendance GmbH)

The Sensora

The Sensora was born out of the research I have been conducting with my associate Ma Premo since the 1980s. We define it as a multisensorial system of integrative therapy, and it is among the chromotherapy systems that bridge the dimensions of the body and the psyche. Although it is based on instruments that manipulate physical light with great precision, its function is to interact with the global state of the person through his or her sensory perceptions. It works within what I consider the domain of the subjective influence of light (a subject we'll cover in chapter 11), and it constitutes the essence of my professional work.

The Sensora has the advantage of being the fruit of the interaction between two complementary specialties: on the one hand, my own scientific background and electronics expertise as a physicist; and on the other hand, the fine energetic sensitivity and psychotherapeutic experience of my colleague Ma Premo. This complementarity has guided us through over thirty years of exploration and experimentation in sound spatialization, brain-wave entrainment, and light; integrating these three led to the development of the Sensora in 1995. Since then multiple generations of improved versions have been produced.

The Sensora is designed to offer an immersive sensorial experience; it is a whole environment rather than a simple instrument. It consists of equipment and software that is installed in a dedicated projection room. It includes a special chair, a light projector and screen, a surround-sound audio system, and a control computer (see fig. 9.32). The room, as much as possible, is insulated from external noise and light, and its walls are

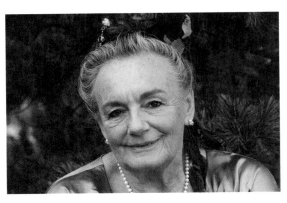

Figure 9.31. Ma Premo

nonreflective in order to maximize the purity of the colors projected on the screen. This assembly acts in a multisensorial way by integrating three dimensions: a visual aspect consisting of a colored light projection (chromotherapy), an auditory aspect with music (musicotherapy), and a tactile aspect supplied by the chair that produces physical sensations derived from the music soundtrack (kinesthetic transduction). Once these three dimensions are correctly harmonized, a powerful sensorial synergy unique to the Sensora is experienced.

The dominant aspect of the system remains that of light and is based on a technology that I call *light modulation*. It enables the creation of complex light patterns capable of acting simultaneously within several chromotherapy modalities: that of the specific effects of colors,

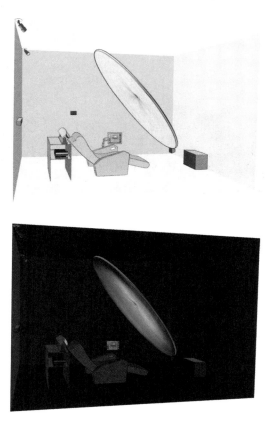

Figure 9.32. Schematic view of the Sensora space at rest (top), and during a session (bottom) (© Sensortech Inc.)

naturally, but also of brain laterality, as well as the entrainment of internal rhythms, including brain waves and slower physiological rhythms. These light patterns are projected onto a large screen suspended over the person lying in the treatment chair so as to cover most of the field of vision. The resulting sensation of being immersed in a field of pure, vibrant colors is remarkable, and the visual impact significantly contributes to the therapeutic effectiveness of the system.

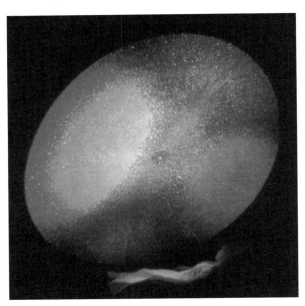

Figure 9.33. The large Sensora projection screen
(© Sensortech Inc.)

A Sensora session is multisensorial and typically lasts between twenty and forty-five minutes. It is in itself an enjoyable experience of deep relaxation, personal attunement, and well-being. In addition, it has a far-reaching therapeutic potential. According to the set of colors and the frequencies of pulsation used, one can generate a whole range of sensorial influences, from relaxing to stimulating, that can support wellness and the therapeutic process. For a therapist, the Sensora is a powerful tool capable of amplifying and accelerating psychological treatment.

The Sensora is used worldwide as a complementary tool in psychotherapy, hypnotherapy, massage, postoperative convalescence, and palliative care settings. It has proven to be a particularly effective support in the treatment of depression, burnout, post-traumatic stress disorder, anxiety, insomnia, chronic fatigue, chronic pain, fibromyalgia, addiction, and certain instances of tinnitus.

The SensoSphere

To make light modulation accessible to a greater number of people, in 2014 I released the SensoSphere. It is a therapeutic lamp that creates a harmonizing ambience in the room it is placed in. Derived from the same technology as the Sensora, the lamp features similar chromotherapeutic properties in a compact, portable form—its globe measures either 30 or 40 centimeters in diameter depending on the model (see fig. 9.34).

The SensoSphere contains seventeen independent trichromatic LED light sources that generate complex 3-D light patterns in one of three modes: relaxing, stimulating, and balancing. The algorithms that control the light constantly introduce subtle random variations into the patterns. The SensoSphere can run indefinitely without ever repeating itself, a feature that particularly pleases me—one never tires of contemplating its beauty.

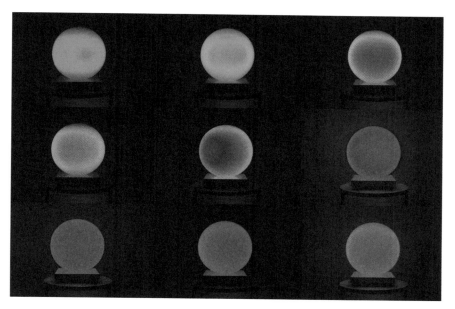

Figure 9.34. The SensoSphere (© Sensortech Inc.)

Sensora Case Study

(from Edwige Chasselon and
Céline Fabre, psychotherapists)

Presenting problem: Long-term depression

Case details: The subject reported experiencing severe depression for about two years. His problems began when the relationships with his brother and sister were severed after a conflict over the sale of the family home. At the same time he felt he was a victim of various injustices at work. These accumulated stresses led to a deep depression, with sadness, fatigue, and lack of energy, along with insomnia, psychomotor retardation, low self-esteem, inappropriate sense of guilt, trouble concentrating, and negative ruminations resulting in withdrawal from nearly all aspects of life. He was on sick leave from work and would stay in bed all day until his wife returned home from her job. Prescription antidepressants had not had any significant effect. He showed great discomfort: lowered eyes, withdrawn shoulders, little facial expression, and an irregular gait. These symptoms might be associated with a form of alexithymia, a personality construct characterized by the subclinical inability to identify and describe emotions in the self.

Treatment: Since monthly visits to a psychiatrist had so far not proven helpful, the subject's wife, in desperation, brought him to the "Le 3CE" center* specializing in treatment for trauma, depression and burnout (we had met her at an event where she learned about the Sensora technology). The man was unable to drive or even orient himself in the streets, so his wife had to do the driving. Upon arriving he was immediately brought to the Sensora space, where he was given an explanation about the technology. The protocol first used was aimed at reducing his insomnia. It was the Sensora program called "Reverse Hi" (using psycholeptic lateral light) followed by "Night light." After this first session, the man came out with his head slightly raised, his eyes more open, and a more stable gait. His insomnia disappeared after two sessions.

We then worked on alleviating his depression with the program "Direct Hi" (psychostimulating lateral light), followed by a program for balancing body and mind. Following this we alternated between the program to

*The Centre de Cryothérapie Corps Entier in Aix-en-Provence, France.

aid sleep and one favoring balance. He received sixteen sessions lasting between forty and fifty minutes each. These took place two times a week for the first three weeks, followed by one session a week for the next three weeks, and as of this writing we are seeing him once every three weeks. **Outcome:** After six sessions the subject regained his desire to live. He was able to reduce his medication and began to do sports and improve his nutrition. He sleeps well. His wife is tremendously grateful—her husband is now able to go to the movies, meet with friends, and enjoy his life once again.

Resources

www.sensora.com

www.stresslighttherapy.com

Mary J. Ross, Paul Guthrie, and Justin-Claude Dumont. "The impact of modulated color light on the autonomic nervous system." *Advances in Mind-Body Medicine* 27, no. 4 (2013): 7–16.

The Sound Learning Centre

The Sound Learning Centre, located in London, is an excellent example of the clinical application of audiovisual stimulation for the well-being of children suffering from learning difficulties and behavioral problems such as those stemming from autism, dyslexia, and ADHD (attention deficit hyperactivity disorder). The center was established by Pauline Allen in 1994. Allen, a specialist in sound therapy, light and color therapy, and neurodevelopmental therapy, offers treatments based on the therapeutic effects of light and sound, and she and her team often obtain astonishing results.

Here is how Allen describes her approach:

We have been working in the field of learning and sensory difficulties for many years and have extensive experience in the different ways that sound, light, color, and physical exercises can be used to bring the mind-body system back into balance. We have developed a unique mix of effective, noninvasive ways of treating the whole person and are often able to bring about transformational change where before there was little prospect of improvement.

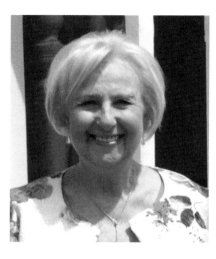

Figure 9.35.
Pauline Allen

The light modality used at the Sound Learning Centre is based on light-wave stimulation, or LWS, as developed by Dr. John Downing, who himself was inspired by Harry Riley Spitler's syntonic phototherapy. This technique makes use of Downing's visual stimulation devices the Lumatron and the Photron. The sound modality is based on the auditory integration training* developed by Dr. Guy Bérard, which aims to rebalance the auditory system by listening to sounds filtered according to the person's needs.

These methods do not have complete clinical validation and are thus not recognized by the medical establishment. Most of the time children are brought to the Sound Learning Centre after their parents have exhausted the standard treatment options. The multiple successes in cases with children for whom all hope has been abandoned is what motivates Pauline to persevere in this work.

---

*For more information on the auditory approach of Dr. Bérard see www.berardaitwebsite .com. The origin of his technique goes back to the work of otolaryngologist and inventor Dr. Alfred Tomatis and his "electronic ear."

Sound Learning Centre Case Study
(from Pauline Allen)

Presenting problem: Child with learning difficulties

Case details: Isabelle was unable to study effectively, and the results of the school exams she was due to take in six months' time were predicted to be disastrous. After hearing a talk by Pauline Allen about how sensory issues frequently underlie many learning difficulties, Isabelle's mother decided to take her to Allen. The mother believed that there was a big, unexplained gap between Isabelle's dismal academic performance and her demonstrated intelligence; she had a "light-bulb moment" when she realized that there could be a missing link that explained her daughter's underachievement.

Later, Isabelle herself wrote, "Before I went to the Sound Learning Centre I was struggling with everything: memory, concentration, tiredness and processing of information. I also had problems with stuttering and used to have lots of outbursts because I was so frustrated with everything. I knew I was not performing like my friends and I wondered why. I had been tested in school and been told they had found nothing. I had been to the doctor several times and been told the same."

It turned out that Isabelle had difficulties with binocular vision, visual perceptual difficulties, and sensitivity to light, and her color visual fields of awareness were very constricted, which is quite common with stressed-out, light-sensitive people. Although there was some high-frequency hearing loss, her hearing thresholds were within the range generally considered normal, although not perfect. Such auditory, visual, and developmental profiles have significant detrimental effects on performance and negatively affect the integration of physiological and sensory functions, balance, moods, concentration, and eating and sleeping habits. Apart from her academic and social difficulties, Isabelle's breathing rate was also rapid.

Treatment: Based on this assessment, we recommended a therapy that used light therapy, light-wave stimulation (LWS) for twenty minutes twice per day, and sound, Bérard's auditory integration training for thirty minutes twice per day. Both approaches were delivered independently over a period of ten days.

Outcome: At the end of the ten days of therapy, Isabelle's visual field had expanded significantly, and her hearing profile showed much more balanced responses in both ears, while her auditory processing showed improvement. She was sleeping better and was more focused and "switched on." She was happier and less stressed. Her memory, mood, coordination, and speed of running had all improved. At a follow-up assessment six months later her mother wrote, "She is much, much happier and a more settled child. She is now in the middle of her exams and her approach is methodical, her comprehension is much improved, and she is managing her stress levels *much* better." Isabelle herself wrote, "It is now nearly six months since I had my treatments and I have been back for some retests. I have noticed that a lot of things have changed, all for the better. I am about to sit my exams, and I think that thanks to the treatments I should be alright now and should get the grades that I need to allow me to go to college. I think if I had not had treatment I would not be where I am right now."

Perhaps the final word should go to Isabelle's sister, who told Isabelle, "I always thought you were stupid, but Mum was right, you're intelligent!"

Resources

www.thesoundlearningcentre.co.uk

Van Obberghen Color Therapy

Color therapy and color psychology expert Pierre Van Obberghen, whose background includes acupuncture, homeopathy, psychotherapy, and holotropic breathwork, has developed one of the most evolved and coherent systems for the psychological and symbolic interpretation of color that I have ever encountered. His color therapy method is comprehensive, both in terms of how the appropriate color for a treatment is chosen and the diversity of ways in which it is applied. The Van Obberghen method is a remarkable synthesis of the chromotherapeutic knowledge coming from various traditions, including Western, Chinese, and Vedic. He uses colored light at all these levels:

* In the visual field
* On the whole body
* Locally on affected areas
* On reflex points of the ears, feet, hands, eyes, nose, and teeth
* On the energetic circuits of the acupuncture meridians

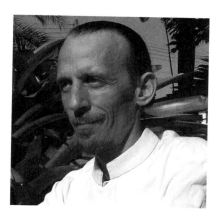

Figure 9.36.
Pierre Van Obberghen

In his 2014 book, Van Obberghen described his color therapy method as:

a set of therapeutic techniques using the properties of colored light to induce physiological reactions that are favorable to the

241

maintenance or the reestablishment of health. This system is based on simple principles of biology and physiology and the laws of light, optics, and electromagnetic phenomena. Colors induce a process of self-healing. The organism, triggered by the wavelength of the color, will regulate itself by stimulating the areas where the energy is lacking, or conversely, by calming areas where the energy is excessive.

Working together with Dr. Dominique Bourdin, another pioneer of chromotherapy, Pierre has put different instruments together for colored light projection. These include spotlights, light pens, and panels designed to be driven by his "Bio-Color" control module. More recently he directed the development of a new generation of tools called Lumencure, which are controlled by a mobile app on a user's phone (see fig. 9.37).

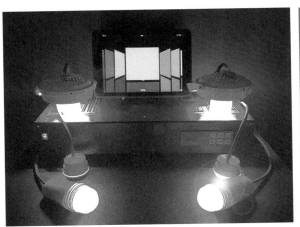 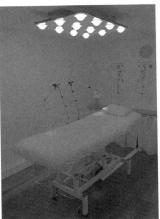

Figure 9.37. The Lumencure instruments: the PhysioLED set (left) and light panel (right) (© Color Institute)

One of the most outstanding creations of Van Obberghen is his unique color test, which he calls the *personal chromatic profile*. He says,

Chromotherapists are also interested in our perception of color and in the ways in which we gather visual information, which they consider to be manifestations of the deepest states of being. The color test allows us to examine the emotional relationship that we have with colored objects. It uses the phenomenon of attraction and aversion to colors in order to evaluate a person's health. It is also a tool for analyzing personality. . . .

If one presents a series of colors arbitrarily placed on a grid to an individual, and if we ask him to keep half the colors and dispose of the other half based on his preferences, the result of his selection can be plotted on a graph. On the graph we will see peaks and valleys and balanced areas. This graph is like a person's chromatic identity card, and it reflects precisely the person's view on the world of colors.

I first met Pierre in the 1990s in India, at the Osho ashram, where many explorers of energy medicine were to be found. That is where he showed me his recently created color test, and I immediately appreciated its soundness. In addition to providing an accurate profile of the person's physical, emotional, and mental well-being, the test can also be used to generate a color-balancing session targeting any identified chromatic deficiencies and their related physical, emotional, and mental states (see fig. 9.38). We have found this function to be so effective that in collaboration with Pierre we have integrated it into the Sensora.

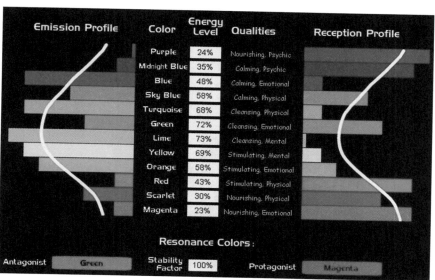

Figure 9.38. An example of a personal chromatic profile obtained by means of the Van Obberghen color test (in this case, using its Sensora version)

Every time I meet Pierre he never ceases to amaze me with his latest innovations. One of his most recent is what he calls "organic color," a light-synthesis method that generates colors with constant subtle variations rather than in a static way, as is usually the case in chromotherapy. It reflects his conviction that natural colors in our surroundings are usually dynamic and fluctuating—a conviction that I share and have always applied in the Sensora.

Van Obberghen has trained hundreds of practitioners in his method. He regularly offers workshops and trainings at his Institut de la Couleur (Van Obberghen Color Institute), in Switzerland.

Resources

www.color-institute.com (in French, though an English version may be available in the future)

Pierre Van Obberghen. *Traité de Couleur Thérapie Pratique* (Practical Color Therapy Handbook) Paris: Guy Trédaniel éditeur, 2014.

The Spectrahue Method

Spectrahue is based on the rich heritage of traditional Chinese medicine, color psychology, and energetic medicine. It bridges the physical and energetic aspects of light and is based on spiritual principles that combine color and sacred geometry. Canadian Julianne Bien is the founder of this color delivery system, which can be used in a number

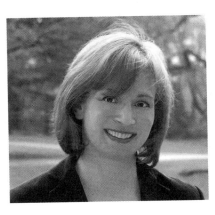

Figure 9.39.
Julianne Bien

of holistic modalities for both humans and animals. Like many innovators in this field, Bien has been guided by her own love of light, a passion she communicates in interviews, seminars, videos, and accredited course manuals, books, and webinars.

The principal tool of Spectrahue is a light stick known as the Lumalight. Bien's exploration led her to create and refine the Lumalight light sources. This flexible tool consists of a small, portable, ergonomically designed lamp that can be coupled with a variety of colored filters. From the original set of seven colors, the Spectrahue collection has grown to over sixty specialized filters, including models with geometric inserts (see fig. 9.40).

Although most manufacturers of chromotherapy light sources now use LEDs to generate a quasi-monochromatic light, the Lumalight uses an incandescent light source. For Bien, the wide spectrum of this white thermal source is far more biocompatible. It is also neutral, so it can completely adapt to the properties of the various filters. This is particularly important in the use of crystal-quality color filters (such as gemstones), because the subtler properties of the colored beam of light can transmit the particular signature of the filter.

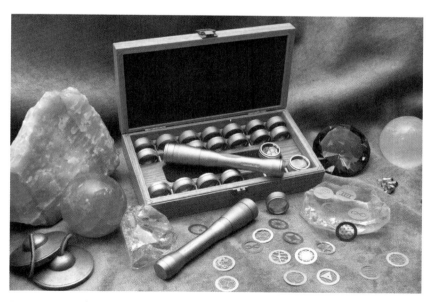

Figure 9.40. The Lumalight by Spectrahue (© Spectrahue Light and Sound Inc.)

Bien describes her approach to working with light:

> The Lumalight user works off the body, never touching it, and moves within the electromagnetic field—the pulsating aura—in the aural rhythm. The hand-held penlight sends out color frequencies, guided by geometrically designed inserts, toward the traditional acupuncture points aligned along the meridian system. These gentle polychromatic light emissions allow the organism to absorb the frequencies it requires—to disperse stagnant energy or cool down harmful excitation. The idea is to gently let the body take the color frequency values out of the light being offered and let it do what it knows best—recreate balance and thrive.

Spectrahue supports people in their pursuit of holistic well-being and spiritual self-discovery, self-realization, and self-healing. Its tools are affordable and readily available, and there are thousands of these units in use worldwide.

Resources

www.spectrahue.com

Julianne Bien. *Golden Light: A Journey with Advanced Colorworks.* Spectrahue Light and Sound Inc., 2004.

———. *Color Therapy for Animals.* Spectrahue Light and Sound Inc., 2014.

Samassati Colortherapy

Samassati Colortherapy works more at the level of the mind than the body. Its name refers to one of the final maxims spoken by the Buddha: "Be a light unto yourself" (*samassati* in Sanskrit). At its foundation is the wonderful capacity of colored light to bring about the sensation of renewal and awareness. This method involves several different ways of interacting with light, taking into account the integration of body, emotions, and spirit. It entails knowledge of the reflex points of acupuncture as inspired by, among others, Peter Mandel's Colorpuncture.

The Samassati technique was created by Nishant Matthews, a therapist and teacher whom I've known for many years who specializes in psychotherapy-based meditation practice. Born of Matthews' extensive experience with meditation and his intimate knowledge of the properties of color, this work exemplifies the most subtle therapeutic work with light possible. Nishant describes his method in these words:

> Samassati Colortherapy is a graceful way of regaining contact with the natural health within ourselves. First it dissolves the fields of stress, tension, and confusion that are in the body and mind. Then it goes deeper into the person to stimulate the natural resources that are there. Light will turn them on. In the field of light, negative energetic patterns resolve in the direction of healthy energy flows, unclear psychological issues find their way back to clarity, and emotions tend to balance in a graceful, nonviolent way. We get to be ourselves again. . . .
>
> There are fields of consciousness within all of us. These fields respond brilliantly to the warm presence of a practitioner and the resonant tones of color light. Profound and simple.

Samassati Colortherapy is offered in individual sessions by therapists trained in the technique. In practice, the light is administered

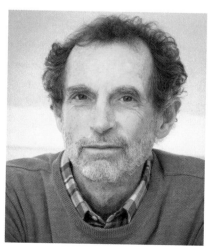

Figure 9.41. Nishant Matthews, founder of Samassati Colortherapy

by a small handheld source with colored filters, such as the Lumalight torch described previously. The therapist is in constant interaction with the client and can illuminate his or her whole field or specific points according to recommended sequences. The approach is intuitive and is based on observation of the subtle reactions of the client to various colors.

Samassati Colortherapy is used in psychotherapy settings, personal transformation practices, and as a support to physical health. To date over a thousand practitioners worldwide have been trained in this method.

Samassati Color Therapy Case Study
(from Nishant Matthews)

Presenting problem: Recurring liver pains after hepatitis

Case details: Four years after suffering severe hepatitis in India, client complained of recurring pains in liver area and a general sense of sluggishness through the whole body.

Treatment: Client was asked to describe the color fields as she perceived them in her liver. She reported a liver with muddy green exterior and red spots inside. Therapist applied a mid-tone green light to the liver region and asked for reports on the shifting colors around the liver. Client reported a field of stress and lingering inflammation around the liver. Treating her field with a green field of light and steady presence rapidly brought about a complete shift in the presenting issue. Client further reported that the muddy green of her liver became a lighter color, like spring green, as the treatment progressed. The painful red spots in the liver dissolved into a pink tone. Symptoms of pain and stress cleared away.

Outcome: Following this single treatment client described herself pain- and symptom-free after the treatment. At a follow-up appointment six months later she reported same result. Three years later she is still reporting no signs of stress.*

*From the ILA Light Therapy Case Studies Report (2013): 42.

Resources

www.nishantmatthews.com

www.garden-of-light.info

Nishant Matthews. *The Friend: Finding Compassion with Yourself.* U.K.: O Books, 2010.

Aura-Soma

It was in India in the 1980s, at the Osho ashram, that I first observed the Equilibrium collection of the Aura-Soma system. This consists of little bottles containing two colored liquids perfectly separated by their distinct densities. I was immediately fascinated by the visual magic of the color combinations, some of which especially attracted me. Just holding a bottle in my hand and looking at it seemed to induce a mysterious sense of comfort. One could also inhale its perfume or apply its contents to the skin.

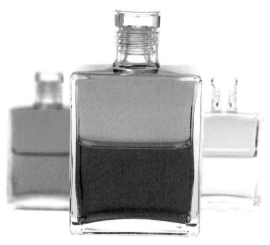

Figure 9.42. Aura-Soma Equilibrium bottles
(© Aura-Soma Products, Ltd.)

That particular set of Equilibrium bottles must have been one of the very first, because Aura-Soma had just been created in 1983 by Vicky Wall, who was then already age sixty-six. She had spent her youth apprenticed to an old master apothecary who had initiated her in the use of herbs, oils, and essences. After an accident that left her almost blind, she developed an intuitive perception of the colors emanating from the people and objects surrounding her. She felt called to create these precious objects, veritable chromatic jewels composed of essential oils and natural coloring extracted from plants and crystals. Vicky Wall has since passed, but here is how she tells it in her autobiography:*

> Once I had started to put together my colored jewels, I seemed impelled to make many variations, each one appearing to have its own vibrations. It was as if I worked under some strong compulsion, and various combinations of colors began to form under my fingers. I was completely absorbed in them. . . .
>
> Aura-Soma Equilibrium seems to have a magic of its own. It appears to relate to the personal needs of the individual. For some, the power is purely visual. For others, it acts as a personal barometer, reflecting like a mirror the moods, situations, and physical needs of the moment. Equilibrium offers a feeling of living energies giving supply and meeting demand . . . As one handles the Equilibrium bottles, the desire to go deeper becomes almost compulsive.
>
> [We] were realizing that Aura-Soma was not just color therapy depending on the healing vibrations of color, but a powerful new-old concept that held within it the ancient alchemy of the apothecary wherein lay the secrets of field and forest, the herbs, the flowers, the resins. (Wall 2005)

Aura-Soma is a good example of the subtler aspects of chromotherapy. This method does not claim to have any therapeutic action at the level of the body. It is rather described as a technique that helps modify consciousness and aids the growth of awareness.

---

*Aura-Soma: Self-Discovery through Color, © Mike Booth (2005).

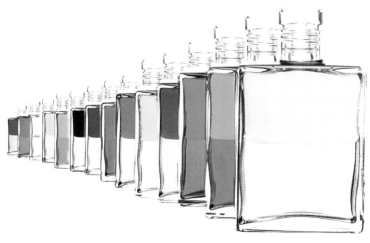

Figure 9.43. Aura-Soma "Equilibrium" collection:
"You are the colors that you choose"
(© Aura-Soma Products, Ltd.)

Resources

www.aura-soma.net

Vicki Wall. *Aura-Soma: Self-Discovery through Color.* Rochester, Vt.: Healing Arts Press, 2005.

In part 3 of the book we've looked into a dimension of our interaction with light that goes beyond the purely physical aspects, touching on our energy fields. In so doing, we've discovered a multitude of innovative light therapy techniques based on the unique properties of colors. We are now ready to explore light's most subtle dimension, its ability to awaken our own consciousness.

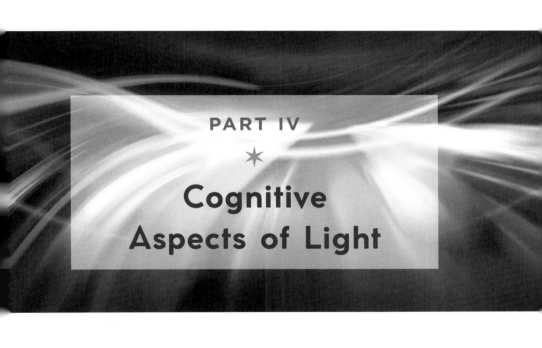

PART IV

✳

Cognitive Aspects of Light

10

SYNC AND RESONANCE

How Light and Sound
Cause Biological Balance

Unlike many other phenomena, the witnessing of [the spectacle of sync] touches people at a primal level. Maybe we instinctively realize that if we ever find the source of spontaneous order, we will have discovered the secret of the universe.

STEPHEN STROGATZ

IN 1665, DUTCH PHYSICIST AND MATHEMATICIAN Christiaan Huygens, being unwell, had been bedridden for a few days. In the room where he lay came the steady *tick-tock* from two clocks he had developed, clocks that, for the time, were marvels of utmost precision. After a while he noticed that the pendulums of the two clocks oscillated in synchrony, swinging toward and away from each other in perfect unity. The clocks were a meter apart and there was no contact between them. When Huygens would disturb one of the pendulums, the perfect synchrony was restored again in less than half an hour.

Intrigued, Huygens began a series of experiments in an effort to explain this strange temporal relationship. He eventually found the cause: infinitesimally small vibrations spread from one clock to the other though the wall on which the two clocks were

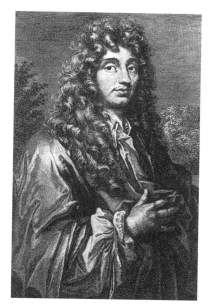

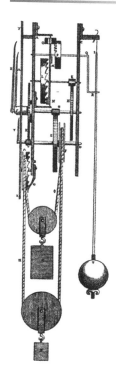

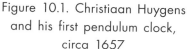

Figure 10.1. Christiaan Huygens
and his first pendulum clock,
circa 1657

mounted.* This seventeenth-century scientist was one of the first to make
the methodical observation of a universal phenomenon—that of the natural tendency of groups of oscillating objects to enter into synchrony, a discovery that foreshadowed what specialists today call *the science of sync.*

Although this tendency seems natural to us, there is nothing banal
about it. The threatened collapse of a bridge being crossed by a regiment of soldiers marching in step is a tale well known. The most recent
example is that of the Millennium Footbridge in London, which was
forced to close the very day of its official opening in 2000 because of
lateral swaying initiated by the resonant steps of pedestrians. It reveals
that order and organization are spontaneously generated, as opposed
to a progressive and inescapable disorder dictated by the second law of
thermodynamics for any physical system left to itself.

---

*Mathematical analysis recently confirmed that the synchrony observed by Huygens is
explained purely by the transfer of sound waves between the two pendulums (Oliveira and
Melo 2015).

WHAT IS SYNCHRONY?

Oscillation, or vibration, is omnipresent in all planes of reality. Its origin is easy to conceptualize. All systems under tension tend to come back to their initial state after they are disturbed. In doing so a system acquires a certain inertia that causes it to go somewhat beyond its initial state so that it then swings back in the other direction, thus creating a back-and-forth movement, the rhythm (or frequency) of which depends on the tension.* This image applies equally to a guitar string vibrating on a musical note, to a planet orbiting the sun under the tension of the force of gravity, and to an electromagnetic wave propagating under the tension of the vacuum permittivity of free space.

Not only does everything vibrate, but all these vibrations have an inevitable tendency to synchronize. This universal tendency toward synchrony is found at all levels of our world, from inanimate objects to living systems. It affects quantum particles entering into a state of coherence, giving rise to seemingly miraculous phenomena like superconductivity, in which trillions of electrons are unified, or laser light, in which a multitude of photons are combined. This tendency also manifests at the cosmic level, where the synchrony between the rotation of the moon and its orbit around the Earth prevents us from ever seeing its dark side. This tendency intervenes at all levels of life, an example being when millions of fireflies start to flash in complete oneness, offering us a magnificent spectacle miles wide, as can be seen on the shores of some rivers in Asia.

The Science of Sync

American mathematician Steven Strogatz (2003), known for his work on theories of chaos and complexity, maintains that it is only recently, in the 1990s, that mathematical formalism and computer simulations have allowed us to begin to analyze the phenomenon of synchrony. Because of

---

*In even more technical terms: at the root of all mechanical oscillation there is a cyclical exchange between a form of kinetic energy related to the speed of the object and a form of potential energy related to the distance of the object from its initial state. This is a universal phenomenon that often gives rise to a sinusoidal vibration, which is a fundamental curve in nature.

the nonlinear nature of the equations involved in its analysis, currently only simple examples can be generated, such as those using sets of weakly coupled, nearly identical oscillators. But from these models invariably emerges this remarkable tendency toward spontaneous synchrony.

This science has potentially major applications. For example, it can help us understand how the ten thousand pulsating cells that comprise the sinoatrial node, the heart's natural pacemaker, attain a consummate and constant harmony during the billions of heartbeats that occur in an average lifetime. Likewise, we can also understand what pathological mechanisms can detract from this synchronizing, leading to fatal heart arrhythmia.

BRAIN WAVES

Perhaps the most extraordinary example of synchrony can be found in the brain, where each of its ten billion neurons is in itself a tiny oscillator capable of producing ongoing electrical discharges. Vast

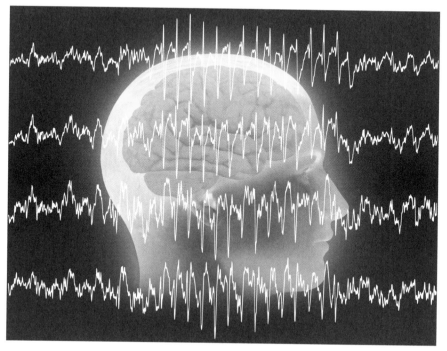

Figure 10.2. Our brain is continually emitting EEG waves.

assemblies of synchronized neurons fire almost in unison, while their minuscule electrical fields overlap in a coherent manner, generating a global field strong enough to be detected around the skull.

It was in 1924 that for the first time German psychiatrist Hans Berger was able to measure this field, one consisting of about 10 microvolts (abbreviated μV), which became known as the *electroencephalographic wave,* or EEG (see fig. 10.2 on page 257). This realization would offer a great deal of information about the activity of the brain, as each type of mental state is correlated to a specific EEG wave oscillating in specific frequency bands.

Photic (Visual) Entrainment

In 1934, electrophysiologists Edgar Adrian and Brian Matthews observed that EEG waves could be influenced by visual stimulation. In this phenomenon, known as *photic entrainment,* it became apparent that the brain, when exposed to the external stimulus of a pulsating light, has a natural tendency to generate an evoked potential of the same frequency, in resonance with the external stimulus. This resonance initiates in the thalamus and after a few minutes extends to the cortex, inducing a mental state corresponding to the particular frequency.

This experience has long been known. In 300 CE, Ptolemy, a disciple of Aristotle, described the sensation of contentment induced by the observation of the sun's rays through a rotating wheel. And at the very beginning of the twentieth century Dr. Pierre Janet, at the Salpêtrière Hospital in Paris, reproduced the same sort of effect. By focusing on pulsating light from a kerosene lamp placed behind a rotating wheel, his patients found relief from their states of depression, tension, and agitation.

A wonderful early example of photic entrainment is the Dream Machine created by British artist Brion Gysin. It consists of a simple cylinder with a central light placed on a turntable revolving at 45 or 78 turns per minute. The cylinder is pierced in such a way as to generate stroboscopic pulsations in the alpha EEG wave band. Starting in the 1960s, Gysin and American poet William Burroughs together explored altered states of consciousness induced through focusing on or contemplating this device.

EEG Brain Wave Types

A wave with frequencies from 8 to 13 Hz, in the *alpha range*, appears when the brain is in a neutral state, a bit like the motor of a car when it is turning over in neutral. It is therefore associated with relaxation or a mental state of rest, without attention being focused on anything in particular. When there is mental concentration or attention focused on something in the outside world there is an acceleration of the EEG wave into the *beta range,* the frequency of which varies from 14 to 30 Hz. The brain slows down to its least active state in deep sleep, with an EEG wave in the *delta range,* which has a frequency from 1 to 4 Hz. A wave from 4 to 7 Hz, which is found between the delta of deep sleep and the alpha of the neutral state, is in the *theta range,* which manifests in intermediary hypnagogic states such as those that happen between sleep and wakefulness. This is a particularly rich state of consciousness often associated with visualization, creativity, and learning.

Until the 1990s it was estimated that these four types of EEG waves, from 1 to 30 Hz, covered the whole range of cerebral functions. We now have considerably expanded the register with some newly discovered waves: *gamma* (from 30 to 100 Hz), *lambda* (from 100 to 200 Hz), and *epsilon* (under 1 Hz). The roles and functions of these ranges are still only partially understood. The gamma wave seems to be connected with the experience of consciousness, particularly when registering approximately 40 Hz, and also in certain states of synchrony and coherence when there is a temporal cognitive fusion unifying the whole of the cerebral activity. Gamma waves are found in abundance in meditators who are doing practice at an advanced level, or during lucid dreaming. Recent research has detected these waves particularly in the visual cortex. The functions of the lambda and epsilon bands found at the extreme ends of the register are still poorly understood. They seem to appear simultaneously during exceptional experiences of a mystical nature or during out-of-body experiences.

Audio Entrainment

The cerebral entrainment phenomenon is not limited to visual stimulation. There exists a variation of this that is driven by auditive

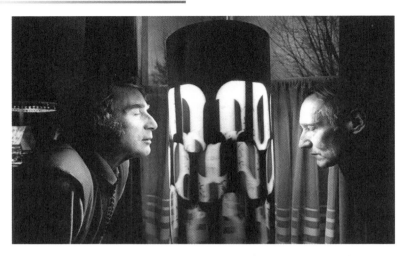

Figure 10.3. The Dream Machine of Brion Gysin (left),
seen here with William Burroughs in 1972
(courtesy of the Bancroft Library, University of California, Berkeley)

resonance, called *audio entrainment*. It can be induced either by sounds pulsating at the sought-after entrainment frequency (isochronic sounds) or by presenting to each ear a tone with slightly different frequencies (binaural sounds, for example, that use 300 Hz and 310 Hz to generate a 10 Hz beat frequency in the alpha range). The binaural principle was discovered in 1839 by Prussian physicist Heinrich Wilhelm Dove, but it was not until the 1960s that there was systematic investigation of the phenomenon, notably in America by Robert Monroe via his Monroe Institute, which is devoted to the exploration of altered states of consciousness.*

Having experimented with both of these two classes of entrainment, visual and audio, I have come to the conclusion that the visual version is more effective than the audio—which is not surprising when one takes into account that the sense of vision is considered to be responsible for 80 percent of our total sense stimulation and therefore

---

*Recent studies have indicated that the binaural sound technique induces relatively low evoked potential levels, which would imply that the many psychoactivating effects observed by Monroe were in fact not caused by brain-wave entrainment (Stevens et al. 2003). This is a good example of the dynamic nature of research in this field.

has greater impact than the sense of hearing. Since then this observation has been corroborated by various clinical studies. Frederick et al. (1999) measured the effects of visual entrainment in comparison with those coming from sound: they are about twice as strong. In my research using my own instruments, including the Sensora, I have favored the photic (visual) entrainment.

One of the more noteworthy phenomena is obtained by the stimulation of both senses in *audiovisual entrainment,* or AVE. Several generations of AVE devices have come on the market since the 1970s (including the DAVID and the PSiO, described in chapter 9). For the most part these consist of goggles equipped with pulsating light and a set of earphones.

AN EXPLORATION OF RESONANCE

Resonance has always played a central role in my own research into light therapy. From the very beginning of my exploration into the effects of sound and light on consciousness starting in the 1980s, brain waves have provided the parameter that has enabled me to measure the impact of different types of sensory stimulation, especially since there were few ways to objectively evaluate or quantify slight variations of an internal state, which are often the only effects resulting from subtle audiovisual interventions.

Around the time I first started my research I heard about a revolutionary instrument called the Mind Mirror. Designed by Geoff Blundell, an engineer, and the research scientist Maxwell Cade, it was capable of detecting EEG brain waves (see fig. 10.4). The Mind Mirror was the first portable device offering direct visualization of the distribution of all the bands of frequencies for each cerebral hemisphere. In his book *The Awakened Mind: Biofeedback and the Development of Higher States of Awareness,* Cade was able to identify a series of curves associated with different mental states; this discovery enabled him to distinguish with remarkable finesse the different kinds of meditation (Cade and Coxhead 1979).

Of course, today devices exist that are far more complex and precise, capable of offering detailed EEG images of the multiple cerebral areas. But the simplicity and the clarity of the curves of the Mind Mirror remain unsurpassed for depicting the mental state of a person in a global and direct way. I met with Blundell in the '80s at his laboratory near London and had an opportunity to buy one of his devices, which was of great use in my own explorations at the time.

As I then spent several months a year in India at the ashram of my spiritual master, Osho, I had at my disposal a rather exceptional laboratory to conduct the types of experiments that were of interest to me. I had access to several hundred meditators coming from all corners

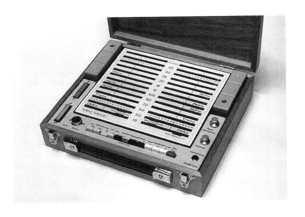

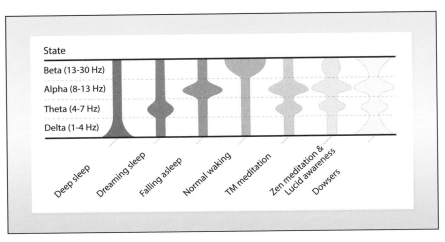

Figure 10.4. The Mind Mirror EEG device (top), with examples of the brain-wave curves displays (bottom)

of the world, delighted to be guinea pigs and join in the investigation of the mind. This field of research was only in its infancy, with few established facts, and thus was also wide open to explorations of an empirical nature, which I carried out with my psychotherapist friend and colleague Ma Premo. At that exhilarating time we both felt that we were making new discoveries every day.

At First Sound, Then Light

From the very beginning of my studies in electronics I had been interested in sound through my work in developing sound synthesizers, at first analog, then digital when that technology appeared in the 1970s. This brought me to an exploration of sound spatialization—sound that exploits localization—and to the development of a series of spatialization devices marketed by my friend Paul Devlas (whom I had met in India) through his California-based company, Omnisound: the SP-1, SSP-100, SSP-200, and OPS-1 models.

Although Paul and I never made a fortune with this project, the devices were used by many well-known artists and even by NASA for their research in psychoacoustics long before the worldwide expansion of surround-sound devices now commonly found on the market. I am often surprised to find that these first SP-1s, although long ago surpassed by the technology of today, have sometimes been preserved by those who continue to appreciate their unique functions (see fig. 10.5).

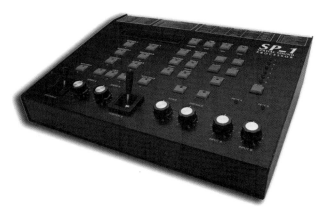

Figure 10.5. The SP-1 sound spatializer, circa 1984

Ma Premo and I worked together to increase the effects of the psychotherapeutic methods she used through the addition of sound. Two of these methods were holotropic breathing and bioenergy. We found out that sound, when spatialized along circular trajectories, acquires a particular power at certain rotation rhythms.* This brought us into contact with the phenomenon of resonance, as we strove to validate this finding through EEG measurements.

This interest in brain waves naturally brought me to an exploration of audio entrainment, then photic, and then to the development of appliances that use light. It seemed quite natural to me to apply my understanding of sound synthesis based on oscillators to the control of light pulsations. I was surprised to observe that though the use of simple oscillators was frequent in AVE, it appeared that no one had yet applied to light the more complex oscillating structures found in sophisticated sound synthesizers.

Light Modulation

This period marked the beginning of my study of what I now call *light modulation,* a generic term depicting the use of oscillators to modulate (which is to say, vary) the properties of a light source. Principally, two types of modulation exist: amplitude modulation (AM), which corresponds to a cyclical modification of the intensity of the light; and frequency modulation (FM), corresponding to a cyclical alteration of the color, since it is the frequency of light that determines its color.

Of course the rules for the application of modulation are very different for light than for sound, notably in relation to their respective frequency ranges. The development of light modulation that has occurred since then has both refined and optimized these rules. Starting my work with just one oscillator, I then moved to structures with three oscillators and, more recently, with twelve intermodulating oscillators, increasing at

---

*I continue to this day to apply this observation when creating multisensorial programs. A sensation perceived as rotating in a clockwise direction has a rather stimulating influence, encouraging extroversion, whereas a sensation perceived as rotating in a counterclockwise direction provides a calming influence, encouraging introversion. This seems to be the case not only for audio sensations but for visual and kinesthetic ones as well.

each stage the modulation possibilities. When one takes into account the properties of each one of the oscillators (such as amplitude, frequency, phase, wave shape, symmetry, duty cycle, etc.), such a structure would offer more than a hundred parameters of control.

Since such an abundance of possibilities could easily become diz-zying, the goal of this part of the exploration was to find out the most interesting combinations and those that were most efficient in terms of psychophysiological effects—an expertise patiently built up over twenty years of experimentation.

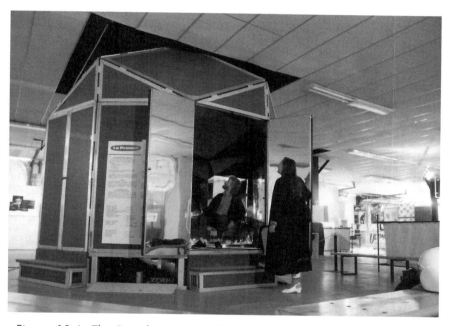

Figure 10.6. The Pyradome, one of our early multisensorial experiments created with a group of artists and researchers. It received 20,000 visitors at the Images of the Future expo in Montréal during the summer of 1986 (left, the author; right, Ma Premo).

Experiments in India

My initial experimental period in India in the '80s was particularly pro-lific. Our project received the total approval of Osho, who, always the visionary, made this memorable pronouncement: "Sound and light will be the therapy of the future." From then on we kept his encouragement in mind, particularly during the 1990s when our intensive personal involvement in this research found no real echoes in the world at large. Few people had any interest in working with therapeutic light (it was before the recent discoveries brought about through light medicine), and we often came to a point where we were about to give up. But then each time we found ourselves immersed in the extraordinary purity of the colors with which we worked, we were somehow convinced we should persevere.

So it was at the ashram in Pune where for the first time the opportunity arose to systematically test the whole gamut of modulations that the prototypes of my light modulators were then able to generate. This was possible thanks to our ashram volunteers, whose perceptions had become sensitized as a result of the practice of meditation, enabling them to describe and tell us what they felt. We discovered that certain light patterns were very harsh, others delicious, some neutral, and yet others hilarious.

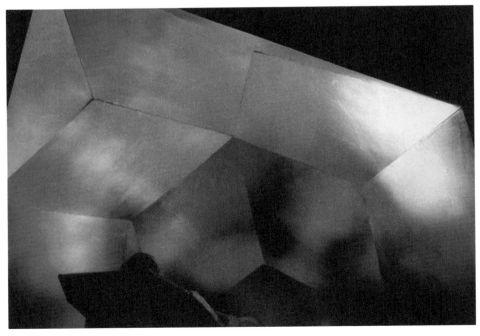

Figure 10.7. Early Sensora prototype, circa 1991
(© Sensortech Inc.)

Some Observations on Light Pulsations

Gradually, some general outlines emerged from this period of experimentation, and certain key frequencies became apparent. To name some of the more significant ones:

* **The majority of people find stroboscopic pulsations used traditionally by AVE devices too intense and aggressive.** Although there is no doubt that they maximize the brain potential that they evoke, it is at the price of a kind of violation of the brain, which is forced to react to an external stimulus of high potency. My light modulators offer a much finer control of the pulsation, where the variation in luminous intensity can be adjusted down to a very small range (generally from 1 to 5 percent of the total intensity, in contrast to others' stroboscopic versions, where the modulation is total at 100 percent). The effect created from the light is a shimmering one that is very soft, almost at the edge of perception—the opposite of that produced by stroboscopic pulsation. Rather than provoking a protective reaction against what is felt as sensorial aggression, the light instead becomes fascinating and seductive, initiating a spontaneous invitation to merge with the psyche. We believe that this soft modulation has the potential to create a deeper and more lasting therapeutic effect than that of the classical AVE.

* **The sensitivity to pulsations is not uniform in our visual field.** The central region of the visual field, rich in cones, is that area that is most precise and that reacts most rapidly, whereas the peripheral visual regions that are rich in rods are optimized for weak intensities and are slower. Having understood that the perception of rapid cerebral pulsations is weaker at the peripheral visual field, we then adjusted the depth of the light modulation in such a way that the pulsations were increased in that region in order to equalize global perception. The field that resulted was much more adapted to our visual system. This type of improvement clearly illustrates the level of refinement that we look for in the creation of the complex patterns that are used in therapeutic light. It requires a system of projection operating with several zones that are controlled in an

independent manner. Our Sensora system, for example, makes use of five separate zones.

* **In the same way that each of us has preferences and even aversions to certain colors, the reaction to particular brain pulsations (those from 1 to 30 Hz) is very personal in that some frequencies appear to us more agreeable than others.** However, it seems that one frequency was universally enjoyed by just about all of our subjects: 7.8 Hz, at the border between the theta and alpha bands. And it is certainly no coincidence that this frequency is that of a natural phenomenon of great importance: the *Schumann resonance.* This is the frequency of the stationary electromagnetic field surrounding our planet, which circulates between the ionosphere and the surface of the Earth, kept in perpetual activation through the electrical discharges from lightning at one place or another in the atmosphere. As early as the end of the 1800s the existence of this natural resonance had been suspected by Nikola Tesla, who had been trying to transfer electrical energy over long distances through the atmosphere. But only in 1952 did physicist Winfried Otto Schumann determine its fundamental frequency of 7.83 Hz. Higher-frequency harmonics also exist. This planetwide field is weak but measurable in the order of 10^{-3} μW/m^2 (microwatts per square meter), and all life on Earth has evolved under its primordial presence. It is therefore not surprising that its frequency is felt as being wonderfully harmonious. We use it in many of the multisensorial programs of the Sensora to induce a state of balance and integration.

* **The range of frequencies that are used in the practice of light modulation cover the range from 1/100 to 50 Hz.** The limit at the higher frequency broadly corresponds to the critical fusion frequency of the eye (the maximum frequency that our visual system is able to perceive before the pulsation disappears and the light becomes static at an averaged intensity).* The limit at the

---

*Higher frequencies certainly have notable biological effects and are used in other modalities such as frequency-specific therapy, but they do not target the visual system, which interests us here.

lower frequency corresponds to very slow cycles of over a minute, or about 100 seconds, because lower than that we cease to be able to perceive them as a continuous oscillation.

* **If light pulsations from 1 to 30 Hz can provoke resonance with brain waves, other frequencies can interact with many other physiological processes of a cyclical nature when their range is accessible through light modulation.** One of the most important resonances is that of the heartbeat, in the order of 1.2 Hz at its normal rhythm, to which no one is insensitive. The shamans of different peoples across the world are most likely very conscious of this frequency because we have come to understand that the hypnotic rhythm of the percussion instruments used in rituals can often be found at one or another harmonic of that frequency. Other examples of physiological frequencies are those of breathing (with a cycle of approximately three seconds), the movement of peristalsis (five seconds), the craniosacral pulsation (ten seconds), and slow oscillations of arterial pressure known as Mayer waves (ten seconds) (Julien 2006).

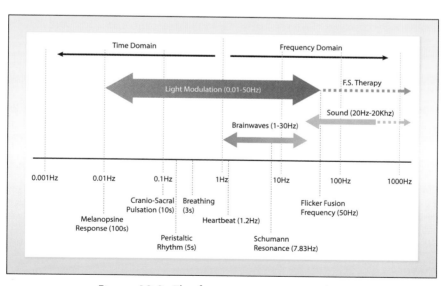

Figure 10.8. The frequency ranges used in light modulation

These examples are good illustrations of the rich quality of the psychophysiological interaction fields accessible through the means of low-frequency light pulsations. Scientists are still at the beginning of their exploration of these domains, but I am convinced that this area of study will experience a much greater expansion in the new science of vibratory medicine.

The Risks and Perils of Pulsation

In every form of the therapeutic use of light pulsation, close attention must be paid to the potential risks arising from psychophysiological reactions. We all know that powerful stroboscopes such as those sometimes seen at music and dance venues can be disturbing. In fact, their impact can be quite dangerous for certain people who are subject to photosensitive epilepsy (Fisher et al. 2005). In this type of photosensitivity, luminous flashes, particularly when they are in the range of 5 to 30 Hz, can provoke an epileptic reaction or seizure. There are abundant instances of such crises being triggered by ongoing flashes of light on a highway, for example, or from television sets displaying images involving intense pulsations. The most notorious case is that of the "Pokemon Shock" that was triggered in Japan in 1997 as a result of the effects of a televised cartoon that sent 685 viewers to the hospital for seizures or other troubles of an epileptic nature (*Yomiuri Shimbun* 1997).

This risk seems to have dampened the attraction to AVE, and it is one of the facts that from the start of our research caused us to orient ourselves toward a safer approach, based on two principal factors. The first, which we have already mentioned, is the softening of the light pulsations themselves. The second is the utilization of an open mode of diffusion; rather than delivering light through AVE goggles, where intense flashes of light can trigger claustrophobia in certain people, we chose to work with a large screen in an open area, which is both inviting and offers an ambience of security. From the thousands of Sensora sessions that have been given to date, no one has experienced an epileptic seizure. Furthermore, what came as an unexpected surprise was our observation that the opposite was in fact true: in cases where people had even serious epileptic conditions, the soft pulsations of the light of the Sensora led them to an agreeable pacifying of their photosensitivity, giving them greater confidence and a gradual desensitization to such pulsations.*

RESONANCE, A UNIVERSAL PHENOMENON

Resonance is a universal phenomenon found at all levels of existence, from the atomic to the galactic. It enables important exchanges of energy through the influence of very weak fields or stimuli. This is accomplished by the capacity of resonance to bring about a cumulative transfer of the energy of these fields with almost perfect efficiency.

With regard to mechanical vibrations, this transfer is produced by the gradual accumulation of kinetic energy transmitted at each cycle, as in the case of Huygens's pendulum clocks or with a resonating guitar string in which the vibration is generated by air molecules carrying sound. In electronics a resonant circuit starts to oscillate with the input of the slightest current. The ultimate demonstration of resonance can be found at the quantum scale, where the absolute precision of the levels of energy in atomic layers manifests as highly specific resonant frequencies during all interactions or energy exchanges.

The Signature of the Sun

The extreme precision of resonance is revealed in a multitude of ways, including an example involving sunlight that I find particularly fascinating. In 1814, Bavarian optician Joseph von Fraunhofer was the first to observe the solar spectrum in detail through an improved version of Newton's prism. Fraunhofer found hundreds of mysterious dark lines that have since been dubbed *Fraunhofer lines* (see fig. 10.9).

But it was necessary to wait until 1859 before Gustav Kirchhoff and Robert Bunsen, considered to be the inventors of spectroscopy, were able to explain the origin of the lines. Kirchhoff and Bunsen first noticed that each element, when it is vaporized by a flame, emits certain

---

*This approach is consistent with that of cognitive behavioral therapy for epilepsy, which allows that "being able to recognise the early symptoms preceding an epileptic fit brings the ability to take counter-measures towards preventing it" (Petitmengin 2006).

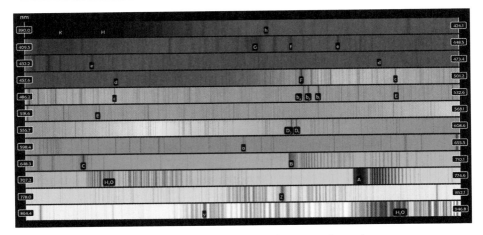

Figure 10.9. Fraunhofer lines dispersed across the solar spectrum
(© Opto-Knowledge Systems Inc.)

characteristic lines of color. They then found an exact correspondence between many of these colors and those of the Fraunhofer lines. The conclusion was inevitable: the lines must be caused by the presence of these same elements in the atmosphere of the sun. Fraunhofer lines thus constitute a kind of "signature of the sun" that reveals the intimate properties of its internal composition.

And resonance appears again here: the lines of any element that is transmitted in a light beam can interact in a cohesive way with the atoms of the same element contained in a target at a distance. Through its particular spectroscopic signature, could the light of our sun, the source of all life on our planet, have a subtle influence on the biochemical balance of those elements that make up living matter?

This is the contention of researchers such as my colleague Alexander Wunsch, who considers that none of our artificial light sources are capable of perfectly reproducing the beneficial therapeutic effects coming directly from the light of the sun itself (refer also to chapter 6).

The Infinitesimal Energies of Life

To be surprised that such minute aspects of the solar spectrum can have some measure of importance is to fail to be aware of the acutely sensitive links between living matter and resonance.

The techniques of interferometry, based on the measurement of extremely small shifts between resonating waves, are capable of attaining a precision of one part in 10^{17}.* It has recently been confirmed by Holmes et al. (2015) that the rods of the retina can detect signals as weak as three photons, whereas a typical candle emits 10^{19} photons per second. And even if official medicine has established the biologically significant limit of electromagnetic microwaves (those of our cell phones) at 10,000,000 µW/m^2, which is the North American standard, many researchers have observed adverse responses from living cells with microwaves fields as little as 3 µW/m^2 (Bioinitiative Report 2012).

I have no doubt that the new medicine will excel at working with the infinitesimal levels of energy that are the source of the organization of all living matter.

The Cosmic Octave

We can't speak of resonance without mentioning the concepts of *harmonic* (the exact multiple of a frequency) and octave (the doubling of a frequency). All vibratory phenomena having a frequency of resonance are sensitive to an influence of that same frequency, or of the frequency of one of its harmonics. The equivalence of these influences is familiar to us in music. To our ear, the note that we call an A remains an A regardless of whether it is played in a higher or lower octave. For certain artists and researchers this law of the octave is universally applicable, enabling communication to be established between separate domains in nature. I have always been intrigued by the natural law of the cosmic octave put forth by the Swiss musicologist Hans Cousto, which suggests a harmonic relation between colors and musical notes.

Since the time of Newton and Goethe, many scholars have tried to establish a link between light and sound, investigations that have led to some delightful creations, like that of British artist Alexander Rimington. In 1893, Rimington invented one of the first color organs, a keyboard instrument that transformed a music recital into

---

*To get an idea of what this level of precision means: it is equivalent to measuring the distance between the Earth and the moon within a few nanometers (a billionth of a meter).

a spectacle of light (see fig. 10.10). In 1910, the Russian composer Alexander Scriabin included a part for a light-keyboard of his own invention, called the Luce, in the score of his opera *Prometheus*.

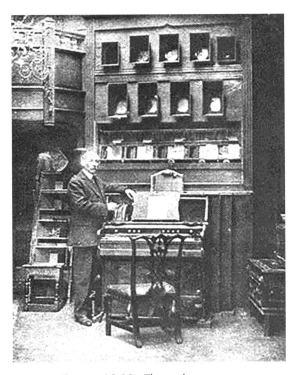

Figure 10.10. The color organ
of Alexander Rimington, circa 1893

Cousto's method appears to me to be the most elegant. He divides light frequencies by a sufficient number of octaves (it takes about forty) in order for them to be brought down to the range of audio frequencies, and in this way he obtains a correlation between colors and notes.* For example, red is a faraway harmonic of the note G, green is a harmonic of C, and blue is a harmonic of D (see table 10.1).

I remain convinced that it is not by chance that the whole range

*Cousto goes further in his method of octaves to obtain correlations between the planets (based on their period of rotation) and sounds and colors. German music producer Joachim-Ernst Berendt put this combination together in his remarkable album *Primordial Tones*.

of visible light frequencies, from the darkest red to the faintest violet, covers exactly one octave, just as one finds in the musical scale. Even if it is difficult to conceive a physical link between frequency domains so disproportionately distant from one another (by a factor of 1,000 billion), this harmonic relationship has an intrinsic beauty that for me amply justifies its use, and I have taken pleasure in creating multisensorial programs with the Sensora wherein sound, light, and kinesthetic frequencies are in harmonic coherence.

TABLE 10.1. THE CORRESPONDENCE BETWEEN NOTES AND COLORS ACCORDING TO COUSTO'S OCTAVE METHOD

SOUND			LIGHT		
NOTE	Hz	x OCTAVES	COLOR	nm
do (C)	262	41	Green	521
re (D)	294	41	Blue	464
mi (E)	330	41	Indigo	414
fa (F)	349	41	Violet	390
sol (G)	392	40	Red	696
la (A)	440	40	Orange	620
ti (B)	494	40	Yellow	552

Vibrational Medicine

Resonance is at the very heart of vibrational medicine, which one could say is the action of resonance on living matter. It is important to realize in vibrational medicine that it is the frequency of a signal rather than the kind of substance from which it originates that matters. This is because the vibration of a substance can always be converted into that of another by means of resonance—for example, from sound to light (acousto-optic), from light to electric (opto-electronic), and from electric to mechanic (piezoelectric).

Living systems overflow with the means of energetic transduction, as do all of our senses that convert mechanical, electrical, or luminous signals into nerve impulses. The essence of vibrational medicine consists then of decoding the innumerable vibrational patterns that animate us, and interacting with them through appropriate resonances. In whatever way the successful outcome of this medicine of the future will ultimately manifest, it seems certain that light, being one of the most pure of all vibrational forms available to us, will play a pivotal role.

Through the universal phenomenon of resonance, light reaches to the elusive spaces where matter, energy, and our own awareness meet. Let us now take a closer look at how light can assist us in the transition from the material and objective world to our inner perception and subjective realm, thereby facilitating healing at a deeper level.

11

OBJECTIVE LIGHT, SUBJECTIVE LIGHT

Using Light to Promote a Harmonious State of Being

Meditation is the inner sun,
The source of inner light.

Osho

RIGHT FROM THE VERY START of my interest in light in the 1980s what intrigued me most was to find out whether it could contribute to enhancing altered states of consciousness—specifically, the higher state of meditative consciousness. This propelled my interest in developing new techniques for the control of light based on its modulation. I started out by studying its effects directly on myself, and then I examined its effects on others. This process, which was of an empirical nature, showed clearly that certain types of light could indeed have profound effects on the mind and on the psyche.

At the same time it was obvious to me that no technical method could create a state of meditation. Meditation is being present to oneself, a conscious awareness of our experience *in the moment*. No machine, no technology, can give us this state of awareness. However, nothing prevents us from using technology to contribute to the creation of an interior space that is favorable to meditation, and in so doing helping it to occur—which is what we intended to do by means of visual stimulation. When we accomplished this we discerned that this sort of sensorial approach could have other applications as well. Ma Premo and I both realized that light could have considerable potential for psychotherapeutic applications. However, though we could clearly recognize its effects, we were still incapable of fully comprehending *why* they were taking place; it was very difficult to understand this correctly by simply relying on the scientific or psychological facts that were available to us at that time.

We discovered in our early experiments that the light we were using seemed to intervene in an intermediate zone between the physiological influence of color in its most concrete biophysical aspect and its purely cognitive impact through its capacity to evoke a rich interior universe. The conventional scientific references at the time took into account only one of these two influences, and this seemed inadequate to us. In fact, it was only gradually, over the course of about twenty years, that we developed a model to better understand the nature of this intermediary domain, and as a result we were able to identify the scope of therapeutic applications of this type of light.

THE POWER OF COLOR ON THE MIND

One of our early inspirations came as a result of the first studies about the way the brain reacts to the perception of color. Generations of researchers had already explored the cerebral structures connected to vision, the most important of all our senses. They had started to identify a complex organization capable of decoding information coming from the retina by means of a successive sequence of cerebral centers, each one processing a particular aspect of the visual field, with the major part of the visual cortex found at the back of the brain, where the optic nerve extends to the occipital lobe.

But it was only in 1989 that Lueck et al. identified the anatomical center that specifically processes information about color. This study was accomplished with positron emission tomography (PET), which enabled scientists to see the metabolic activity in the brain in a very direct way. The technique consisted of having subjects view two analogous images, one a set of rectangles in multiple colors (known as "Mondrians" because they evoke similar-looking images made by painter Piet Mondrian) and the other the same set of rectangles in achromatic shades of gray (see fig. 11.1). They took care to preserve equal luminosity in both types of images in order to create the same level of nervous stimulation in the brains of the test subjects. Then they tested to see which cortical zones reacted differently. In this seminal study, which was later published in the journal *Nature,* they demonstrated that they were able to isolate the brain's color center* in a region of the visual cortex called the V4 area (Lueck et al. 1989).

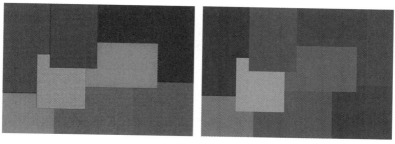

Figure 11.1. "Mondrian" images in their chromatic (left) and achromatic (right) versions

A particular detail that stood out when I read this study was a graph that depicted the levels of activity in the different cerebral areas when subjects viewed the color images and the achromatic images. Naturally, the color center in the brain reacted more actively to the colored version of the image, while another area, called the *frontal eye fields,* showed a clear suppression of activity with the colored image (see fig. 11.2). This area is to be found in the frontal cortex, the cerebral lobe generally associated with evolved mental activity, such as language, motivation, and planning.

---

*The color center located in the V4 area of the visual cortex includes the lingual gyrus and the fusiform gyrus.

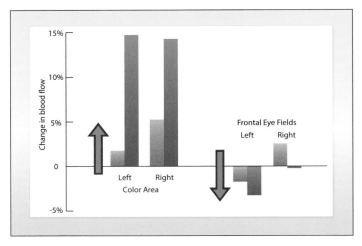

Figure 11.2. Differential stimulation of cerebral zones (Lueck et al. 1989): chromatic (colored bars) and achromatic (gray bars)

The logical implication is that color appears to reduce mental activity while simultaneously stimulating the visual cortex. It is as though pure color consisted of complete information in itself, in such a way that the brain is not obliged to pursue any further mental analysis. This was in stark contrast to the same image in black and white, in which the frontal eye fields—i.e., higher cortical functions—are stimulated by the absence of color. Could color be a stimulus permitting the increase of global cerebral energy, yet calming the mind at the same time? This was a seductive possibility, because such a function is precisely what meditation does.

This close relationship between color and the mind was again emphasized in an astonishing study carried out by Kosslyn et al. (2000). He applied the same technique as Lueck (PET measurements resulting from viewing the Mondrian images); however, Kosslyn used subjects who were highly suggestible and placed them under hypnosis.* He discovered that in this case the color center reacts less to the actual coloring of the test image than to the suggestion under hypnosis that the image is colored (or not). Not only does color perception influence the mind, as Lueck had shown, but mind influences color perception: the two are intimately linked.

―――――――――

*According to Kosslyn's study about 8 percent of the general population is highly suggestible to hypnosis.

THE DOMAINS OF INFLUENCE OF LIGHT

Let's examine more closely two important areas where color exerts its influence: the objective domain (working through the physiological and biophysical channels) and the cognitive domain (animating our thoughts and our consciousness).

In this book we have explored a number of influences coming from the objective domain, which are influences mediated by the purely physical properties of light. This includes all those influences to be found in the new light medicine. So we have photobiomodulation, through which light acts directly at the cellular level, stimulating the mitochondrial respiratory chain and modulating the production of ATP, our metabolic energy source. Also influenced is the nonvisual optical pathway, through which light governs the endocrine system by means of the retinohypothalamic tract. Notably, this includes a profound influence on our central internal clock and consequently on circadian rhythm. Another objective effect of light is that of photic entrainment, which we explored in the previous chapter. Here, pulsating light interacts with brain waves to directly induce different mental states.

Many modalities of alternative light medicine come from the objective domain as well. For example, in syntonic optometry the visual field of the subject is exposed to precise colors in order to obtain specific autonomic effects. In Colorpuncture, the colors are chosen and applied according to the stimulated reflex points. The common characteristic of all of these objective influences is the systematic manner in which their action takes place, independent of the will or of any cognitive involvement of the subject.

The cognitive domain of light is that which passes through the sense of vision; this influence is one of the most profound we can have in life. Through vision, we build an interior representation of our entire world. Vision informs our superior cognitive faculties; it can evoke all the emotions, sensations, and thoughts that define us.

We've all heard that old truism, "An image is worth a thousand words." The arts of painting and photography, television, and cinema are visual forms that can give meaning to our existence. In their most exalted manifestations such as sacred geometry or mandalas, images are capable of exerting influence of a higher spiritual nature. When light interacts in such a way with our mental universe, it is not only acting through its physical properties; it becomes a vehicle for the transfer of information through images that are formed by our visual system. The influence of light in this cognitive domain is characterized by the complexity of its form and by its rich informational content.

The Subjective Domain, the Third Area of Influence

So we possess many ways of using light, which can act on either one or the other of these two domains, the objective and the cognitive. But what happens at the boundary between these two? Essentially, in this intermediate domain we try to induce perceptions of a superior cognitive order by using the objective properties of light. For this reason I call this third domain of influence the *subjective domain* because it intervenes at the level of our interior perception, which is subjective. We will see that it concerns one of the most fertile of regions, and this has profound implications for the therapeutic application of color.

What do we mean when we say "perceptions of a superior cognitive order"? This has to do with all cognitive activity capable of inducing within us a harmonious and positive state of being. Such activity can take several forms: any emotion that evokes beauty or pleasure; the sensation of unity with the flow of life; deep relaxation; or, again, an impression of immense peace and security. Why would such perceptions be of particular therapeutic interest? Most of us understand this intuitively: they permit us to rediscover our natural equilibrium, and they open the door to an intrinsic mechanism of healing always ready to move into action when we give it the opportunity.

Homeostasis, the Key to Life

Homeostasis is the process of autoregulation by which a living organism maintains its integrity in the midst of the surrounding chaos in which it exists. In fact, for many medical researchers homeostasis is even considered to be the essence of life, its defining factor. All pathological states result from an inability of the body to maintain homeostasis in one aspect or another. In the holistic view of medicine it is thought that an organism naturally creates its own healing when the obstacles to homeostasis have been removed. And it is here that cognitive activity can play a central role.

This view of healing is presently shared by a significant number of people. It is upheld, of course, by energetic medicine practitioners, but also to a certain extent by conventional medical parties. The idea in fact goes back all the way to origins of medicine: for Hippocrates, the "Father of Medicine," the body was its own healer. And this is increasingly true due to certain discoveries that are gradually being integrated by conventional medicine—a development that has been instrumental in paving the way for a more open-minded approach to healing.

One of these recent discoveries is epigenetics, which reveals that the activity of DNA, even though it is considered to be the ultimate proof of the supremacy of biochemistry in health matters, is subject in its genetic expression to the influence of one's mental attitude.

Another recent discovery is the realization of the importance of the placebo effect, wherein the capacity to control purely physiological phenomena through the power of the mind has been confirmed in numerous studies—a subject we'll return to in the final chapter of this book.

Neuroplasticity

If homeostasis is subject to the influence of positive cognitive activity, the nervous system and the brain are even more so. This should not be surprising since mental activity is one of the primary functions of the brain.

All perceptual or mental processes occur by means of electrochemical cascades that travel through the immense network of neurons in the brain. This network is the very substrate that conditions their existence. But this interrelationship between mental activity and the neurons is not unidirectional. It has now been clearly established (notably, as a result of the work carried out by neurophysiologist Eric Kandel, who was awarded the Nobel Prize in Medicine in 2000) that perceptual and mental processes are capable of modifying the structure of the neurons themselves, multiplying their synaptic connections according to their need.

Neurons generate thought—however, thought is also capable of forming neurons. Although for centuries we considered that the brain, once it had formed, remained static and was unable to regenerate itself, we now know that it is much more malleable and dynamic. It is what we call *neuroplastic*, signifying its ability to reorganize itself through the formation of new neuronal connections throughout the length of a person's life.

Canadian physician Norman Doidge (2007, 2016), in his excellent work of making this field accessible to the nonprofessional world, enumerates a number of important pathologies (some of which are considered incurable) that were improved or even completely healed by means of neuroplastic methods, including chronic pain, cranial trauma, stroke, autism, multiple sclerosis, Parkinson's disease, and depression.

Psychoneuroimmunology

A new branch of medicine, psychoneuroimmunology, studies the intimate link between our thoughts and the immune system. Because there is no obvious connection between the central nervous system and the immune system's traditional messaging system, which is the lymph system, it was unexpected to find that the former can significantly influence the latter—but this is just what the pioneers in this new field have established.

There are many examples of how our psychological climate has a direct bearing on the state of our health. To name a few well documented ones: elevated stress exacerbates asthma or eczema; diminished social support accelerates the progression of HIV infection or cancer; wounds, whether surgical or chronic, heal slower in patients experiencing increased levels of fear or distress.

Psychoneuroimmunology is starting to paint a clearer picture of which neural pathways put the cells of the immune system—as well as our master glands and our hormonal balance, which are closely related to immune health—under the influence of our mind (Ziemssen and Kern 2007).

Toward a Subjective Light

Epigenetics, the placebo effect, neuroplasticity, psychoneuroimmunology—many avenues offer different ways of viewing how cognitive activity influences health, both physical and mental. However, one thing is clear: it does not happen with just any old cognitive activity. While we almost never stop thinking during our lifetime, we cannot heal out problems or illnesses just by thinking! So if cognitive activity is to have an effect of a therapeutic nature, it would necessarily have to be other than that of our usual mental processes, distinct from the "noise" of the habitual, ongoing cerebral animation.

This is what I was alluding to when I previously spoke of "perceptions of a superior cognitive order." The following approaches would be favorable to maximizing the healing capability of cognitive activity:

* Offering a stimulus of sufficient intensity to fully awaken our attention
* Generating attention that is defragmented and perceived as unifying
* Sustaining an uplifting and moving perceptual quality
* Encouraging the absence of negative or stressing thoughts

How can light be helpful in inducing the above perceptions? To begin with, it activates our principal sense channel, that of vision; a visual stimulation correctly balanced can generate ample perceptual intensity and thereby captivate our attention. Then light capitalizes on our innate appreciation of color; evolution has programmed us to be attracted to pure colors, which we perceive as entrancing. Who among us does not marvel at the surreal beauty of a rainbow? Thirdly, light can be shaped into presenting a signal to the mind that is harmonious and guides us toward a unified perception, remaining at the same time dynamic enough to avoid becoming boring or monotonous.

One can now understand why light belonging to the objective domain or the cognitive domain is *not* optimal for these functions. The objective domain is not necessarily programmed for visual stimulation, as in the case with photobiomodulation, nor is it designed to awaken a cognitive perception, as in the case of bright light therapy. When using color, as in syntonic optometry, it is typically with the presentation of one color at a time, a visual stimulus that would be too simple to evoke an uplifting cognitive perception. And light belonging to the cognitive domain, such as that originating from a work of art or a film, would have a tendency to simply awaken the usual thought patterns that we normally experience and not bring about therapeutic effects.

Thus we have a special interest in this intermediate subjective light, which seeks to combine the sensorial power of objective light with the wakeful consciousness of cognitive light. It is of course no easy task to achieve this, and the researchers of today are only starting to address this challenge with the help of the latest information and various means now at their disposal. It is highly possible that it can be approached by a wide range of techniques.

THE SENSORA

My personal research in this area brought me to a specific approach using subjective light. This is the Sensora system, described in the previous chapter. It is based on a technique of light modulation in which an array of low-frequency oscillators controls the intensity and the color from the light sources. Over a period of time we developed a number of strategies to help bring us closer to an ideal light, one capable of inducing therapeutic transformation by using the objective properties of light to generate a positive cognitive influence.

Strategy 1: Sensorial Immersion
The light projections from the Sensora are made on a large screen, the size and position of which are designed to cover most of the visual field of the subject, who is seated beneath the screen in a zero-gravity chair (one that reclines in such a way that the legs and feet are raised higher than the torso). One is literally immersed in a field of pure color, which maximizes the sensorial impact of the light.

Over time we refined certain aspects of the screen, adding to its efficiency: It is inclined at a forty-five-degree angle to further the impression of total immersion. It is "vaporized" with a finish of silver-colored microparticles, offering a texture that increases the perception of spatial depth coming from the luminous projection. It is equipped with a small central light source, a focal reference point serving to anchor the visual experience as it is lived. And it is of a circular form, inspiring the feeling of greater unity.

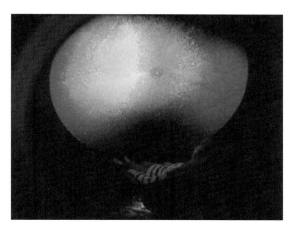

Figure 11.3. The immersive screen of the Sensora
(© Sensortech Inc.)

Strategy 2: Optimization of the Complexity of the Light Patterns

Experimentation led us to choose a light system with five independent sources because we determined this number is an optimal compromise to work with subjective light. This permitted the creation of light patterns of just the right degree of complexity capable of evoking the intermediate area between the objective and cognitive domains.

To arrive at our goal of stimulating "perceptions of a superior cognitive order," i.e., the area of subjective influence, we took into account the disadvantages of both the strictly objective domain of influence and the strictly cognitive. In the objective domain of influence one generally uses a single source of colored light, which precludes offering any dynamic visual aspect to the projection. Such a light source becomes boring after a few minutes because it does not offer any real cognitive interest.

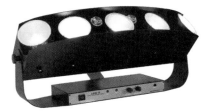

Figure 11.4 The Sensora LPA-2 projector with its five light sources (© Sensortech Inc.)

On the other hand, in the domain of cognitive influence one would typically work with video screens composed of many millions of pixels. Their complex images would be interpreted by the brain as being of the same order as reality, and they would therefore activate the same mental processes that constitute the normal habits of our everyday life. With their many interpretations, memory references, and projections into the future, the mental processes awakened by stimulation of the cognitive field of influence would have little chance of creating the kind of cerebral reorganization we strive for. Subjective influence provides a complexity sufficient to introduce a visual vitality capable of captivating the attention; at the same time it remains beneath the threshold beyond which the pattern ceases to be purely abstract, thereby unleashing interpretive mental activity—similar to the "Mondrians" discussed earlier in this chapter. Such light patterns result in stimulating attention and awakening while reducing mental activity, precisely the combination induced by meditation.

Strategy 3: Applying Cerebral Laterality

In the Sensora projectors the five light sources are distributed in a linear fashion and oriented from left to right along the width of the projection screen. This arrangement corresponds to the lateral structure of our visual system, with its two eyes, and the nervous system, with its two cerebral hemispheres, both of which prioritize the horizontal orientation. By controlling the phase (or timing) of the oscillators assigned to each of the five light sources, the system of light modulation is capable of generating apparent movements in the projected luminous patterns. It is these movements that bring the sought-after visual vitality to the subjective light. Because the movements are generated by oscillators they are cyclical and possess a specific frequency that can be adjusted to induce different psychophysiological resonances. When spread across the frequency range of light modulation shown in figure 10.8 on page 269 such resonances can entrain brain waves, settle the heart rhythm, or pacify the breath cycle.

The lateral structure of the luminous movements permits us to adjust their influence according to the needs of the treatment. One can generate, for example, lateral sweeping movements in the left or the right direction, or movements that extend outward or inward from the central zone, reminiscent of the opening or closing of a colored flower. In general, the sweeping movements to the right as well as the outward movements that come from the center have a tendency to stimulate and awaken: they are of an extroverted nature. The sweeping movements toward the left, as well as the inward movements toward the center, have the opposite effect: they tend to relax and calm and are of an introverted nature. With the Sensora, the light from one side of the visual field stimulates the visual centers of the crossed brain hemisphere, and the continuing alternation between the two sides is reflected in a flow of nerve signals passing from one brain hemisphere to the other (see fig. 11.5). All types of lateral sweeping movements therefore contribute to the interhemispheric communication of the brain—a highly beneficial factor in maintaining homeostasis.

In addition, with the Sensora we routinely use lateral light (developed by Dr. Anatoly Chuprikov, mentioned in chapter 9) in our light-therapy programs. This is enabled by projecting complementary colors on each half of the visual field, one being stimulating and the

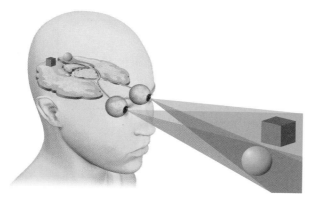

Figure 11.5.
Cerebral laterality
of the visual system

other sedating. This powerful light therapy modality allows us to rebalance the arousal levels of the two brain hemispheres, which are typically skewed in conditions such as depression or insomnia.

Strategy 4: Low-Energy Photic Entrainment

Photic entrainment, which is based on light pulsations at frequencies conforming to those of brain waves, within a range of 1 to 40 Hz (refer as well to the discussion of the delta, theta, alpha and beta brain waves ranges in chapter 10), is a powerful method for the objective influence of light, allowing for induction through resonance of the mental state associated with the frequency of the cerebral stimulation. As we have seen, the benefits of this type of audiovisual entrainment (AVE) have been amply validated in clinical studies. Briefly, they include support in treating various forms of affective, sleep, and stress-related disorders, as well as learning difficulties.

It is possible to redirect this class of light influence into the subjective domain by a very simple method: by reducing the depth of the light pulsations to the extent of rendering them almost imperceptible. In classic AVE the light pulsations are stroboscopic, with a pulsation amplitude of 100 percent. In the Sensora, however, we have reduced this pulsation amplitude to much, much lower levels, on the order of

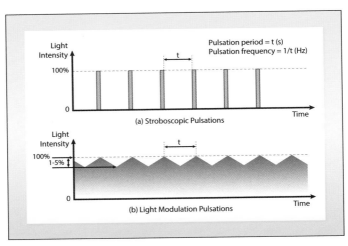

Figure 11.6. Comparison of stroboscopic (top) and light modulation (bottom) light pulsations

1 to 5 percent, thereby eliminating the aggressive aspect of stroboscopic pulsations (see fig. 11.6).

Very early on in our exploration of subjective light we saw the importance of this approach, which is much softer. We are not trying to maximize the cerebral *evoked potential,* the brain's natural tendency to resonate with the external stimulus, but are hoping instead to increase the effects from a much higher cognitive process. Instead of a mechanical entrainment of the brain waves, we obtain cognitive appreciation from an agreeable sensation induced through the delicate, shimmering light. The vibrational information from the low-energy pulsation is of course still present, but it now functions through an experience of well-being or pleasure. As mentioned earlier, we have found this subjective influence to have a deeper therapeutic effect than the purely objective one of classic audiovisual entrainment.

Strategy 5: Very Slow (Subdelta) Modulation

The technique of AVE normally uses the frequency range of cerebral waves, beginning with the low frequencies of the delta band, from 1 to 4 Hz, which are the waves of deep sleep. Our research has shown us the importance of light modulation at frequencies that are even lower than that, in the *subdelta range.* These subdelta oscillations are so slow that one no longer sees them as pulsations. They are received more as a continuous flow; perceptually, they pass from the frequency domain to the temporal domain. Their gentle ebb and flow helps to generate a sensation of floating, which greatly facilitates cognitive abandon and a feeling of deep relaxation that is characteristic of subjective light. We consider this so important that I dedicated in the light modulation architecture of the Sensora a complete bank of subdelta oscillators for each luminous source. With time (seconds) and frequency (Hz) inversely proportional, they operate at rhythms that last from 1 second (1 Hz) to 100 seconds (1/100 Hz).

It is difficult to say exactly at what physiological or cognitive level these subdelta modulations work. Perhaps they contribute to resonances with the numerous rhythms of our body that belong in the same range, such as the breath or arterial pressure waves. In recent years, neurologists interested in the EEG aspect of this phenomenon have called these frequencies "slow" (from 1 to 1/10 Hz) and "infraslow" (from 1/10 to 1/100 Hz) oscillations, and they are also aware that they have their origin in the thalamus, the so-called gray matter of the brain (Hughes et al. 2011). They do not yet understand their function but believe that they play a role in the "regulation of behavioural performance" (Lörincz et al. 2009). Another class of subdelta EEG signals is the slow cortical potentials (slow current shifts in the EEG originating from the upper cortical layers), the therapeutic promise of which is being explored in biofeedback procedures in order to help children with ADHD (Strehl and Birbaumer 2006).

Whatever it may be, I was very intrigued by an observation made by Dave Siever, one of the pioneers of AVE, about subdelta oscillations. In a pilot study carried out in 2001 he concluded that the subdelta pulsations (between 0.5 and 1 Hz) have a marked effect on the reduction of hypertension—in fact, to a higher degree than that from medication normally prescribed for this problem, and of course without any side effects (Mullen, Berg, and Siever 2001) (see fig. 11.7). Siever also noted a marked improvement in the symptoms of fibromyalgia using subdelta. Of course, this study was carried out on a relatively small group of participants—twenty-eight, for a period of a month. Nevertheless, the results agree with our own observations of the beneficial effects of the Sensora for various forms of chronic pain.

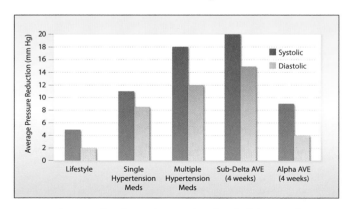

Figure 11.7. The result of a pilot study of subdelta on hypertension, showing that the maximal blood pressure reduction is obtained from subdelta AVE (Mullen, Berg, and Siever 2001) (© Mind Alive Inc.)

Strategy 6: The Purity of the Luminous Signal

One of the keys to understanding the action of subjective light is its capacity to evoke a sense of wonderment. Many things have to be in place in order for this to happen, but one of the most significant is the purity of the light projected. This purity is important on many levels.

To begin with, there must be chromatic purity: the colors of the luminous patterns have to be as saturated as possible to maximize their visual impact. The technique most adapted to the creation of multi-colored light is that of additive color mixing, which consists of mixing the light from primary sources in different proportions. In general, there are three primary sources: a red, a green, and a blue.

In the 1980s and '90s I developed projectors with halogen light sources equipped with dichroic filters with a very sharp spectral profile. The high-intensity LEDs that appeared in 2000 are what I now use in the new generation of Sensora projectors (LPA-2 and LPA-3), as well as in the SensoSphere. As light sources, the colored LEDs are inherently relatively monochromatic (with a bandwidth of 20 to 40 nm), close to the pure colors of the rainbow, and a trio of red, green, and blue LEDs can offer a mixture of pure color spanning the greater part of the visible spectrum. The weakness of such an arrangement is in the yellow part of the spectrum, which is difficult to reproduce through the mixing of red and green LEDs, the wavelengths of which are too far apart from each other. One can fix this by adding a fourth, amber-colored primary source, intermediate between the red and green (see fig. 11.8). In the latest generation of the Sensora light projectors I have gone further and now use LED sources with six primary colors (red, amber, green, turquoise, blue, and violet), greatly alleviating the limitations of the classic red-green-blue additive color synthesis method.

Apart from the purity of the color, it is also necessary to consider the "cleanliness" of the luminous signal, the absence of "noisy" instabilities in its intensity. We return here to the question of the flickering of LEDs (which we considered in chapter 6's discussion of the potentially harmful effects of light). This flickering intervenes as soon as the command circuit of the LED is not uniform; conventional LED light sources frequently exhibit substantial flickering. The command circuit

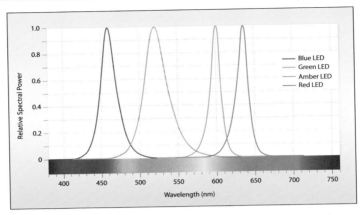

Figure 11.8. Spectrum profiles of the four primary colors
of the Sensora projectors

of the majority of commercial light products uses a digital "chopping" of the current in the LED. This technique, known as *pulse-width modulation* (PWM), has been adopted because it is easy and inexpensive to produce, but it does lead to substantial flickering (see fig. 11.9).

Even if the flickering is actually invisible as a result of using a frequency that is too high to be perceived by the eye (which does not respond much beyond 50 Hz), it will still interfere with the much more subtle modulation that we are attempting to introduce in the light signal to achieve the desired therapeutic benefits. It is a little like trying to superimpose the delicate song of a cricket above the noise of a rock concert.

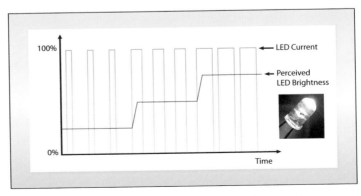

Figure 11.9. Pulse-width modulation of the light signal as typically
used to control the average apparent brightness of an LED

It is not easy to develop a command circuit for LEDs that is totally free from any flickering, especially if one looks for precise control of the mixture of colors and the gradation of brightness. It requires linear circuits with a precision capacity in the order of 0.01 percent, unusual in electronics. But it is the only way to attain the purity of the luminous signal required in subjective light.

Strategy 7: Multisensorial Stimulation

The sensorial voyage offered through subjective light can be intensified by the integration of other senses that complement the visual. This is the reason we add a surround-sound component in the Sensora, as well as a kinesthetic component. This latter is to be found in a special chair equipped with an array of eight sound transducers that convert an audio signal into a kinesthetic vibration that is felt through contact with the chair. In an extension of my research on sound spatialization I developed an audio processor capable of synthesizing kinesthetic patterns circulating along sthe length of the surface of the chair—a process that I call *dynamic sound transduction* (see fig. 11.10).

These two audio systems (surround-sound and transduction) enable us to extend the modulation applied to the light signal to similar modulations for the auditive and tactile levels. When it is well designed, the interplay of these harmonized modulations contributes to creating a remarkable multisensorial synergy felt as deeply unifying and harmonizing.

We even experimented by including an olfactory component to this synergy. We came to the conclusion that it brought a wonderful fusion with the other senses, but we had to let go of this avenue because of

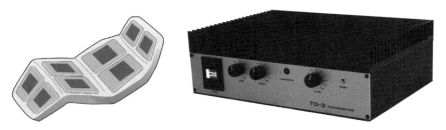

Figure 11.10. The dynamic sound transduction chair of the Sensora (left) with its TD-3 processor (right) (© Sensortech Inc.)

practical problems connected to the persistent odor of scents in the treatment space.

Subjective Light on a Video Screen?

The light projectors developed for the Sensora are complex pieces of equipment, expensive because they are built on a small scale. Occasionally I am asked why we do not use commercial video equipment instead (projectors or TV screens) to do our light projections in the subjective light domain, and thus benefit from the lower cost of their mass production. I would be delighted to be able to do so, all the more since it would facilitate a wider distribution of the Sensora programs using standard video or internet formats. Unfortunately, it is not a viable alternative for the following reasons.

Video technology is based on a succession of rapid images, with a frame rate from twenty-four to some hundred images per second, depending on the model. This fixed pulsation interferes with the subtle modulation of subjective light, just as the flickering from common LED projectors does. In addition, a video image is composed of up to several million pixels, and its transmission requires a signal of very high frequency. The global light signal emanating from such a massive number of pixels is very noisy—a little like the visual equivalent of white noise to be found in an audio system.

These sources of noise inevitably disturb the luminous purity and stability that are sought after for therapeutic applications. One can easily feel the difference between the light from the Sensora and that coming from a video source, which would not be able to offer the same relaxing and regenerative qualities.

Clinical Validation

It has always been difficult for those of us who explore the frontiers of the energetic use of light to validate their work in an acceptable scientific manner. Apart from the financial aspect involved in undertaking such studies, the effects of energy interventions, which are often quite subtle, are difficult to quantify; we simply do not have adequate instruments to measure them. How can we manage to quantify the delicate changes taking place in an interior state of being, or the rebalancing of vital life-force energy?

Yet this seeming limitation has not stopped researchers from continuing to pursue this line of research, and many strategies to apply such measurements, even though somewhat indirect, have been developed by professionals who are open to these ideas. One such scientist is psychologist Mary Ross. Following our request for a study on the Sensora, she proposed we carry out an evaluation based on its influence on the autonomic nervous system (ANS). The balance or equilibrium of the two branches of the ANS (the sympathetic nervous system and the parasympathetic nervous system) is a fundamental element of homeostasis, and we suspect already that it is sensitive to certain forms of light (which is the central premise of syntonic optometry.)

Mary developed a study protocol based on a combination of measurements that are both physiological and psychological. One of the ways of evaluating the equilibrium of the ANS is to measure heart-rate variability. This consists of taking samples of the precise rhythm of a subject's heartbeat over several minutes. A remarkable amount of information can then be ascertained from the analysis of subtle variations in the rhythm, from one beat to another. Whereas an overly static rhythm is unhealthy, small variations in the rhythm are indicative of our capacity for autoregulation. The technique had originally been developed for cardiac diagnostic use, but its pertinence in our field has been expanded through the analysis of specialized measures such as cardiac coherence, a measure of the order, stability, and harmony in the heart rhythm, to include more global psychophysiological aspects related to positive emotions and well-being (McCraty and Shaffer 2015).

In 2013, Ross led a study that involved a group of 117 subjects, one group in Texas and the other in Quebec (Ross, Guthrie, and Dumont 2013), the purpose of which was to evaluate the effects of light modulation on the ANS. Each participant received a light session for a period of twenty minutes. The sessions were randomly chosen from four types: three chromotherapy sessions of light modulation from the Sensora using specific combinations of colors and frequency modulations to obtain either relaxation, energy, or balance; plus a fourth, a placebo session using static white light. The results confirmed that the effects of Sensora sessions corresponded to their intended function, while there were no comparable results from the placebo session. The three chromotherapy sessions reduced the cardiac rhythm and skin conductance and increased the *heart rate variability*, whereas the white-light (placebo) session produced no significant changes (see fig. 11.11).

All chromotherapy sessions produced significant lowering of the total mood disturbance index in the Profile of Mood States (POMS), a psychological rating scale used to assess transient, distinct mood states. This indicates a general improvement in the overall state of mind (or mood), as well as a reduction of fatigue, depression, and anger indices. For all these categories, the placebo session resulted in either a low or negligible impact (see fig. 11.12).

What is noteworthy is that this study corroborates our original observation: that light modulation sessions reveal a double effect, wherein a deep and profound relaxation is obtained simultaneously with an increased state of awareness. This combination corresponds to what is commonly called being "in the zone"—a state denoting peak performance. This state has certain things in common with meditative states and is recognized as having great therapeutic potential. What is most remarkable is that this particular combination of increased awareness and relaxation is induced by means of therapeutic light, without any conscious effort on the part of subjects.

LIGHT AND NEUROTRANSMITTERS

It is possible to create a beneficial therapeutic effect on the physiological as well as on the psychological level through the influence of positive sensorial stimulation. In 2010, Ma Premo and I had a chance to meet an expert in the functioning of the brain, who clarified our understanding of this approach. This was Lise Lippé, a consultant in emotional and stress management who was one of the most sought-after specialists in Quebec for the treatment of post-traumatic stress disorder (PTSD). She has considerable experience in neurophysiology, which she uses when working with those most at risk for this problem, including policemen and firefighters.

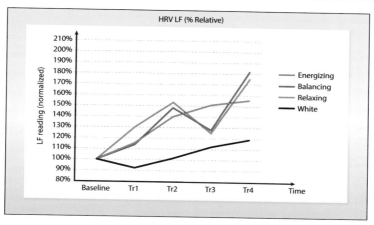

Figure 11.11. The LF, or low-frequency, component of the variability of cardiac frequency, associated with an increased psychophysiological coherence (from Ross, Guthrie, and Dumont 2013)

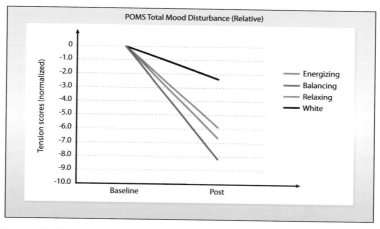

Figure 11.12. The index of total mood disturbance: a lower rating corresponds to an absence of disturbance according to the Profile of Mood States (POMS) test (from Ross, Guthrie, and Dumont 2013)

Lise has the rare gift of being able to perceive the specific action of diverse *neurotransmitters* directly in her own body, having trained herself to attain a high degree of sensitivity in identifying subtle cognitive changes. These chemical compounds are liberated by the neurons to ensure and regulate communication throughout the brain.

At the extremity of each neuron, the terminal knob at the end of the axon joins with the dendrites of the next neuron in vast cerebral networks containing hundreds of billions of neurons. The neurotransmitter molecules are released by the transmitting neuron at the junction, the synaptic cleft, and circulate to the various post-synaptic receptors of the targeted neuron (see fig. 11.13). Numbering about a hundred, these neurotransmitters create an interneuronal language. Each has a particular role related to its chemical composition. As with musical instruments with very distinct tones, they compose the symphony of sensations and perceptions that play within the brain.

When Lise sat down beneath the luminous projections of the Sensora she marveled at the veritable intersynaptic fireworks display she was feeling. She described how the intense beauty of such pure color liberated a flush of the neurotransmitter dopamine, producing a sudden sensation of delight—a "wow!" moment—and how the delicate pulsations released a flood of endorphins, offering a softer but somewhat longer sensation. For her, the cerebral impact of this subjective light, both physiological and psychological, was beyond doubt.

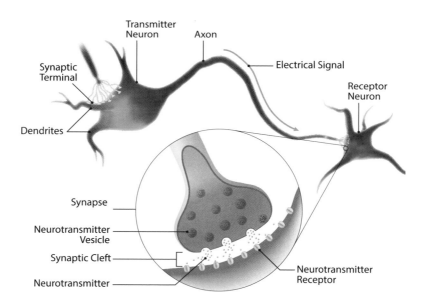

Figure 11.13. Representation of intersynaptic communication between neurons, achieved through the release of the neurotransmitters

Light That Is Pleasurable

According to the modern way of looking at neurophysiology as elaborated by people like French surgeon Henri Laborit and American neuroscientist Antonio Damasio (2010), the brain can ultimately follow one of two specific biochemical orientations: that of pleasure and that of discontent. Each of these two has an associated response within the ANS. A situation of displeasure or stress activates the sympathetic nervous system. That which is soothing or pleasurable turns on the parasympathetic nervous system.

Situations of chronic stress as well as traumatic shock result in more or less permanent overactivation of the sympathetic nervous system. The neurotransmitters that are associated with this state of mind, including acetylcholine, bring stimulation to the adrenal glands, which in turn emit the adrenaline and glucocorticoids that fuel the fight-or-flight response. When this mechanism does not succeed in resolving the situation of displeasure, a behavioral inhibition system will eventually take over that stimulates neuroendocrine responses. Over time, an exhaustion of the reserves of the neurotransmitters takes place, as well as a weakening of the immune system. Psychologically, the prospect of facing the ongoing impossibility of carrying out an efficient or successful response to chronic stress can result in depression. Biochemically, the formation of free radicals, the highly reactive molecules produced from the degradation of the neurotransmitters, damages the nerve cells.

In a depressed person a deficit in the neurotransmitters of pleasure (catecholamines such as dopamine, and the opioid peptides such as endorphins) becomes chronic. The person is simply no longer able to feel pleasure. Pharmaceutical remedies try to correct this by introducing artificial molecules to compensate for the depletion, but this inevitably leads to undesirable side effects as well as to drug dependency.

All this enables one to see the possible impact that the sensorial influences of subjective light can offer at the biochemical level. When positive stimulation is sufficiently intense, it may manage, if only for a short time, to awaken the sensation of pleasure. This unblocking, even if temporary, can contribute to the reawakening of the dormant circuits for the neurotransmitter secretions of pleasure. And *pleasure is an antidote for the pathological behavioral inhibition response of depression.* Crucially, this is accomplished by means of completely natural sensorial channels, without risk of side effects.

Together with our efforts for the clinical validation and understanding of the mechanisms involved in effective light therapy, Ma Premo and many other therapists who are now using the Sensora, continue to explore its therapeutic applications. The most encouraging results are to be found in the psychotherapeutic domain, especially concerning depression, PTSD, anxiety, and insomnia. The experiences of these practitioners are sometimes surprising, revealing effects that can be quite unexpected. For example, how does one explain that the light of the Sensora has a soothing effect on tinnitus, as we observed on several occasions? Could it be because the pathways of the auditive and visual nerve circuits cross over each other in certain regions of the brain?*

Another unforeseen effect has to do with the reduction of chronic pain; for example, in cases of degenerative osteoarthritis, fibromyalgia, and pain of neuropathic origin. One can assume that it would be connected to the subdelta modulation, mentioned above. But the effect is not systematic and does not function in the same way for everyone—a characteristic limitation of an intervention with a quality as "soft" as this one. Nevertheless, for certain people the experience of pain reduction can be quite remarkable.

In closing I want to mention one of our most memorable cases, which involved a woman with an inflammatory form of advanced breast cancer that caused intense, chronic pain that could only be controlled through the use of powerful pain-killing drugs. A session of light therapy from the Sensora every two or three days enabled her to substantially reduce her pain medication. By eliminating four of the five pain-killing drugs that had been prescribed, she reduced their debilitating side effects at the same time. The light radically changed the quality of her last few months of life, for which she was infinitely grateful.

---

*These regions include the superior colliculus, which merges information coming from the senses of both vision and hearing.

12

LIGHT AND CONSCIOUSNESS

An Intimate Association

Lead me from the unreal to the Real
Lead me from darkness to Light
Lead me from the momentary to the Eternal

BRIHADARANYAKA UPANISHAD (700 BCE)

THE STUDY OF CONSCIOUSNESS should be our primary preoccupation, since consciousness* is at the root of all other studies. It is a vast subject, extending well beyond the scope of this book. So why look into this now, in the context of its relation to the therapeutic applications of light? Because ultimately the highest form of healing that is capable of bringing light is that which passes through consciousness. Between light and consciousness there exists a privileged link, which we will try to clarify in this final chapter.

---

*Because of the ill-defined interpretations given to the terms *consciousness* and *mind,* we will not distinguish them here for the purpose of simplifying this presentation.

BEYOND THE INFLUENCE OF PHYSIOLOGY

I recently had a conversation with Jacob Liberman about the relationship between light and consciousness, an area in which he is considered an authority. He told me that during his long career as a therapist he has observed moments of profound personal transformation on numerous occasions during the application of therapeutic colored light. To him, the remarkable and rapid appearance of such states could not be explained by the simple physiological action of light, which is otherwise slow and gradual; it would seem that such a reaction would necessarily imply a direct interaction with consciousness.

I came to the same conclusion about the light of the Sensora, which occasionally facilitates deeply moving experiences of expanded consciousness in a completely spontaneous and unexpected manner. To give one memorable example: a participant at one of our public presentations became aware of memories that had been hidden since the time of her childhood, enabling her to experience this realization in a liberating way. And this occurred simply by focusing on the patterns from our projections of modulated light.

Beyond the powerful influences that light can exert on our body such as those described in the first part of this book, it appears that light can indeed act in ways perhaps even more profound—at the level of consciousness itself.

WHAT DO WE KNOW
ABOUT CONSCIOUSNESS?

A biologist or neurologist will tell us that consciousness is the apparent activity of that special biochemical computer that is the brain—a composite of the coordinated play of our billions of neurons, with their almost incalculably numerous synaptic interconnections (which are estimated to be from 100 to 1000 trillion). Through some form of magic that for the moment remains unexplained—though likely not for long, considering the advances in neurology and genetics—the brain specialist would explain that this gigantic clustered heap is the source of our wondrous feeling of beingness from which it seems to flow spontaneously. Our specialist might add that this feeling would likely be a by-product of the more important capacity of intelligence to help a person plan the future, a quality essential for human survival in earlier times. After all, when one sees what can be done today with computers, with their mere few billion transistors, all this appears to be fairly straightforward; one simply has to see some of the numerous "conscious" robots and androids in our science-fiction films to believe that this is so.

This way of looking at things put forth by our dominant materialist-reductionist paradigm is the only viewpoint that is considered acceptable by the scientific establishment. All variations from this viewpoint can be none other than arbitrary religious dogma or spiritualist fantasy of the New Age type, right?

I would like to underscore here that even from the purely scientific perspective there exist viewpoints regarding consciousness that sharply diverge from conventional notions, as we shall see in the following.

Theories of Consciousness

Philosophers, and more recently physicists, neurobiologists, and other scientists, have developed various theories on the nature of consciousness. They fall into three basic categories:

Materialism says that consciousness is a by-product of the electrochemical functioning of the neurons of the brain. It results from the process of evolution, which has led to the development of more and more advanced nervous systems. Reaching beyond a certain level of complexity, consciousness appears because it has certain advantages for the survival of the species. In some of the most extreme versions of physicalist theory such as eliminative materialism, consciousness is simply an illusion, a "heterogeneous assembly combining a series of poorly understood mental processes" (my translation of the words of French anthropologist Jean-Philippe Bocquenet (2010) describing the viewpoint of the American philosopher Daniel C. Dennett). This is the theory of consciousness favored by the present-day scientific community, following ideas that have dominated since the rise of the reductionist position that took hold of the intelligentsia starting from the seventeenth century.

Dualism says that consciousness, by its very nature, is fundamentally different from matter but coexists with it in the universe. In other words, the mind and body are distinct and separate. The origin of this idea about dualism is usually attributed to seventeenth-century French philosopher René Descartes, the "Father of Modern Western Philosophy." Cartesian dualism has profoundly influenced all scientific thought up to the present.

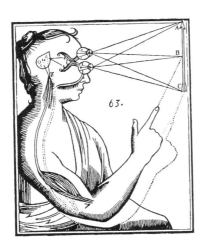

Figure 12.1. According to the dualistic vision of René Descartes, the nonmaterial soul is connected to the body through the pineal gland, the "third eye" (illustration taken from his work "Traité de l'homme," 1648)

This way of looking at consciousness paved the way for the materialism that subsequently developed. The thinking goes that since the body can function very well in an independent manner without a nonmaterial soul, which is the case for all animals other than humans according to Descartes, and since this hypothetical soul cannot be detected through any means of scientific measuring, why continue to maintain that it exists? Why not drop the whole idea?

Numerous contemporary versions of dualism have appeared that correspond to the different ways of conceptualizing the nature of consciousness, the so-called mental aspect of reality, and its ways of interfacing with matter. Many physicists belong to this school and explore quantum models of consciousness from a dualistic point of view. A case in point is the hypothesis of orchestrated objective reduction (abbreviated as Orch-OR), which says that consciousness is born through the quantum effects within subcellular structures contained in the neurons, the microtubules.

It is there that ongoing collapses of the brain's quantum wave function take place, at a rhythm of approximately 40 Hz, which corresponds to the gamma brain-wave range (Hameroff and Penrose 2014).

Idealism says that consciousness is the fundamental constituent of reality, and matter is simply an illusion appearing in the field of that consciousness. This viewpoint is in agreement with the wisdom of various spiritual traditions including certain schools of Hinduism in India such as Advaita ("nonduality"), and the Neoplatonism that arose in third-century Greece. It may seem perplexing at first—how can we imagine the Earth and the galaxies existing purely through consciousness? However, if we examine this in depth it is quite logical: all that we know of reality can only be the fabrication of our minds through the perceptions gathered from our senses. Nothing permits us to establish either philosophically or scientifically the existence of anything that could be found outside that which is of the mind. Both time and space themselves are creations of consciousness. If this is not evident to us, then it's because we are caught in the pattern of conditioning that allows us to function in this reality without really looking at it too closely.

This is a profound way of thinking about things—difficult perhaps to understand, but rich in conceptual consequences that match those found in some interpretations of quantum mechanics. According to these interpretations everything exists in a virtual state, and it is only through the collapse of the quantum wave function provoked by the conscious act of observation that this potentiality can be realized.

This view also connects with some of the most recent work in theoretical physics, which sees in elementary particles, or the basic constituents of matter, a manifestation of the principles of mathematical symmetry. Ultimately, the elementary particles would be solely composed of information, which is the property of consciousness.

Physicists in the Medley

No matter to what extent the scientific community is resistant to reintroducing consciousness to its representation of the world, it is nevertheless obliged to do so because of the discoveries of quantum mechanics. Physicists have known ever since the beginning of the twentieth century that a fundamental transition is taking place when an observer contemplates nature, for it is only in such a situation that the field of virtual quantum probabilities emerges as the macroscopic reality that we know. It is the enigmatic *measurement problem* that generations of theorists have tried to clarify.

Physicists on Consciousness

Many of the greatest physicists who have been pondering the nature of consciousness, some of whom are Nobel Prize winners, consider consciousness to be more fundamental than matter:

Max Planck: "All matter originates and exists only by virtue of a force. . . . We must assume behind this force the existence of a conscious and intelligent Mind. This Mind is the matrix of all matter."

Sir James Jeans: "The stream of knowledge is heading towards a non-mechanical reality; the universe begins to look more like a great thought than a great machine."

Erwin Schrödinger: "In all the world, there is no kind of framework within which we can find consciousness in the plural; this is simply something we construct because of the spatiotemporal plurality of individuals, but it is a false construction. . . . the self-consciousnesses of the individual members are numerically identical both with [each] other and with that Self which they may be said to form at a higher level."

David Bohm: "Deep down the consciousness of mankind is one. This is a virtual certainty because even in the vacuum matter is one; and if we don't see this it's because we are blinding ourselves to it."

Sir Arthur Eddington: "The stuff of the universe is mind-stuff. . . . The mind-stuff of the world is something more general than our individual conscious minds; but we may think of its nature as not altogether foreign to feelings in our consciousness."

"It is difficult for the matter-of-fact physicist to accept the view that the substratum of everything is of mental character. But no one can deny that mind is the first and most direct thing in our experience, and all else is remote inference."

"Physics is the study of the structure of consciousness."

Freeman Dyson: "Atoms are weird stuff, behaving like active agents rather than inert substances. They make unpredictable choices between alternative possibilities according to the laws of quantum mechanics. It appears that mind, as manifested by the capacity to make choices, is to some extent inherent in every atom. The universe is also weird, with its laws of nature that make it hospitable to the growth of mind. I do not make any clear distinction between mind and God. God is what mind becomes when it passes beyond the scale of our comprehension."

Eugene Wigner: "When the province of physical theory was extended to encompass microscopic phenomena through the creation of quantum mechanics, the concept of consciousness came to the fore again. It was not possible to formulate the laws of quantum mechanics in a fully consistent way without reference to the consciousness."

Albert Einstein: "We physicists believe the separation between past, present, and future is only an illusion, although a convincing one."

As experiments on quantum entanglement* continue to deepen the significance of this phenomenon, the quantum universe is becoming increasingly strange for physicists. Inspired by the original principle of Young's double-slit experiment (described in chapter 2) to produce entangled particles, physicists have devised experimental settings of greater and greater refinement that reveal not only the link between nonlocalized particles separated in space, but also connections that appear to transcend time. This can be seen in *delayed-choice* experiments, where a photon "chooses" its quantum state according to what will happen to its entangled partner in the future.

Faced with such recent discoveries, our ideas about time and space and the relationship between matter and consciousness are now very much put to the test. For many physicists the only viewpoint that is

---

*Quantum entanglement is a phenomenon by which two or several particles remain connected, even when they are separated from each other by great distances. A measurement of one of the particle's quantum state instantly determines the state of its entangled companions, however far apart they may be.

completely coherent with quantum mechanics is that which admits the crucial role of consciousness in physical reality.*

In fact, for some time now alternative ideas about consciousness have been embraced by physicists at the top of their field—a minority[†] perhaps, but a very significant one.

The "Hard Problem" of Consciousness

Researchers who are involved in the serious study of consciousness are concerned with two fundamental problems. The first involves how information travels through the immense cluster of neurons in the brain to form our perceptions and thoughts. This is what is called an "easy problem" of consciousness, not because it is simple to resolve, but because it belongs to the category of those dealing exclusively with mechanisms that can be specified. It is important to understand that problems of this type are the only ones being studied by neurology or by those working on the development of artificial intelligence.

The second problem is what philosopher David Chalmers (1995) calls the "hard problem." This is the mind-brain question that philosophers have been pondering since antiquity. In very simple terms it can be expressed this way: how can something that is to all evidence immaterial—mind—manage to interact with matter? For example, I have the idea of wanting to have a drink, and my hand then starts to move toward a glass. How did that original spark appear within my consciousness? How did it manifest? This question is by its very nature completely different from anything in the "easy problem" category. It has been with the hope of understanding this fundamental question that the diverse theories of consciousness have evolved. But in the end, beyond the patter of abstruse philosophical jargon and strange as it may seem, no one has any idea how to answer this question.

---

*This is the von Neumann-Wigner interpretation (in honor of its initiators, American physicists John von Neumann and Eugene Wigner), which continues to be one of the most important interpretations of quantum mechanics today.

[†]According to a 1998 study published in *Nature,* 93 percent of the most influential American scientists consider themselves nonreligious and nonspiritual, therefore subscribing to the materialist viewpoint (Larson and Witham 1998).

Matter and Consciousness:
Toward a Unified Vision

New approaches offering a more unified vision beyond the division between matter and consciousness are starting to appear. Perhaps the most coherent of these, called *panpsychism,* has been advanced by philosopher of science Ervin László (2004), among others. In this way of thinking, matter and consciousness have existed together, simultaneously, since the origin of the universe. But where this theory separates from dualism to offer a more unified vision is where it considers matter and spirit as not being radically separate, but rather two aspects of a single reality, in that matter is what we apprehend when we look at the body of a living being, and spirit is what we perceive while looking at it from the interior.

A parallel approach is that of biocentrism as expounded by American scientist Robert Lanza (and Berman 2009). Lanza says that consciousness is none other than the actual nature of all forms of life—in fact, he considers it their determining characteristic. In a reversal of the materialistic perspective, he posits that the universe was created by life itself, as a manifestation of consciousness. This identification of the unity of life and consciousness is in agreement with the conclusions of scientists studying its quantum aspects. According to physicist Mae-Won Ho (2008), life consists of a state of quantum coherence that is extended throughout an entire organism.

Other daring physicists speculate on the consequences of the unification of matter and consciousness, sketching new models of reality. Theoretical quantum physicist Amit Goswami (2001) bases his ideas on the intimate relationship between the collapse of the quantum wave function and consciousness. French physicist Philippe Guillemant (2015) has studied how the introduction of consciousness enables us to clarify the difficult paradoxes of quantum mechanics, such as those of nonlocality and indeterminism. I had the pleasure of receiving him at my home on Lake Violon when he was passing through Quebec, at which time he delighted me with his explanations of phenomena as strange as the importance of the influence of the future on the present (retrocausality) and its consequences for free will.

The nature of our own consciousness remains an enigma, maybe even more so in our age because we have a tendency to imagine that science has already explained it.*

The Mystical Experience

There is a fundamental flaw in the scientific approach to the question of consciousness: that consciousness cannot reflect on itself. Naturally, philosophers are well aware of this self-reference paradox, another aspect of the "hard problem," but they do not know how to resolve it. And in reality there is only one solution, which has been taught by sages since antiquity: Consciousness cannot be approached through thought, but it is possible to be totally immersed in it. One cannot really examine consciousness, but one can become it. This is the mystical experience, the experience of the mystic.

The only real exploration of consciousness is that which is accomplished by diving into its very source. It is an exploration that demands infinitely more determination and courage than that of the scientific approach because it implies an interior transformation. The thinker is content with an examination of the external forms and manifestations, without ever touching the essence of the mystery—an easy solution when one prefers to sidestep the deeper question.

That a plunge into the source of consciousness might at all be possible is difficult to conceive, and it remains the role of those rare persons who have managed to do so to provide testimony. Here, words and thoughts are of limited value: a direct transmission from the state to which it corresponds is by far preferable. Such a transmission can awaken an interior awareness that is already present in essence within each of us. And that is the function of the spiritual master, well known in the East but less understood in the West.

---

*Notably, many psychiatrists, considered to be professionals on the subject of consciousness, do not subscribe to the prevalent materialist viewpoint. A recent study involving 600 psychiatrists carried out in Brazil shows that nearly half of them, 47 percent, did not believe that consciousness is the product of cerebral activity. That proportion grew to 60 percent following a debate on the mind-brain question (Moreira-Almeida and Araujo 2015).

The master whom I had the unique opportunity to work with in India, Osho, shared this awareness with total impeccability, and I will be forever grateful for the extraordinary privilege available to me through this transmission. It becomes impossible to conceive of consciousness in the same way after spending those years by his side. Osho had an exquisite way of contrasting the materialist viewpoint with that of pure consciousness. He said,

> "The mystics in India have declared,
> 'Aham Brahmasmi—I am God.'
> And Skinner declares, 'I am a rat.'"

This koanlike statement alludes to the philosophy of behavioral psychologist Burrhus Frederic Skinner, for whom our consciousness can be reduced to an assembly of behaviors programmed through the brain, in the same way that it occurs in a rat. The implication is obvious: let each person choose the vision of life he or she prefers.

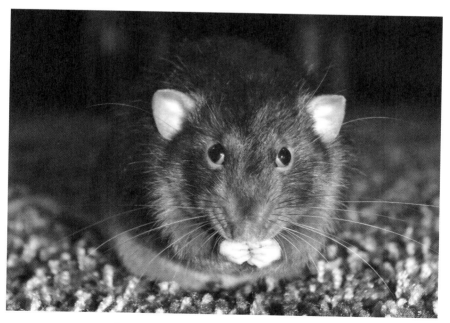

Figure 12.2. The choice is yours . . .

Encounter with Dr. Mario Beauregard

When I had occasion to meet cognitive neuroscientist Mario Beauregard in 2007, he was working at the Centre de Neuroimagerie at the University of Montréal. He had started his research on the relationship between the brain and consciousness, which led him to publish several books on the subject (Beauregard 2012). He became one of those rare researchers to scientifically study the mystical experience. He soon found himself on the frontline of what he calls the "brain wars," opposing idealist fighters and the established forces of materialism. And like many such warriors he had to pay the price. He eventually lost his employment at the University of Montréal, which did not appreciate his unorthodox research. Luckily, other centers of learning have a more open spirit, and he was welcomed at the psychology department of the University of Arizona, a forward-looking institution where the Center for Consciousness Studies is now established.

I asked Dr. Beauregard to study the effects of the Sensora on the brain, and with his assistants he proceeded to take preliminary electroencephalographic (EEG) measurements. We were not able to complete the project, but I was afforded a chance to see just how demanding research can be in this field. Basic factors such as the necessity for the subject to keep his eyes open in order to take in the light of the Sensora session interfered with the EEG measuring process, because of a phenomenon known as *alpha-blocking.* And the inconvenient and bulky electrodes of the EEG monitor, which the subject had to keep on his head all the while, were the antithesis of the gentle effects of relaxation that the light of the Sensora was trying to induce.

For Dr. Beauregard, researchers involved in neurological explorations that deal with decoding cognitive processes have to keep in mind that everything they can measure is what is known as the "neuronal correlates of consciousness," the reflection of consciousness as it appears in the brain. No one can say whether these correlates are the source of consciousness in themselves, which would reflect the materialist point of view, or merely a physical echo of a primordial cause which is nonmaterial. A frequently used analogy is that of a radio transmission (coming from consciousness) taken in by a receiving device (the brain). In this case it would be futile to try to find out where the program announcer of the radio show, whose voice originates so clearly from the appliance, is to be found among the neurons of the receiving brain.

In the opinion of most people and the majority of neuroscientists, the extraordinary images of cerebral activity obtained through functional magnetic resonance imaging (fMRI) demonstrate the material nature of consciousness since it can be photographed so clearly. But a more extensive examination of this technique (which in fact merely illustrates the density of the flow of blood in the brain) indicates that in reality this link is far from being unequivocally established (Shifferman 2015).

The Power of the Placebo

My goal in this discussion of consciousness is to awaken the reader to the concept of its precedence over matter. If consciousness is nothing other than a secondary effect or by-product of matter, as stated by the materialist viewpoint, what point is there in studying its effects on health? Surely in such a case it makes more sense to analyze biochemical processes that ultimately would be the only significant vital agents. But if we admit to the fundamental role of consciousness, then the door is open to ways of healing involving forces that are not material.

One of the most obvious examples of the capacity of our thoughts to influence healing is that of the placebo effect. In the placebo effect a person can benefit from the results of a treatment by simply being convinced of its positive influence, even if the treatment has no intrinsic value at all, such as a sugar pill. This phenomenon has another version in reverse, that of the nocebo effect, where a subject submits to a treatment that is also neutral but has a negative effect solely because the person is convinced that it is harmful.

For the pharmaceutical industry, the placebo effect is mostly seen as an annoying failing interfering with clinical research that evaluates medications—a justified view, since, for example, placebo treatments have frequently turned out to be just as effective as the best antidepressant drugs available in cases of depression (Fournier et al. 2010).

However, these implications are of major importance, incontrovertibly demonstrating the influence of our consciousness on the body—to such an extent indeed that a new branch of medicine centered on such questions has recently emerged.*

Certain placebo studies have obtained results that are quite astonishing. One of the most outstanding is that of orthopedic surgeon Bruce Moseley et al. (2002). In the 1990s, Moseley administered a fake procedure involving an arthroscopy to the knees of patients with osteoarthritis, a degenerative illness of the joints. This intervention normally consists of scraping and removing bits of cartilage by means of an incision at the knee joint, but in the fake version only the incision was carried out. Despite the highly mechanical nature of the operation, which would render it unlikely to be susceptible to subjective influence, Moseley's study showed that patients who received the fake version obtained exactly the same benefits as those who had undergone the real operation!

In another recent study the power of conviction was very clearly illustrated. Kaptchuk et al. (2010) gave a placebo to subjects with irritable bowel syndrome, and instead of concealing this from the subjects he informed them of the fact that it was indeed not real medication, telling them simply that placebo treatments have been clinically recognized as effective. This treatment, despite the disclosure, offered significant benefit to the subjects.

Color has also been found to be capable of influencing the placebo effect. In a study where three versions of the same pill, a tranquilizer colored either red, yellow, or green, were given to patients with anxiety, the green pill had significantly better results than the other ones, while patients with depressive symptoms felt better with the yellow pill (Schapira et al. 1970).

Spiritual Healing

While the placebo effect forces medicine to accept the power of the mind, it represents just the tip of the iceberg with regard to the influence

---

*The Beth Israel Deaconess Medical Center of Harvard Medical School now has a program of studies on the placebo effect.

of consciousness on health. For many spiritual practitioners the highest form of healing is spiritual, where treatment consists solely of interventions of a cognitive nature. It is practiced in many different ways across the world, and the results undoubtedly vary considerably with regard to effectiveness. At times, however, the results are almost miraculous, and the number of clinically verified cases of spiritual healing is substantial.

I myself have had occasion to experience one of the best documented of these healing practices, inspired by Bruno Gröning. This German healer, who died in 1959, carried out many healings during his lifetime. His teaching offers a spiritual technique practiced today in many countries; it consists simply of experiencing or being open to a universal healing force that connects with one's body, while at the same time relinquishing all references to illness or negative thoughts. The person must constantly maintain a positive mental attitude and a firm belief in the healing. The Bruno Gröning Circle of Friends has accumulated thousands of case studies, each one medically validated, giving testimony to spontaneous healings of a vast range of maladies and troubles of both physical and psychological origin, including illnesses considered incurable. The most noteworthy of these for me had to be the healings that occurred with people in my own immediate environment, which enabled me to believe in the reality of spiritual healing.

In this domain, where there is too little scientific validation, it is encouraging to discover the work of pioneers like Dr. Bernard Grad of McGill University, who beginning in the 1960s applied clinical protocols to the study of healing energy—a series of scientific studies that deserve to be better known.* Others have taken up the challenge, like Dr. William Bengston (and Fraser 2010, 2012), whose research shows the effectiveness of healing through the laying on of hands.

A RETURN TO LIGHT

If I allowed myself to indulge in this rather lengthy discourse on consciousness, it was only to return to our main subject, light.

---

*A forthcoming biography of Dr. Bernard Grad is due out in 2018.

Since light has such an important sensorial impact on us, we can easily understand its capacity to direct our attention and to focus our consciousness in particularly efficient ways. Techniques based on the power of light can optimize cognitive processes that have a beneficial therapeutic influence, including the placebo effect.

From the beginning of time and among all people, light has been intimately associated with consciousness. It is in itself the symbol of pure intelligence, of clarity in understanding, and of plenitude. Its immaterial quality and its fluidity are of the same nature as spirit. American physicist-philosopher Arthur Zajonc expresses it in this beautiful way: "Seeing light is a metaphor for seeing the invisible in the visible, for detecting the fragile imaginal garment that holds our planet and all existence together. Once we have learned to see the light, surely everything else will follow" (Zajonc 1993).

It is most likely that these characteristics are connected to the overriding importance of our primary sense, that of vision. Light is involved in our major source of sensory information; it is in fact our most vital link with the world of the senses. But it is also endowed with a transcendent significance that surpasses its purely sensorial role. This fact is well illustrated in a remarkable phenomenon known as the near-death experience.

The Heavenly Light

The *near-death experience* (NDE) happens when people have undergone a trauma that brings them to the point of death, after which they return once again to life. In many of these cases this occurs during a critical medical intervention that causes a temporary cessation of the metabolic activity of the brain, accompanied by the total disappearance of the EEG waves, which in principle denotes the cessation of all conscious activity.

American psychiatrist Elisabeth Kübler-Ross began research on such experiences in the 1970s, work that was subsequently assumed by researchers like Dr. Raymond Moody. These investigators accumulated numerous testimonies, many of which contain factual verifications that defy the usual explanations given to deny the nonmaterial aspect of

NDEs (Kübler-Ross 1991; Moody 1984). According to statistics, NDEs are surprisingly frequent: they have been reported by more than 4 percent of the population of the United States and Germany.

Typically, the subject of an NDE watches himself floating above his body and is able to see and hear what is happening around him. Subsequent phases may include meetings with welcoming and reassuring beings (sometimes they are parents or other family members who have died), as well as an accelerated review of the person's entire life. For many the experience culminates with the sensation of being attracted through a tunnel leading to an intense light that brings them into a different, nonphysical reality. Inevitably the NDE finishes with an abrupt return to the physical body and the reanimation of the person who has just "died."

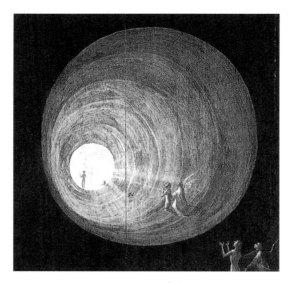

Figure 12.3. Visions of the hereafter:
The Ascent of the Blessed (detail), by Hieronymus Bosch,
1500 (Palazzo Grimani, Venice)

Whatever the interpretation of such experiences may be, the salient point for us is the identification of an experience of a transcendent nature with light, through which light acquires a numinous quality greatly surpassing that of the simple sense of vision. The testimonies are often very moving, like that of Vicki Umipeg, who nearly died in an emergency room following a car accident. She found herself out of her body, in an idyllic scene at the other end of the tunnel leading to light: "Everybody there was made of light. And I was made of light. What the light conveyed was love. There was love everywhere. It was like love came from the grass, love came from the birds, love came from the trees" (Ring and Cooper 1999). What is most amazing is that Vicki had been blind since birth! For the thirty blind subjects interviewed by psychologists Kenneth Ring and Sharon Cooper for their book *Mindsight: Near-Death and Out-of-Body Experiences in the Blind,* the perception of light from "the beyond" was very similar to that experienced by normal NDE subjects. The authors call this vision that seems to be totally separate from that of the eyes "mindsight."

Few of us are given a chance to live such a near-death experience, but all of us have deep feelings for that aspect of light that represents what is most sublime in us.

Light and Death

The majority of NDEs have a transformational effect on those who have lived through them, often altering their most intimate values at a profound level. Many of these people lose their fear of death. This acceptance is particularly rare in Western society, where there is a tendency to mask and avoid all references to death, regarded as the last taboo. But this denial of death is not universal. Many cultures consider it healthy to be fully conscious of it in everyday life. In Bhutan, a Buddhist country famous for its "gross national happiness" rating, it is considered appropriate to think of death five times a day. This may seem strange to us, but psychologists now recognize the value of such an attitude. In a recent analysis, Michael Wiederman (2015) reported that contemplating our death appears to reduce the existential anxiety we may have about it, and at the same time also brings more meaning to life.

In many spiritual traditions death is considered a key moment in our existence, which we have every interest in passing through in the most conscious way possible. Tibetans especially have developed a whole science with regard to the transition period between life and death, which is called the *bardo*. Light plays a very important role in this spiritual science, representing various aspects of existence through different colors.

A Conversation with Dr. Raymond Moody

In the summer of 2015, during a conference in Montréal, I met Raymond Moody, whose work on near-death experiences has always fascinated me. Being now more than seventy years old, he had come to a certain detachment with regard to all he had experienced through his forty years of research, and he endeavored in his presentation to give us the essence of what he had been able to take away from his many years of study.

He told us that he was totally convinced, based on everything he had learned, of the reality of a life after physical death. And as he continued his presentation he mentioned that with the methods currently at our disposal there is as yet no definitive way to establish a completely undeniable scientific proof of this reality, because for him the nature of the plane of existence reached after death is too different from that which we live in now.

At the end of his presentation I asked him the following question: "If no real proof is possible, what enabled you to be convinced beyond a doubt that this reality actually exists? Was there some special trigger factor that persuaded you?" I found his answer intriguing. "Yes, for me the trigger element in this research was the fact that some of the testimonies came from people I knew well enough to be absolutely confident about their integrity. Quite simply, I could never question what they had recounted."

I understood this situation very well, because it was the same sort of thing that enabled me to plunge into an inner adventure with a spiritual master. There are areas of life, often the most significant, where we can only find the right path through the living example of those in whom we have the greatest confidence.

I have always felt a deep affinity with Tibetan spirituality, and I was fortunate to have had close contact with two Rinpoches, the honorific title given to the teachers of that tradition. One of them,

Latri Nyima Dakpa Rinpoche, is of the original Bön tradition that existed before the arrival of Buddhism in Tibet. Being aware of our interest in light and its colors, he helped us create a session for the Sensora inspired by the Bön Bardo of Dying, which touches on the moments preceding the imminent death of the physical body. In this process the person passes through a certain number of states that correspond to the dissolution of the various layers of our being, each one presented to our perception through a particular color. It therefore lends itself ideally to a simulation in the multisensorial environment of the Sensora, where one can beautifully reproduce these colored atmospheres.

Certain people might find the idea of undergoing a therapeutic session dealing with death morbid. Is it simply that they could not understand the reason for such a process? Such a meditative experience has to do with enabling a person to clarify her own understanding when looking at death and be able to befriend its approach at the appropriate time, consciously and with ease. The session familiarizes the person with those signs that occur just before the last moments, enabling her to be more present and not be in the grip of fear when death actually comes—which of course it does inevitably! For us, such a session represents a beautiful example of the marriage between light and consciousness.

The Light of the Mind

In its most subtle aspects, light can help us at levels of our being that a purely physical treatment could not even begin to approach. At these levels we no longer seek to heal only the body, which is the domain of medicine; the emphasis is to bring healing to our connection with life itself, our most profound existential equilibrium. These levels are reached through meditation, prayer, and spiritual practice.

All of us have a certain awareness of the nonmaterial dimension of light within us. It is the same as the "mindsight" of the near-death experiences. Many ancient cultures created refined techniques based on inner visualizations of light and color and benefited from this important link between consciousness and light. My first contact with this type of technique took place shortly after my arrival in India. During a meditation retreat it was suggested that we do a series of exercises consisting of visualizing currents of colored light and to then have them circulate within the body. The technique appeared to be very sophisticated, using colors and internal channels that had been chosen with precision. The origin of this technique is not very well known, but it probably came from the Essenes, who most likely learned it from the ancient Egyptians. I remember my delight while perceiving the beauty of the colors that could be evoked in this special way, and the elegant efficiency of this energy circulation.

Techniques of a similar kind can be found in many traditions, both Eastern and Western. The yoga of India, for example, speaks of kundalini, a vital energy coiled at the base of the spine that is perceived in the form of light that travels upward through the *nadis* (energy channels distributed throughout the body, with the main ones circulating the length of the spinal column) and the *chakras* (mandala-like energy centers represented as having specific colors, numbering five or seven, or sometimes more depending on the system). The Tibetans taught me

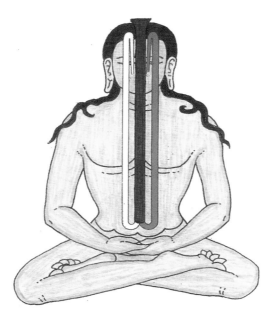

Figure 12.4. The circulation of internal energy through the visualization of colored light in the interior channels, according to the Tibetan model of the Bön tradition

wonderful techniques for the circulation of light within us, activated by means of the breath, such as the Ninefold Breath practice, which brings vitality and clarity to the spirit.

We could consider these cognitive approaches to be the purest form of light therapy. I would like to think of the Sensora as a technological attempt to materialize some of this light that is essentially of a nonmaterial origin, thereby making it accessible to a greater number of people.

Seeing Impossible Colors

Working for decades with the palette of colors synthesized through my instruments of light projection has given me occasion to learn about the different variations of color in such an intimate way that I sometimes find that our color range is too limited. This causes me to dream about new colors that until now are not known. Scottish philosopher David Hume asked the same question in 1739: Is it possible to perceive new colors? In fact, it happens to many of us that we can sense the existence of such "super colors." Occasionally in dreams one is witness to colors that are so subtle and marvelous that they appear to not belong to the material world. And sometimes in a state of meditation our interior vision manifests colors of unequaled astral purity. More directly, psychedelic drugs can stimulate the visual cortex in such a way as to create sensations that surpass the normal color range perceived by means of retinal stimulation. And intense stroboscopic pulsations such as those used in audiovisual entrainment, AVE (see chapter 10), can also generate hallucinations of iridescent colors on occasion.

Such super colors do not necessarily have an equivalent on the physical plane because they are the result of a cognitive process of a purely interior nature. However, I discovered that some researchers have managed to create some new colors. Biophysicists Vincent Biliock and Brian Tsou (2010) showed such "impossible colors" to their subjects, colors simultaneously composed of yellow and blue, or red and green—complementary pairs normally mutually exclusive for our visual system. To succeed in this endeavor it requires stringent conditions, which explains why these unusual colors are normally not perceived. These researchers used light projections composed of two adjacent colored fields, using either the yellow-blue pair or the red-green pair. To begin with they made sure that each field was isoluminous, that is, of an equally perceived intensity, which requires adjustment for each individual. Then the projection is stabilized in the visual field through a gaze-tracking electromechanical system. It is only then that the majority of subjects see, appearing before them, at the border between the two zones, colors that are totally unknown.

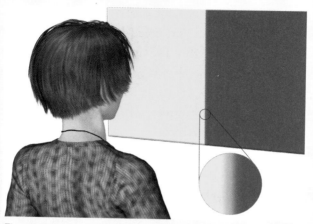

Figure 12.5. A new "impossible color," neither yellow nor blue, appears at the border between two colored zones.

Of course such experimental configurations are difficult to achieve in practice. However, to evoke almost astral-like colors from within has proved to be more accessible, and the Sensora light system now achieves this regularly with increasing success. This effect is due to a combination of factors. The use of light sources with deeply saturated colors (pure colors), soft pulsations in the brain-wave range, and fluid movements in the colored zones all contribute to generating a visual ensemble where it is easy to let oneself go and move into a more abstract world, one that is more interior. This contact with an almost heavenly dimension brings us for a moment to the *Realm of Ideas* as envisioned by Plato in his theory of forms—the idea that nonphysical (but substantial) forms (or ideas) represent the most accurate reality. We believe that such a contact, even if ephemeral, has healing powers of unsuspected depth.

Some Metaphysical Speculation

Why does light appear to us to be so close to consciousness? We can allow ourselves to speculate on the origins of this affinity, starting with what we know about the nature of light.

From the viewpoint of physics, a particle of light, a photon, is one of the only particles with no mass.* It is therefore of a purely energetic nature, without material components. And in this it already contains a mystery: how can a particle having zero mass, no material support, ever acquire energy? Einstein's theory of relativity tells us that the only way to achieve this is to move at the speed limit of our physical reality— what we call the speed of light. This speed of light is not an ordinary speed; one must not imagine that it is the same as familiar speed, just a much faster version of the speed at which material objects travel. In fact, it creates a mysterious boundary in our universe where time and space come together and split according to the equations of relativity. It transforms the very nature of physical reality.

The theory of relativity states that the closer an object gets to reaching the speed of light, the more time slows down and distances start shrinking, from its viewpoint. And if it actually attains the speed of light, something incredible happens: for the object, time stops and distances are no longer. And it is in this inconceivable reality that the photon exists. If time has stopped and distances have disappeared, we could say that the photon is simultaneously everywhere in the universe; at least for itself, time and space no longer exist.

But isn't it just this quality that we assign to consciousness, this existence that does not depend on space and time? Consciousness and light thus appear to share the same existential realm.

ENLIGHTENMENT

For all the peoples of the Earth, light is associated with what they conceive to be the most sublime and the most divine. The "clear light of

---

*The other null-mass particles are gluons, the carrier particles of the strong interaction, but they are forever confined to the interior of the atomic nucleus and inaccessible to our perception. The carrier particle of gravity, the graviton, might also have a null mass, but it remains hypothetical.

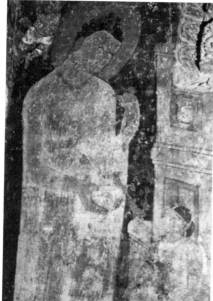
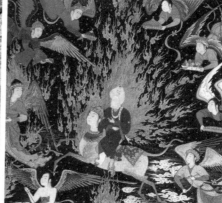
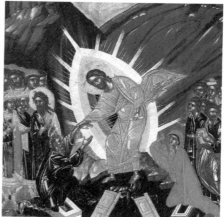

Figure 12.6. Auras and halos, signs of the sacred: (clockwise) some examples from Buddhism (the Buddha with a begging bowl), Islam (the ascension of Mohammed), and Christianity (the apparition of Jesus)

the soul," as it is called in the Tibetan Vajrayana tradition, manifests in the form of auras and halos surrounding the sages and saints of all the traditions.

Tibetans speak of the rainbow body phenomenon, a transfiguration that occurs when great masters die and their physical body transforms into light. It is said that this dissolution takes place over a period of days, during which time rays of multicolored light radiate from where the corpse of the deceased is resting. After some more time no traces of the body can be found. To us this might seem incredible, but for the Tibetans it is quite real. Nyima Dakpa Rinpoche told me that there are still some people in Tibet who have seen such things with their own eyes.

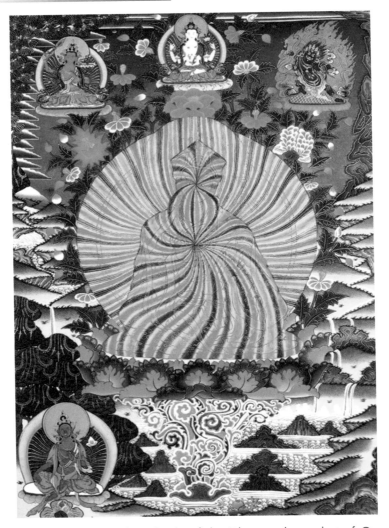

Figure 12.7. The rainbow body of the Tibetans; here, that of Guru Rinpoche ("Precious Guru"), Padmasambhava, who brought Buddhism to Tibet in the eighth century CE (© www.thangkar.com)

The association between consciousness and light can be found most significantly in those traditions that use the word *enlightenment* to describe the highest mystical state of consciousness, a way of always identifying it in terms of light. This identification with light is magnificently expressed in these words by Osho (1985, 1986):

Enlightenment simply means an experience of your consciousness unclouded by thoughts, emotions, sentiments. When the consciousness is totally empty, there is something like an explosion, an atomic explosion. Your whole insight becomes full of a light which has no source and no cause. . . . I must have come across hundreds of mystics describing it as if suddenly thousands of suns have risen within you. That is a common expression in the mystic's language, in all languages, in different countries, in different races.

The experience of ultimate consciousness, then, is one of a "thousand suns."

We all have an innate sense of the divine, which we may have the privilege of touching in special moments. These moments are those that give a real sense of meaning to life. And it is always in these moments that light will accompany us, our precious life-giving source.

POSTFACE

IT ALL STARTED this way:

It acted like a bolt of lightning on my consciousness, a stunning and unexpected experience that's etched in my memory to this very day. It began as a result of reading one simple sentence in a leaflet with a few of the master's sayings, which had found its way to me through a fortuitous sequence of events. I was only sixteen, but I had been given to introspection since childhood. Starting at age twelve, entranced by the cantatas of Bach, who in some way was my first master, I found myself initiated into the ecstasies of the inner world. A little later I discovered a second master in Einstein. I was fascinated by the perspective of a man who by the power of thought alone was able to unlock the fundamental mysteries surrounding the nature of time and space, and by so doing transform the understanding of the material world for all humankind.

It was not surprising, then, that I felt attracted by a calling to study theoretical physics. By then I had started at the University of Montréal. This time of my life was a period filled with contentment, and I had the impression of having at last found my rightful place in academia. The oppressive atmosphere of high school was gone. No longer did I feel isolated and somewhat of a stranger, having been much younger than my comrades.

Influenced by my older brother Eric, I had for some time already developed a passionate interest in the Buddha, who became my third master. He represented the ultimate example of perfection to which a person can aspire. Through the piercing clarity of his inward gaze

330

Buddha reached to the very source of consciousness wherein a state of indissoluble balance and harmony exists without end. As the writings of Zen Buddhist teacher D. T. Suzuki led me to the discovery of the lives and words of great masters such as Hui-Neng, Hakuin, and others, I felt the nostalgia of separation from their penetrating presences that had been created by the distance of centuries. It was precisely that presence that struck me as I read the little leaflet I held in my hands that day. Without being able to explain it I knew with certainty that its author *knew* what he was talking about: that he spoke from a direct experience of reality rather than merely repeating ideas and conjectures taken from mind, as all of us do. Here was a real, living spiritual master, just like those ancient Zen masters, someone I could actually see in person! In an instant I understood without a single doubt that I had to meet him.

It would take me two years to raise the necessary money for a voyage to India, a far from trivial undertaking for a young student. Even if they were unable to completely understand the need for this sojourn, my parents had sufficient confidence in me to respect my determination, and for that I will always admire their remarkable openness of spirit. Although they gave me financial support for my studies, I nonetheless had to take responsibility for financing my pilgrimage.

It was thus that in 1976, at the age of eighteen, I became a disciple of Osho. Until the death of the master in 1990, I alternated between periods spent with him in India and return voyages to the West, where my unusual career started to take form. I applied myself first to my studies in physics, thus acquiring a solid scientific base that was to be indispensable for my later work. Placing particular emphasis on quantum mechanics and general relativity, I specialized in astrophysics.

I completed my master's degree, which dealt with the diffusion of helium gas in stellar atmospheres. I explored in detail the incredible route taken by light, where each photon born of nuclear fusion in the heart of a sun leaps from atom to atom during hundreds of thousands of years within the gigantic mass of the star, to finally emerge at its surface—a journey that would have taken only seconds in the void. Although tempted to begin a doctorate, the path of meditation that I had already embarked on had created too big a distance from conventional values, so that I could no longer conceive of a career in academia, which now felt too restrictive. So I decided to become an independent researcher, dedicating my efforts to a field that life had patiently prepared me for: the application of science and technology to the service of consciousness. An independent researcher is wise to choose an area of endeavor that has only been studied in a limited way, and this would surely qualify as such. At that time I could not have known that this was to bring me eventually to an in-depth exploration of light, since this latter, which lends itself with such ease to manipulation through technology, offers a royal path toward the expansion of consciousness.

> I am seated on the ground, at the feet of the master. After two years of single-minded pursuit, I have reached the long-sought objective. At last I am here in India, in the very courtyard of his home. The evening is heady with the scents of bewitching perfumes. Sweet, unfamiliar natural sounds of the night, so unique to this paradoxical country, gently enfold me. It is May, and the heat is suffocating. In my naivete I had not known that I was arriving at a time when it was at its most scorching, just preceding the eagerly awaited giver of relief, the monsoon. But what difference does it make? In this moment so rich, so full, such details are of no real consequence . . .

That first night in India I came face-to-face with the vortex of energy of the master. His emanation was of such intensity that everything at the periphery of his presence seemed to disappear, as if drawn into the gravitational horizon of a black hole. And when I closed my eyes I was bathed in an ineffable interior iridescence, my first contact with the most mysterious dimension of light . . .

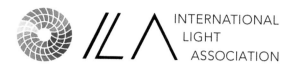

The International Light Association is a nonprofit organization registered in Belgium. It consists of a diverse group of people, some with a professional interest in light and color, and some with a personal or creative connection to light. Some members are light-therapy practitioners and health professionals, while others are scientists and educators. Creative ILA members include artists, architects, and designers. Many have no professional role in using light, but they do have a deep connection with light and color and an appreciation of their effects on our health and well-being, and on the world around us.

Beyond these individual interests, all ILA members have a common desire to share knowledge, skills, and passions; to learn about and apply the latest theories, techniques, and technologies in light and color; and to use this knowledge to promote health, enhance performance and learning, and raise consciousness.

Founded in Belgium at the 2003 Light Medicine Conference, the ILA held its first meeting in a building adjacent to Rubenshuis, in Antwerp. The inspiration for the original logo comes from a beautiful window designed by the seventeenth-century artist Peter Paul Rubens for his house. Overlooking the garden, Rubens's window reflects the sun with mathematical precision and artistic skill, creating a unique metaphor for Antwerp as the "City of Diamonds" and also making a profound statement about the nature of light.

The ILA mission is to share and disseminate information; educate, initiate, and promote research; and create an open-hearted, broad-minded, integrative community in the field of light. A collection of over fifty videos from the ILA conferences on light therapy is available on the ILA YouTube Channel: www.youtube.com/user/ilacolor1.

All those with an interest in light for health are welcome to join by becoming a member of the ILA.

www.international-light-association.org

GLOSSARY

Abbreviations

Hz (hertz)

J/cm² (joules per square centimeter)

K (kelvin)

lm (lumens)

lm/W (lumens per watt)

nm (nanometer, one billionth of a meter)

μV (microvolts)

μW/m² (microwatts per square meter)

actinotherapy: Therapy that uses the ultraviolet part of the light spectrum.

action spectrum: The curve of sensitivity versus wavelength of a light-sensitive biochemical entity (for example, photoreceptors, known as rods and cones, in the eye).

audiovisual entrainment (AVE): Therapy modality combining light and sound pulses to entrain brain waves.

biophoton: A photon (light particle) emitted by a living organism. Biophotons are a manifestation of ultraweak photon emission (UPE).

black body: A nonreflecting object that shines from its own heat.

blue light hazard (BLH): Measure of the risk of damage to the retinal photoreceptors caused by higher-energy photons, particularly those of the deep blue wavelengths ranging from 420 to 470 nm.

boson: In the Standard Model of particle physics, these are the particles that carry the four forces (gravity, electromagnetism, and strong and weak interactions) acting between particles of matter.

brain waves: Small electrical signals emitted by the brain. Brain waves span a range of roughly 1 to 100 Hz. Their frequency bands correspond to specific mental states (delta, theta, alpha, beta, gamma).

bright light therapy: Therapy that uses intense light sources to influence one's chronobiology (often erroneously identified as *light therapy* in common literature).

Chromatothérapie: Therapeutic use of colored light according to a strict protocol based on a diagnosis that is both medical and energetic.

chromophores: Living molecules capable of interacting with light, through either absorbing or reflecting it. Rhodopsin and photopsin contain such molecules.

chromotherapy: Therapies which use the specific influences of different colors from the visual spectrum.

chronobiology: The science of biological rhythms controlled by the cycle of the sun.

circadian: Designates the rhythm of a biological process that follows the 24-hour cycle of the day.

coherence: Occurs when waves from multiple sources are synchronized. This unifies a group of particles from a quantum point of view.

color: A property of light, created by our visual system. It is mainly dependent on the wavelength of the perceived light.

colorimetry: The science of quantifying color and human color perception.

Colorpuncture: Chromotherapy method applying colored light on acupuncture points.

color rendering index (CRI): A measure of the capacity of a light source to accurately reproduce the colors of objects on which it shines. Sunlight has a perfect CRI value of 100, while typical LED bulbs have a CRI of 70 to 85.

color temperature: Applied to a light source, it is the temperature of the black body spectrum closest to the light source spectrum. Also called **correlated color temperature (CCT).**

cones: Photoreceptors of the eye mainly located in the central portion of the retina known as the macula. In the human eye, there are three varieties of cones, each sensitive to a different part of the light spectrum (red, green and blue), enabling us to perceive color.

dissipative structures theory: This theory bridges general systems theory and the second law of thermodynamics and added to the understanding of subtle energy. It states that the only state of equilibrium reached by living beings is that of constant nonequilibrium sustained through ongoing interactions with the environment.

Emotional Transformation Therapy (ETT): A form of psychotherapy based on brain stimulation through the visual pathway that resolves emotional distress within minutes or even seconds.

endogenous phototherapy: Types of phototherapy that make use of the natural interactions light has within the body.

energy medicine: Medicine that views life in terms of its interactions with energy fields (electromagnetic or otherwise), rather than through biochemical interactions as in conventional medicine.

entrainment: The natural tendency of the brain to enter into resonance with a sensorial stimulus.

fermion: In the Standard Model of particle physics, these are the particles that comprise matter.

flicker fusion frequency: The maximum flicker frequency that our visual system is capable of perceiving. Depending on the individual, flicker fusion frequency is in the order of 50 to 90 Hz. Above that frequency, the eye stops perceiving flicker.

Fraunhofer lines: Gaps in the solar spectrum corresponding to absorption of light at specific wavelengths by atomic elements within the sun.

frequency: Number of oscillations per second of a vibrating phenomenon. Applied to light, it is a measure of the number of cycles per second of the electromagnetic wave that is light. Light wavelength and frequency are inversely proportional.

general systems theory: A methodology that attempts to understand complex phenomena based on basic organizing principles, this theory shows how basic inanimate elements can self-assemble into an emergent order, as is the case in living beings.

gluon: A type of boson involved in the strong interaction required for cohesion of the nucleus.

graviton: A type of boson hypothesized to carry the gravitional force.

harmonic: A frequency that is an exact multiple of a base frequency. Waves that are harmonically related can combine and lead to resonance and coherence.

heart rate variability (HRV): Measure of the variations of the heartbeat rhythms, obtained by taking samples of the precise timing of a subject's heartbeat over several minutes. HRV offers measures of psychophysiological aspects related to positive emotions and well-being, such as cardiac coherence.

heliotherapy: Therapy that employs the light of the sun.

homeostasis: The process of autoregulation by which a living organism maintains its integrity in the midst of the surrounding chaos in which it exists. Homeostatis is a key component of health.

hypothalamus: Cerebral area located at the center of the brain, known as "the brain within the brain," that integrates the information originating from all of our main systems: nervous, endocrine and immune.

intensity: Brightness level of a light source, proportional to the number of photons emitted.

intrinsically photosensitive retinal ganglion cells (ipRGC): Ganglion cells of the nonvisual optic pathway that contribute to synchronizing biological activity with the light of the sun.

lateral light therapy: A form of chromotherapy applying complementary colors to each half of the visual field to rebalance the dominance of one brain hemisphere over the other.

light noise: Designates random variations that disturb the purity and stability of a light source; for example, resulting in flickering. Sources having high light noise can cause detrimental side effects in sensitive people, such as migraines or eye strain.

living matrix: The collective assembly of matter, energy, and spontaneous organization that is the source of all living organisms. A living matrix is a network that is simultaneously mechanical, vibrational (capable of oscillation), energetic, electronic, and informational.

luminophore: Phosphorescent materials that convert photons from one part of the light spectrum to another; for example, ultraviolet photons into photons of a visible color as used in fluorescent tubes.

lumen: Unit of luminous flux, a measure of the quantity of visible light emitted by a source.

lux: A unit of illumination equal to one lumen per square meter.

mallilumination: A health concern arising from deprivation of the full spectrum of natural sunlight.

melanopsin: A type of photopigment found in ganglion cells that react mostly to light in the blue part of the spectrum.

MIL therapy: "Magneto Infrared Laser," a form of therapy combining light with magnetic fields to augment the effects of each modality.

monochromatic: Light having photons of the same wavelength.

near-death experience (NDE): Frequently life-altering experiences, these happen when people have undergone a trauma that brings them to the point of death, after which they return once again to life. During NDEs the person remains conscious while seemingly outside of the body.

neuroplasticity: The ability of the brain to reorganize itself through the formation of new neuronal connections throughout the length of a person's life.

neurotransmitter: Chemical compound liberated by the neurons to ensure and regulate communication throughout the brain. There are about one hundred different types of neurotransmitters, some of which are susceptible to the influence of light.

NIF optic pathway: "Non-Image-Forming" visual pathway, the part of the optic nerve linking ipRGCs to the hypothalamus (also known as **nonvisual optic pathway** or **retinohypothalmic tract**).

NILT: "Near-Infrared Laser Transmission," a form of light therapy applying light through the cranium (also known as **transcranial light therapy**).

nonlocality: Two particles issuing from a common source and in interlinked quantum states that can be described by a shared wave function are said to be *entangled*. Observing one of the particles, and therefore identifying its quantum state, instantly determines the state of the other particle independently of their locations.

nonvisual optic pathway: The part of the optic nerve that links the retina to the hypothalamus, responsible for the chronobiological influence of light.

opsin: Proteins in the body that are sensitive to light.

particle physics: A branch of physics that studies the constituents of matter and radiation and their interactions.

photic entrainment: In this phenomenon, the brain, when exposed to the external stimulus of a pulsating light, has a natural tendency to generate brain waves that resonate with the external stimulus.

photobiology: Aspects of biology that are influenced by light.

photobiomodulation: The process that describes the regenerative action of light on our cells.

photon: A type of boson that mediates the electromagnetic force between fermions. Also, a particle of light.

photopic: A process that is related to the properties of the human visual system under normal well-lit conditions.

photopsins: A type of protein sensitive to light that is found in the eye, particularly in the red, blue, and green cones.

phototherapy: Therapy that depends on artificial sources of light.

Planck's constant: The factor of proportionality in the equation that links the energy of a light quanta (photon) with its frequency.

polarization: The orientation of the electric and magnetic fields that make up the electromagnetic wave that is light. This orientation can be linear (in a specific axis) or circular (constantly rotating).

pulse-width modulation (PWM): Electronic method used to control the brightness of LEDs through a digital "chopping" of the LED current. PWM leads to high **light noise**.

quantum electrodynamics: The modern theory of electromagnetic interaction that describes the attraction or repulsion between electrically charged particles caused by the pressure of virtual photons, evanescent particles that quickly emerge and disappear from a surrounding vacuum.

quantum entanglement: a phenomenon by which two or several particles remain connected, even when they are separated from each other in time or space.

quantum field theory: The theory that describes the four forces of interaction between fermions transported by bosons.

quantum mechanics: Quantum mechanics is a description of the world of elementary particles in terms of their probability distribution of all possible states within a given system. The instant a particle emerges from the virtual world of probabilities into our world of the observable, the link between quantum reality and macroscopic reality is established.

resonance: Physical phenomenon wherein a system possessing the ability to vibrate at a certain frequency is stimulated by an external signal of the same frequency.

rhodopsin: A type of protein sensitive to light that is found in the rods of the eyes.

rods: Photoreceptors of the eye that cover the entire surface of the retina, they help us see peripherally and at night.

saturation: The purity of a color. Pure colors contain fully saturated light of monochromatic frequency.

Schumann resonance: The natural phenomenon whereby the frequency of the stationary electromagnetic field surrounding our planet is around 7.83 Hz.

seasonal affective disorder (SAD): A form of depression mostly occurring during winter months, caused by a chronic lack of sunlight. SAD can be efficiently remedied by **bright light therapy**.

Spectro-Chrome: Chromotherapy system created in the 1920s by Dinshah Ghadiali, in which colored light is applied to large areas of the skin.

Standard Model: In particle physics, the current theory classifying all known elementary particles as well as their interactions through force fields.

suprachiasmatic nucleus (SCN): Cerebral area within the **hypothalamus** that governs our internal clock. The SCN is susceptible to the influence of light through the **nonvisual optic pathway**.

synthetic color: A color that does not match with any actual physical color within the rainbow spectrum; also known as **extra-spectral color**. Magenta (obtained by mixing red and blue) is an example of a synthetic color, as it is not found in the rainbow.

synthetic phototherapy: Types of phototherapies that use light as a catalyst in custom-made biological processes.

syntonic phototherapy: A therapy that applies light through the eyes to restore balance within the body's regulatory centers, particularly to correct visual dysfunctions.

thought experiment: A thought experiment considers some hypothesis, theory, or principle for the purpose of thinking through its consequences. It may not be possible to perform it, and even if it could be performed there need not be the intention to do so.

ultraweak photon emission (UPE): A phenomenon that shows living organisms emit light.

visual optic pathway: The part of the optic nerve that links the retina to the visual cortex in the brain, enabling the sense of vision.

wavelength: The distance between two peaks of the electromagnetic wave that is light. In human vision the wavelength of a light source determines its color. Wavelengths in the visible spectrum span a range of 380 to 760 nanometers (billionth of a meter). Light frequency and wavelength are inversely proportional.

REFERENCES

Adey, Ross W. 1990. Electromagnetic Fields and the Essence of Living Systems, in *Modern Radio Science,* 1–36. Oxford, UK: Oxford University Press.

Adolph, Edward F. 1982. "Physiological Integrations in Action." *Physiologist* 25 (2). Suppl.

Agrapart, Christian. 2016. *Se soigner par les couleurs: Guide pratique de la chromatothérapie.* France: Sully.

Agrapart, Christian, and Michèle Delmas. 2011. *Guide thérapeutique des couleurs.* Labege, France: Dangles.

Ahn, Andrew C., Agatha P. Colbert, Belinda J. Anderson, Ørjan G. Martinsen, Richard Hammerschlag, Steve Cina, Peter M. Wayne, and Helene M. Langevin. 2008. "Electrical Properties of Acupuncture Points and Meridians: A Systematic Review." *Bioelectromagnetics* 29 (4): 245–56.

Albarracin, Rizalyn, Janis T. Eells, and Krisztina Valter. 2011. "Photobiomodulation Protects the Retina from Light-induced Photoreceptor Degeneration." *Investigative Ophthalmology and Visual Science* 52 (6): 3582–92.

Alotaibi, Mohammad A., Mark Halaki, and Chin-Moi Chow. 2016. "A Systematic Review of Light Therapy on Mood Scores in Major Depressive Disorder: Light Specification, Dose, Timing, and Delivery." *International Journal of Basic and Applied Sciences* 5 (1): 30–37. Supp. no. l.

ANSES. 2010. *Effets sanitaires des systèmes d'éclairage utilisant des diodes électro-luminescentes (LED).* Maisons Alfort, France: Agence Nationale de Sécurité Sanitaire de l'Alimentation, de l'Environnement et du Travail.

Avci, Pinar, Gaurav K. Gupta, Jason Clark, Norbert Wikondal, and Michael Hamblin. 2014. "Low-Level Laser (Light) Therapy (LLLT) for Treatment of Hair Loss." *Lasers in Surgery and Medicine* 46 (2): 144–51.

Azzouzi, Abdel-Rahmène, Sébastien Vincendeau, Eric Barret, Antony Cicco, François Kleinclauss, Henk G. van der Poel, Christian G. Stief, et al. 2016.

"Padeliporfin Vascular-Targeted Photodynamic Therapy Versus Active Surveillance in Men with Low-Risk Prostate Cancer (CLIN1001 PCM301): An open-label, phase 3, randomised controlled trial.", *Lancet Oncology* 18 (2): 181–91.

Baldwin, Kate. 1927. "Therapeutic Value of Light and Color." *Atlantic Medical Society Journal.* April.

Barrett, Douglas W., and F. Gonzalez-Lima. 2013. "Transcranial Infrared Laser Stimulation Produces Beneficial Cognitive and Emotional Effects in Humans." *Neuroscience* 29 (230):13–23.

Beauregard, Mario. 2012. *Brain Wars: The Scientific Battle over the Existence of the Mind and the Proof That Will Change the Way We Live Our Lives.* New York: HarperOne.

Becker, Robert O. 1991. "Evidence for a Primitive DC Electrical Analog System Controlling Brain Functions." *Subtle Energies* 2 (1): 71–88.

Bello, Y.M., and TJ Phillips. 2000. "Recent Advances in Wound Healing." *JAMA.* 283 (6): 716–18.

Bengston, William. 2012. "Crossing Disciplinary Boundaries: Going Beyond Even Meta-Analysis on Distant Intention." *Journal of Alternative and Complementary Medicine* 18 (6): 525–26.

Bengston, William, and Sylvia Fraser. 2010. *The Energy Cure: Unraveling the Mystery of Hands-On Healing.* Louisville, Co.: Sounds True.

Berson, David M., Felice A. Dunn, and Takao Motoharu. 2002. "Photo-transduction by Retinal Ganglion Cells That Set the Circadian Clock." *Science* 295 (5597): 1070–73.

Bien, Julianne. 2014. *Color Therapy for Animals.* Spectrahue Light and Sound Inc.
———. 2004. *Golden Light: A Journey with Advanced Colorworks.* Spectrahue Light and Sound Inc.

Biliock, Vincent A., and Brian H. Tsou. 2010. "Impossible Colors: See Hues That Can't Exist." *Scientific American* 302: 72–77.

Bioinitiative Report. 2012. "A Rationale for Biologically-Based Exposure Standards for Low-Intensity Electromagnetic Radiation." www.bioinitiative.org.

Bischof, Marco. 2003. Introduction to Integrative Biophysics, in *Integrative Biophysics,* 1–116. The Netherlands: Kluwer Academic Publishers.
———. 2005. "Biophotons—The Light in Our Cells." *Journal of Optometric Phototherapy.* http://zeniclinic.com/zen/articles/Biophotons.pdf.
———. 2008. *Biophotonen: Das licht, das unseren zellen* (in German). Frankfurt, Germany: Zweitausendeins Verlag.

Bocquenet, Jean-Philippe. 2010. Les mèmes et l'émergence de la culture (in French). Essay published at http://post.sapiens.free.fr/?p=187.

Brainard, George C., John P. Hanifin, Jeffrey Greeson, Brenda Byrne, Gena

Glickman, E. Gerner, and Mark Rollag. 2001. "Action Spectrum for Melatonin Regulation in Humans: Evidence for a Novel Circadian Photoreceptor." *Journal of Neuroscience* 21 (16): 6405–12.

Breiling, Brian, ed. 1996. *Light Years Ahead: The Illustrated Guide to Full Spectrum and Colored Light in Mindbody Healing.* Berkley, Ca.: Celestial Arts.

Buhr, Ethan D., Wendy W. S. Yue, Xiaozhi Ren, Zheng Jiang, Hsi-Wen Rock Liao, Xue Mei, Shruti Vemaraju, et al. 2015. "Neuropsin (OPN5)-Mediated Photoentrainment of Local Circadian Oscillators in Mammalian Retina and Cornea." *Proceedings of the National Academy of Science* 112 (42): 13093–98.

Cade, Maxwell, and Nona Coxhead. 1979. *The Awakened Mind: Biofeedback and the Development of Higher States of Awareness.* New York: Element Books.

CELMA-ELC. 2011. "Position Paper on Optical Safety of LED Lighting." LED WG(SM)011 ELC CELMA. https://www.myledlightingguide.com/white papers/CELMA-ELC_LED_WG(SM)011_ELC_CELMA_position_paper _optical_safety_LED_lighting_Final_1st_Edition_July2011.pdf.

Chalmers, David. 1995. "Facing Up To the Problem of consciousness." *Journal of Consciousness Studies* 2 (3): 200–19.

Chang, Anne-Marie, Daniel Aeschbacha, Jeanne F. Duffya, and Charles A. Czeislera. 2015. "Evening Use of Light-Emitting eReaders Negatively Affects Sleep, Circadian Timing, and Next-Morning Alertness." *Proceedings of the National Academy of Sciences* 112 (4): 1232–37.

Cho, Zang Hee, S. C. Chung, J. P. Jones, J. B. Park, Hi-Joon Park, Hong J. Lee, Edward K. Wong, and B. I. Min. 1998. "New Findings of the Correlation between Acupoints and Corresponding Brain Cortices Using fMRI." *Proceedings of the National Academy of Sciences* 95 (5): 2670–73.

Chuprikov A. P., V. N. Linev, and I. A. Martsenkovskii. 1993. "Lateral Photo-therapy in Somatoform Mental Disorders" (in Russian). *Lik Sprava* (10–12): 56–59. https://www.ncbi.nlm.nih.gov/pubmed/8030309.

Chuprikov A. P. et al. 1994. *Lateral Therapy—Guide for Therapists* (in Russian). Kiev: Zdorovja.

Chu-Tan, Joshua A., Matt Rutar, Kartik Saxena, Yunlu Wu, Lauren Howitt, Krisztina Valter, Jan Provis, and Riccardo Natoli. 2016. "Efficacy of 670 nm Light Therapy to Protect Against Photoreceptor Cell Death is Dependent on the Severity of Damage." *International Journal of Photoenergy* 2016: 1–12.

Cifra, Michal, Christian Brouder, Michaela Nerudova, and Ondrej Kucera. 2015. "Biophotons, Coherence and Photocount Statistics: A Critical Review." *Journal of Luminescence* 164: 38–51.

Cooper, Primrose. 2000. *The Healing Power of Light: A Comprehensive Guide to the Healing and Transformational Power of Light.* New York: Piatkus Books/ Little Brown Book Group.

Corongiu, Giorgina and Enrico Clementi. 1981. "Simulations of the Solvent Structure for Macromolecules." *Biopolymers* 20 (3): 551–71.

Damasio, Antonia. 2010. *Self Comes to Mind: Constructing the Conscious Brain.* New York: Vintage.

Darlot, Fannie, Cecile Moro, Nabil El Massri, Claude Chabrol, Daniel M. Johnstone, Florian Reinhart, Diane Agay, et al. 2016. "Near-Infrared Light is Neuroprotective in a Monkey Model of Parkinson Disease." *Annals of Neurology* 79 (1): 59–75.

Davydov, Alexander S. 1987. "Excitons and Solitons in Molecular Systems." *International Review of Cytology* 106: 183–225. http://www.sciencedirect.com/science/article/pii/S0074769608617131.

Delmas, Michèle. 2010. *Quand la couleur guérit: Psychologie et chromothératie.* France: Guy Trédaniel éditeur.

Deppe, Adolph. 2013. *Therapy with Light, a Practitioner's Guide.* Strategic Book Publishing.

Dinshah, Darius. 2012. *Let There be Light.* Malaga, N.J.: Dinshah Health Society.

Doidge, Norman, MD. 2007. *The Brain That Changes Itself: Stories of Personal Triumph from the Frontiers of Brain Science.* New York: Viking.

———. 2016. *The Brain's Way of Healing: Remarkable Discoveries and Recoveries from the Frontiers of Neuroplasticity.* New York: Penguin.

Dowling, John E. 1987. *The Retina: An Approachable Part of the Brain.* Cambridge, Mass.: Belknap Press of Harvard University Press.

Ecker, Jennifer, Olivia N. Dumitrescu, Kwoon Y. Wong, Nazia M. Alam, Shih-Kuo Chen, Tara LeGates, Jordan M. Renna, Glen T. Prusky, David M. Berson, and Samer Hattar. 2010. "Melanopsin-Expressing Retinal Ganglion-Cell Photoreceptors: Cellular Diversity and Role in Pattern Vision." *Neuron* 67 (1): 49–60.

Edelhäuser, Friedrich, Florian Hak, Ulrich Kleinrath, Birgit Lühr, Peter F. Matthiessen, Johannes Weinzirl, and Dirk Cysarz. 2013. "Impact of Colored Light on Cardiorespiratory Coordination." *Evidence-Based Complementary and Alternative Medicine.* Article ID 810876.

Eells, Janis T., Michele M. Henry Salzman, P. Summerfelt, M. T. T. Wong-Riley, E. V. Buchmann, M. Kane, N. T. Whelan, and Harry Whelan. 2003. "Therapeutic Photobiomodulation for Methanol-Induced Retinal Toxicity." *Proceedings of the National Academy of Sciences* 100 (6): 3439–44.

Fisher, Robert S., Graham Harding, Giuseppe Erba, Gregory L. Barkley, and Arnold Wilkins. 2005. "Photic-and-Pattern-Induced Seizures: A Review for the Epilepsy Foundation of America Working Group." *Epilepsia* 46 (9): 1426–41.

Foster, Russel G., Ignacio Provencio, D. Hudson, S. Fiske, W. De Grip, and M. Menaker. 1991. "Circadian Photoreception in the Retinally Degenerate Mouse" (rd/rd). *Journal of Comparative Physiology* 169 (1): 39–50.

Fournier, J. C., R. J. DeRubeis, S. D. Hollon, S. Dimidjian, J. D. Amsterdam, R. C. Shelton, J. Fawcett. 2010. "Antidepressant Drug Effects and Depression Severity: A Patient-Level Meta-Analysis." *JAMA*. 303 (1): 47–53.

Franze, Kristian, Jens Grosche, Serguei N. Skatchkov, Stefan Schinkinger, Christian Foja, Detlev Schild, Ortrud Uckermann, Kort Travis, Andreas Reichenbach, and Jochen Guck. 2007. "Müller Cells Are Living Optical Fibers in the Vertebrate Retina." *Proceedings of the National Academy of Sciences* 104 (20): 8287–92.

Frederick, Jon A., Joel F. Lubar, Howard W. Rasey, Sheryl A. Brim, and Jared Blackburn. 1999. "Effects of 18.5 Hz Auditory and Visual Stimulation on EEG Amplitude at the Vertex." *Journal of Neurotherapy* 3 (3-4): 23–27.

Friedmann, Harry, Anat Lipovsky, Y. Nitzan, and Rachel Lubart. 2009. "Combined Magnetic and Pulsed Laser Fields Produce Synergistic Acceleration of Cellular Electron Transfer." *Laser Therapy* 18 (3): 137–41.

Frölich, Herbert, ed. 1988. *Biological Coherence and Response to External Stimuli.* Berlin: Springer-Verlag.

Gascoyne, Peter R. C., Ronald Pethig, and Albert Szent-Györgyi. 1981. "Water Structure-Dependent Charge Transport in Proteins." *Proceedings of the National Academy of Sciences* 78 (1): 261–65.

Ghadiali, Dinshah. 1933. *Spectro-Chrome Metry Encyclopedia.* Malaga, N.J.: Dinshah Health Society.

Glickman, Gena, John P. Hanifin, Mark Rollag, Jenny Wang, Howard Cooper, and George C. Brainard. 2003. "Inferior Retinal Light Exposure is More Effective Than Superior Retinal Exposure in Suppressing Melatonin in Humans." *Journal of Biological Rhythms* 18 (1): 71–79.

Godar, Dianne. 2011. "Worldwide Increasing Incidences of Cutaneous Malignant Melanoma." *Journal of Skin Cancer* 2011. Article ID 858425.

Golden, Robert N., Bradley Gaynes, R. David Ekstrom, Robert M. Hamer, Frederick Jacobsen, Trisha Suppes, Katherine Leah Wisner, and Charles B. Nemeroff. 2005. "The Efficacy of Light Therapy in the Treatment of Mood Disorders: A Review and Meta-Analysis of the Evidence." *American Journal of Psychiatry* 162 (4): 656–62.

Gooley, Joshua J., Ivan Ho Mien, Melissa A. St. Hilaire, Sing-Chen Yeo, Eric Chern-Pin Chua, Eliza van Reen, Catherine J. Hanley, Joseph T. Hull, Charles A. Czeisler, and Steven W. Lockley. 2012. "Melanopsin and Rod-Cone Photoreceptors Play Different Roles in Mediating Pupillary Light Responses During Exposure to Continuous Light in Humans." *Journal of Neuroscience* 32 (41): 14242–53.

Goswami, Amit. 2001. *Physics of the Soul: The Quantum Book of Living, Dying, Reincarnation, and Immortality.* Charlottesville, Va.: Hampton Roads Publishing.

Gottlieb, Ray, and Larry Wallace. 2011. Syntonic Phototherapy. *Journal of the International Light Association* Sept.: 8–15.

Grashorn, Michael A. and U. Egerer. 2007. "Integrated Assessment of Quality of Chicken Organic Eggs by Measurement of Dark Luminescence." *Polish Journal of Food and Nutrition Sciences* 57 (4A): 191–94.

Guillemant, Philippe, and Jocelin Morisson. 2015. *La physique de la conscience.* France: Guy Trédaniel éditeur.

Gurwitsch, A. G. 1923. Die natur des spezifischen erregers der zellteilung. *Archiv für mikroskopische Anatomie und Entwicklungsmechanik* 100 (1-2): 11–40.

Hadden, Denise. 2010. *New Light on Fields.* Available at http://www.bernell.com /category/s?keyword=denise+hadden.

Haim, Abraham, Adina Yukler, Orna Harel, Hagit Schwimmer, and Fuad Fares. 2010. "Effects of Chronobiology on Prostate Cancer Cells Growth *In Vivo.*" *Sleep Science* 3 (1): 32–35. http://sleepscience.org.br/details/85/en-US/efeitos-da -cronobiologia-no-crescimento-de-c-eacute-lulas-cancer-iacute-genas-da-pr -oacute-stata-in-vivo.

Hamblin, Michael R., and Ying-Ying Huang, eds. 2013. *Handbook of Photo-medicine.* Boca Raton, Fla.: CRC Press.

Hamblin, Michael R., Ying-Ying Huang, Aaron C. H. Chen, James D. Carroll. 2009. "Biphasic Dose Response in Low-Level Light Therapy." *Dose Response* 7 (4): 358–83.

Hameroff, Stuart, and Roger Penrose. 2014. "Consciousness in the Universe: A Review of the 'Orch OR' Theory." *Physics of Life Reviews* 11 (1): 39–78.

Hanford, Nicholas and Mariana Figueiro. 2013. "Light Therapy and Alzheimer's Disease and Related Dementia: Past, Present, and Future." *Journal of Alzheimer's Disease* 33 (4): 913–22.

Hattar, Samer, H. W. Liao, Motoharu Takao, David Berson, and King-Wai Yau. 2002. "Melanopsin-Containing Retinal Ganglion Cells: Architecture, Projections, and Intrinsic Photosensitivity." *Science* 295 (5557): 1065–70.

Hill, Richard M., and Elwin Marg. 1963. "Single-Cell Responses of the Nucleus of the Transpeduncular Tract in Rabbit to Monochromatic Light on the Retina." *Journal of Neurophysiology* 26 (2): 249–57.

Ho, Mae-Won. 2008. *The Rainbow and the Worm: The Physics of Organisms.* Singapore: World Scientific Publishing Co.

Hobday, Richard. 2015. "Myopia and Daylight in Schools: A Neglected Aspect of Public Health?" *Perspectives in Public Health* 136 (1): 50–55.

Hollwich, Fritz. 1979. *The Influence of Ocular Light Perception on Metabolism in Man and in Animal.* New York: Springer-Verlag.

Holmes, Rebecca, Bradley G. Christensen, Ranxiao Wang, and Paul G. Kwiat. 2015. "Testing the Limits of Human Vision with Single Photons." *Frontiers in Optics 2015.* OSA Technical Digest (online) (Optical Society of America, 2015), paper FTu5B.5.

Huang, Ling, Zhanjun Li, Yang Zhao, Yuanwei Zhang, Shuang Wu, Jianzhang Zhao, and Gang Han. 2016. "Ultralow-Power Near-Infrared Lamp Light Operable Targeted Organic Nanoparticle Photodynamic Therapy." *Journal of the American Chemical Society* 138 (44): 14586–91.

Hughes, Stuart W., Magor Lőrincz, Harri Rheinhallt Parri, and Vincenzo Crunelli. 2011. "Infra-Slow (<0.1 Hz) Oscillations in Thalamic Relay Nuclei: Basic Mechanisms and Significance to Health and Disease States." *Progress in Brain Research* 193: 145–62.

Iaccarino, Hanna F., Annabelle C. Singer, Anthony J. Martorell, Andrii Rudenko, Fan Gao, Tyler Z. Gillingham, Hansruedi Mathys, et al. 2016. "Gamma Frequency Entrainment Attenuates Amyloid Load and Modifies Microglia." *Nature* 540 (7632): 230–35.

Ibrahim, Mohab M., Amol Patwardhan, Kerry B. Gilbraith, Aubin Moutal, Xiaofang Yang, Lindsey A. Chew, Tally Largent-Milnes, et al. 2017. "Long-Lasting Antinociceptive Effects of Green Light in Acute and Chronic Pain in Rats." *Pain* 158 (2): 347–60.

IEA (International Energy Agency). 2014. "Energy Efficient End Use Equipment (4E) Solid State Lighting Annex—Potential Health Issues of Solid State Lighting Final Report." Paris, France: International Energy Agency.

IEEE (Institute of Electrical and Electronics Engineers). 2010. "LED Lighting Flicker and Potential Health Concern." http://ieeexplore.ieee.org/abstract/document/5618050/?reload=true.

———. 2015. "Recommended Practice for Modulating Current in High-Brightness LEDs for Mitigating Health Risks to Viewers." http://www.bio-licht.org/02_resources/info_ieee_2015_standards-1789.pdf.

ILA Light Therapy Case Studies Report. 2013. *International Light Association* http://www.international-light-association.org/system/files/ILA%20Case%20Studies%20Report%202013.pdf.

Illarionov, V. E. 2009. *Magnetotherapy* (in Russian). Moscow: Libricom.

Jameson, K. A., S. M. Highnote, and L. M. Wasserman. 2001. "Richer Color Experience in Observers with Multiple Photopigment Opsin Genes." *Psychonomic Bulletin and Review* 8 (2): 244–61.

Julien, Claude. 2006. "The Enigma of Mayer Waves: Facts and Models." *Cardiovascular Research* 70:12–21.

Jurvelin, Heidi, Timo Takala, Juuso Nissilä, Markku Timonen, Melanie Rüger, Jari Jokelainen, and Pirkko Räsänen. 2014. "Transcranial Bright Light Treatment Via the Ear Canals in Seasonal Affective Disorder: A Randomized, Double-Blind Dose-Response Study." *BMC Psychiatry* 14: 288.

Kaptchuk, Ted J., Elizabeth Friedlander, John M. Kelley, M. Norma Sanchez, Efi Kokkotou, Joyce P. Singer, Magda Kowalczykowski, Franklin G. Miller, Irving Kirsch, and Anthony J. Lembo. 2010. "Placebos Without Deception: A Randomized Controlled Trial in Irritable Bowel Syndrome." *PLoS ONE* 5 (12): e15591.

Karu, Tiina I. Complete bibliography at www.isan.troitsk.ru/dls/Publications. html (1980–2015).

———. 1998. *The Science of Low Power Laser Therapy*. Amsterdam: Gordon and Breach Science Publishers.

———. 2007. *Ten Lectures on Basic Science of Laser Phototherapy*. Coeymans Hollow, N.Y.: Prima Books.

———. 2008. "Action Spectra: Their Importance for Low Level Light Therapy." *Photobiological Sciences Online*. photobiology.info/Karu.html.

Kobayashi, Masaki, Daisuke Kikuchi, and Hitoshi Okamura. 2009. "Imaging of Ultraweak Spontaneous Photon Emission from Human Body Displaying Diurnal Rhythm." *PLoS ONE* 4 (7): e6256.

Kosslyn, Stephen M., William L. Thompson, Maria F. Costantini-Ferrando, Nathaniel M. Alpert, and David Spiegel. 2000. "Hypnotic Visual Illusion Alters Color Processing in the Brain." *American Journal of Psychiatry* 157 (8): 1279–84.

Kübler-Ross, Elisabeth. 1991. *On Life after Death*. Berkeley, Ca.: Celestial Arts.

Lam, Raymond W., Anthony J. Levitt, Robert D. Levitan, Erin E. Michalak, Amy H. Cheung, Rachel Morehouse, Rajamannar Ramasubbu, Lakshmi Yatham, and Edwin M. Tam. 2016. "Efficacy of Bright Light Treatment, Fluoxetine, and the Combination in Patients with Nonseasonal Major Depressive Disorder: A Randomized Clinical Trial." *JAMA Psychiatry* 73 (1): 56–63.

Lanza, Robert, and Bob Berman. 2009. *Biocentrism: How Life and Consciousness Are the Keys to Understanding the True Nature of the Universe*. Dallas, Tx.: BenBella Books.

Lapchak, Paul A. 2010. "Taking a Light Approach to Treating Acute Ischemic Stroke Patients: Transcranial Near-Infrared Laser Therapy Translational Science." *Annals of Medicine* 42 (8): 576–586.

———. 2012. "Transcranial Near-Infrared Laser Therapy Applied to Promote Clinical Recovery in Acute and Chronic Neurodegenerative Diseases." *Expert Review of Medical Devices* 9 (1): 71–83.

Larson, Edward J., and Larry Witham. 1998. "Leading Scientists Still Reject God." *Nature* 394 (313).

Lazlo, Ervin. 2004. *Science and the Akashic Field*. Rochester, Vt.: Inner Traditions.

Liberman, Jacob. 1990. *Light: Medicine of the Future*. Santa Fe, N.M.: Bear and Company.

———. 2018. *Luminous Life: How the Science of Light Unlocks the Art of Living.* Novato, Calif.: New World Library.

LightingEurope. 2015. "Quantified Benefits of Human Centric Lighting." www .lightingeurope.org.

Litscher, Gerhard. 2009. "Modernization of Traditional Acupuncture Using Multimodal Computer-Based High-Tech Methods: Recent Results of Blue Laser Acupuncture." *Journal of Acupuncture and Meridian Studies* 2 (3): 202–09.

Liu, Timon Cheng-Yi, Lei Cheng, Wen-Juan Su, Yi-Wen Zhang, Yun Shi, Ai-Hong Liu, Li-Li Zhang, and Zhuo-Ya Qian. 2012. "Randomized, Double-Blind, and Placebo-Controlled Clinic Report of Intranasal Low-Intensity Laser Therapy on Vascular Disease." *International Journal of Photoenergy* 2012. Article ID 489713.

Lörincz, Magor L., Freya Geall, Ying Bao, Vincenzo Crunelli, and Stuart W. Hughes. 2009. "ATP-dependent Infra-Slow (<0.1 Hz) Oscillations in Thalamic Networks." *PLoS ONE* 4 (2): e4447.

Lucas, Robert J. 2013. "Mammalian Inner Retinal Photoreception." *Current Biology* 23 (3): R125–33.

Lucas, Robert J., Stuart N. Peirson, David Berson, Timothy M. Brown, Howard M. Cooper, Charles Czeisler, Mariana Figueiro, et al. 2014. "Measuring and Using Light in the Melanopsin Age." *Trends in Neurosciences* 37 (1): 1–9.

Lueck, C. J., Semir Zeki, Karl J. Friston, Marie-Pierre Deiber, P. Cope, Vincent J. Cunningham, Adriaan Lammertsma, C. Kennard, and Richard Frackowiak. 1989. "The Colour Centre of the Cerebral Cortex in Man." *Nature* 340 (6232): 386–89.

Lüscher, Max, and Ian Scott, trans./ed. 1969. *The Lüscher Color Test: The Remarkable Test That Reveals Your Personality through Color.* New York: Pocket Books.

Magnin, Pierre, and Pascal Vidal. 2017. *De la chromothérapie à la médecine photonique - Un arc-en-ciel de santé.* France: Dangles.

Mandel, Peter. 1985. *Energy Emission Analysis: New Applications of Kirlian Photography for Holistic Health.* Synthesis Publishing Co.

———. 1986. *Practical Compendium of Colorpuncture.* Germany: Edition Energetik.

———. 2006. *Esogetics: The Sense and Nonsense of Sickness and Pain.* Germany: Medicina Biologica.

Matthews, Nishant. 2010. *The Friend: Finding Compassion with Yourself.* UK: O Books.

Mayburov, Sergey. 2011. "Photonic Communications and Information Encoding in Biological Systems." *Quant. Com. Com.* 11 (73). arXiv:1205.4134 [q-bio.OT].

McCraty, Rollin, and Fred Shaffer. 2015. "Heart Rate Variability: New Perspectives on the Physiological Mechanisms, and Assessment of Self-Regulatory Capacity and Health Risk." *Global Advances in Health and Medicine* 4 (1): 46–61.

Meesters, Ybe, Wim H. Winthorst, Wianne B. Duijzer, and Vanja Hommes. 2016. "The Effects of Low-Intensity Narrow-Band Blue-Light Treatment Compared to Bright White–Light Treatment in Sub-Syndromal Seasonal Affective Disorder." *BMC Psychiatry* 16: 27.

Mehta, Ravi, and Rui (Juliette) Zhu. 2009. "Blue or Red? Exploring the Effect of Color on Cognitive Task Performances." *Science* 323 (5918): 1226–29.

Meier, Brian P., Paul R. D'Agostino, Andrew J. Elliot, Markus A. Maier, Benjamin M. Wilkowski. 2012. "Color in Context: Psychological Context Moderates the Influence of Red on Approach- and Avoidance-Motivated Behavior." *PLOS One* 7 (7): e40333.

Mills, Peter R., Susannah C. Tomkins, and Luc J. M. Schlangen. 2007. "The Effect of High Correlated Colour Temperature Office Lighting on Employee Wellbeing and Work Performance." *Journal of Circadian Rhythms* 5: 2.

Moody, Raymond. 1984. *Life After Life*. New York: Bantam.

Moreira-Almeida, Alexander, and Saulo de Freitas Araujo. 2015. "Does the Brain Produce the Mind? A Survey of Psychiatrists' Opinions." *Archives of Clinical Psychiatry* 42 (3): 74–75.

Morlet, Laurent, Véronique Vonarx-Coinsmann, Peter Lenz, M. T. Foultier, Leonor Xavier de Brito, Charles Stewart, and Thierry Patrice. 1995. "Correlation between Meta(Tetrahydroxyphenyl)Chlorin (M-THPC) Bio-distribution and Photodynamic Effects in Mice." *Journal of Photochemistry and Photobiology* 28 (1): 25–32.

Moseley, J. Bruce, Kimberly O'Malley, Nancy J. Petersen, Terri J. Menke, Baruch A. Brody, David H. Kuykendall, John C. Hollingsworth, Carol M. Ashton, and Nelda P. Wray. 2002. "A Controlled Trial of Arthroscopic Surgery for Osteoarthritis of the Knee." *New England Journal of Medicine* 347 (2): 81–88.

Mullen, W., K. Berg, and D. Siever. 2001. "The Effect of Audio-Visual Entrainment (AVE) on Hypertension." mindalive.com/index.cfm/research/hypertension/the-effect-of-audio-visual-entrainment-ave-on-hypertension-july-2001-wendy-mullen-kathy-berg-dave-siever-cet/.

Naeser, Margaret. 2009. "Potential Treatment for Cognitive Dysfunction Using Transcranial Laser/Light Emitting Diodes." www.va.gov/RAC-GWVI/docs/Minutes_and_Agendas/Minutes_June2009_Appendix_Presentation08.pdf.

Najjar, Raymond P., and Jamie M. Zeitzer. 2016. "Temporal Integration of Light Flashes by the Human Circadian System." *Journal of Clinical Investigation* 126 (3): 938–47.

Nilsson, Dan E., and Susanne Pelger. 1994. "A Pessimistic Estimate of the Time Required for an Eye to Evolve." *Proceedings of the Royal Society of London* 256 (1345): 53–58.

Nissilä, Jusso S., Satu Mänttäri, Terttu Säkioja, Hanna J. Tuominen, Timo E. Takala, Vesa Kiviniemi, Raija T. Sormunen, Saarela Seppo, and Markku Timonen. 2016. "The Distribution of Melanopsin (OPN4) Protein in The Human Brain." *Chronobiology International* 34 (1): 37–44.

O'Leary, Daniel K., Alan Rosenbaum, and Philip C. Hughes. 1977. "Fluorescent Lighting: A Purported Source of Hyperactive Behavior." *Journal of Abnormal Child Psychology* 6 (3): 285–89.

Oliveira, Henrique Manuel, and Luís Viseu Melo. 2015. "Huygens Synchronization of Two Clocks." *Scientific Reports* 5: 11548.

Oschman, James L. 2003. *Energy Medicine in Therapeutics and Human Performance.* Edinburgh, Scotland: Butterworth Heinemann.

———. 2015. *Energy Medicine: The Scientific Basis,* 2nd ed. London: Churchill Livingstone.

Oschman, James L., and Nora H. Oschman, 1993. "Matter, Energy and the Living Matrix." *Rolf Lines, the news magazine for the Rolf Institute* 21 (3): 55–64.

———. 2015. "Subtle Energies, Biophotons, and Information Metabolism." *Subtle Energy Magazine* Autumn 26 (2): 30–6.

Osho. 1985. *The Last Testament,* Vol. 1. http://oshosearch.net/Convert/Articles _Osho/The_Last_Testament_Volume_1/Osho-The-Last-Testament-Volume-1 -index.html.

———. 1986. *The Transmission of the Lamp.* http://www.oshorajneesh.com /download/osho-books/world_tour_talks/The_Transmission_of_the_Lamp _(Talks_in_Uruguay).pdf.

Ott, John Nash. 1985. "Color and Light: Their Effects on Plants, Animals and People." *International Journal of Biosocial Research* 7.

Palienko, Igor A. 2000. "Hemodynamic Effects of Lateralized Colored-Light Stimulation of the Brain Hemispheres in Patients with Essential Hypertension" (in Russian). *Ukr. Kardiol. Zh.* Nos. 5/6 (Issue II), 46–48 (2000).

———. 2001a. "Effect of Different Light and Color Stimulation of the Cerebral Hemispheres on Cardiac Rhythm Self-Regulation in Healthy Individuals" (in Russian). *Fiziol Zh* 47 (1): 73–75.

———. 2001b. "Modifications of the EEG Activity Upon Lateralized Stimulation of the Visual Inputs to the Right and to the Left Brain Hemispheres by Light with Different Wavelengths." *Neurophysiology* 33 (3): 169–174.

———. 2001c. "Spectral Analysis of Heart Rate Responses to Light and Color Stimulation of the Cerebral Hemispheres" (in Russian). *Fiziol Zh* 47 (2): 70–73.

Pankratov, Sergei. 1991. "Meridians Conduct Light." *Raum und Zeit* 35: 16–18.

Parker, Andrew. 2003. *In the Blink of an Eye: How Vision Sparked the Big Bang of Evolution.* New York: Basic Books.

Parshad, Ram, K. K. Sanford, G. M. Jones, and R. E. Tarone. 1978. "Fluorescent Light-Induced Chromosome Damage and Its Prevention in Mouse Cells in Culture." *Proceedings of the National Academy of Science* 75 (4): 1830–33.

Paul, Michael A., James C. Miller, Ryan J. Love, Harris Lieberman, Sofi Blazeski, and Josephine Arendt. 2009. "Timing Light Treatment for Eastward and Westward Travel." *Chronobiology International* 26 (5): 867–90.

Perera, Stefan, Rebecca Eisen, Meha Bhatt, Neera Bhatnagar, Russell de Souza, Lehana Thabane, and Zainab Samaan. 2016. "Light Therapy for Non-Seasonal Depression: Systematic Review and Meta-Analysis." *British Journal of Psychiatry Open* 2 (2): 116–26.

Petitmengin, Claire. 2006. De l'activité cérébrale à l'expérience vécue. *Sciences Humaines* 3: 59–69.

Phan, Thieu X., Barbara Jaruga, Sandeep C. Pingle, Bidhan C. Bandyopadhyay, Gerard P. Ahern. 2016. "Intrinsic Photosensitivity Enhances Motility of T Lymphocytes." *Scientific Reports* 6: 39479.

Pienta, K. J., and D. S. Coffey. 1991. "Cellular Harmonic Information Transfer through a Tissue Tensegrity-Matrix System." *Medical Hypotheses* 34 (1): 88–95.

Pollack, Gerald. 2013. *The Fourth Phase of Water: Beyond Solid, Liquid and Vapor.* Seattle, Wash.: Ebner and Sons.

Poplawski M. E., and N. M. Miller. 2013. "Flicker in Solid-State Lighting: Measurement Techniques, and Proposed Reporting and Application Criteria." https://goo.gl/fM9ABa.

Popp, Fritz-Albert. 1999. "About the Coherence of Biophotons." Published as *Macroscopic Quantum Coherence* in "Proceedings of an International Conference on the Boston University," edited by Boston University and MIT, World Scientific. Available online. www.academia.edu/1901658/About_the _Coherence_of_Biophotons_Fritz-Albert_Popp_International_Institute_of _Biophysics_Biophotonics_Raketenstation_41472_Neuss_Germany.

Popp, Fritz-Albert, and Ke-hsueh Li. 1993. "Hyberbolic Relaxation as a Sufficient Condition of a Fully Coherent Ergodic Field." *International Journal of Theoretical Physics* 32 (9): 1573–83.

Popp, Fritz-Albert, W. Nagl, K. H. Li, W. Scholz, O. Weingärtner, and R. Wolf. 1984. "Biophoton emission: New Evidence for Coherence and DNA as Source." *Cell Biophysics* 6 (1): 33–52.

Popp, Fritz-Albert, and Y. Yan. 2002. "Delayed Luminescence of Biological Systems in Terms of Coherent States." *Physics Letters A* 293: 93–97.

Prigogine, Ilya, and G. Nicolis. 1977. *Self-Organization in Non-Equilibrium Systems.* Hoboken, N.J.: Wiley.

Provencio, Ignacio, Ignacio Rodriguez, Guisen Jiang, William Hayes, Ernesto F. Moreira, and Mark D. Rollag. 2000. "A Novel Human Opsin in the Inner Retina." *Journal of Neuroscience* 20 (2): 600–05.

Rea, Mark S., Mariana G. Figueiro, Andrew Bierman, and R. Hamner. 2012. "Modelling the Spectral Sensitivity of the Human Circadian System." *Lighting Research and Technology* 44 (4): 386–96.

Ribak, Erez, Amichai Labin, Shadi Safuri, and Ido Perlman. 2015. "Sorting of Colors in the Retina." *American Physical Society*. http://adsabs.harvard.edu /abs/2015APS..MARS47002R.

Ribeiro, Martha Simões, Daniela De Fátima Teixeira Da Silva, Carlos Eugênio Nabuco de Araújo, Sérgio Ferreira de Oliveira, Cleusa Maria Raspantini Pelegrini, Telma Maria Tenório Zorn, and Denise Maria Zezell. 2004. "Effects of Low-Intensity Polarized Visible Laser Radiation on Skin Burns: A Light Microscopy Study." *Journal of Clinical Laser Medicine and Surgery* 22 (1): 59–66.

Ring, Kenneth, and Sharon Cooper. 1999. *Mindsight: Near-Death and Out-of-Body Experiences in the Blind,* 2nd ed. Palo Alto, Calif.: William James Center for Consciousness Studies, Institute of Transpersonal Psychology.

Rojas, Julio C., Aleksandra K. Bruchey, and F. Gonzalez-Lima. 2012. "Low-Level Light Therapy Improves Cortical Metabolic Capacity and Memory Retention." *Journal of Alzheimer's Disease* 32 (3): 741–52.

Rosch, Paul J., ed. 2015. *Bioelectromagnetic and Subtle Energy Medicine,* 2nd ed. Boca Raton, Fla.: CRC Press.

Rosemann, A., M. Mossman, and L. Whitehead. 2008. "Development of a Cost-Effective Solar Illumination System to Bring Natural Light into the Building Core." *Solar Energy* 82: 302–10.

Rosenberg, Barnett, and Elliot Postow. 1969. "Semiconduction in Proteins and Lipids: Its Possible Biological Import." *Annals of the New York Academy of Science* 158 (1): 161–90.

Rosenthal, Norman E., David A. Sack, J. Christian Gillin, Alfred J. Lewy, Frederick K. Goodwin, Yolande Davenport, Peter S. Mueller, David A. Newsome, and Thomas A. Wehr. 1984. "Seasonal Affective Sisorder: A Sescription of the Ayndrome and Preliminary Findings with Light Therapy." *Archives of General Psychiatry* 41 (1): 72–80.

Ross, Mary J., Paul Guthrie, and Justin-Claude Dumont. 2013. "The Impact of Modulated Color Light on the Autonomic Nervous System." *Advances in Mind-Body Medicine* 27 (4): 7–16.

Roth, Mark. 2006. "Some Women May See 100 Million Colors, Thanks to Their Genes." *Pittsburgh Post Gazette,* September 3.

Rowen, Robert J. 1996. "Ultraviolet Blood Irradiation Therapy (Photo-Oxidation): The Cure that Time Forgot." *International Journal of Biosocial Research* 14 (2): 115–32.

Ryberg, Karl. 2010. *Living Light: On the Origin of Colours*. Sweden: Typografia.

Rybnikova, Nataliya, Abraham Haim, and Boris Portnov. 2015. "Artificial Light at Night (ALAN) and Breast Cancer Incidence Worldwide: A Revisit of Earlier Findings with Analysis of Current Trends." *Chronobiology International* 32 (6): 757–73.

Saltmarche, Anita E., Margaret A. Naeser, Kai Fai Ho, Michael R. Hamblin, and Lew Lim. 2017. "Significant Improvement in Cognition in Mild to Moderately Severe Dementia Cases Treated with Transcranial Plus Intranasal Photobiomodulation: Case Series Report." *Photomedicine and Laser Surgery* 35 (8): 432–41.

Schapira, Kurt, H. A. McClelland, N. R. Griffiths, and D. J. Newell. 1970. "Study on the Effects of Tablet Colour in the Treatment of Anxiety States." *British Medical Journal* 1 (5707): 446–49.

Schiffer, Fredric, Andrea L. Johnston, Caitlin Ravichandran, Ann Polcari, Martin H. Teicher, Robert H. Webb, and Michael R. Hamblin. 2009. "Psychological Benefits 2 and 4 Weeks after a Single Treatment with Near Infrared Light to the Forehead: A Pilot Study of 10 Patients with Major Depression and Anxiety." *Behavioral and Brain Functions* 5: 46.

Schikora, Detlef, Rita Klowersa, and Sandi Suwanda. 2012. *The Laserneedle Therapy Handbook*. Laneg Gmbh Wehrden, Germany. Available for purchase at http://www.blum-akupunktur.de/products/Fachliteratur/Lasertherapie/The-Laserneedle-Therapy-Handbook.html.

Schlebusch, Klaus-Peter, Walburg Maric-Oehler, and Fritz-Albert Popp. 2005. "Biophotonics in the Infrared Spectral Range Reveal Acupuncture Meridian Structure of the Body." *Journal of Alternative and Complementary Medicine* 11 (1): 171–73.

Schoenemann, Brigitte, Helji Pärnaste, and Euan N. K. Clarkson. 2017. "Structure and Function of a Compound Eye, More than Half a Billion Years Old." *Proceedings of the National Academy of Sciences* 114: 13489–94.

Scientific Committee on Emerging and Newly Identified Health Risks (SCENIHR). 2012. "Health Effects of Artificial Light." https://ec.europa.eu/health/scientific_committees/emerging/docs/scenihr_o_035.pdf

Scott, James A. 1984. "The Role of Cytoskeletal Integrity in Cellular Transformation." *Journal of Theoretical Biology* 106 (2): 183–88.

Shifferman, Eran. 2015. "More than meets the fMRI: The Unethical Apotheosis of Neuroimages." *Journal of Cognition and Neuroethics* 3 (2): 57–116.

Sit, Dorothy K., James McGowan, Christopher Wiltrout, Rasim Somer Diler, John (Jesse) Dills, James Luther, Amy Yang, et al. 2017. "Adjunctive Bright Light Therapy for Bipolar Depression: A Randomized Double-Blind Placebo-Controlled Trial." *American Journal of Psychiatry* 10.

Soh, Kwang-Sup. 2004. "Bonghan Duct and Acupuncture Meridian as Optical Channel of Biophoton." *Journal of the Korean Physical Society* 45 (5): 1196–98.

Soh, Kwang-Sup, Kyung A. Kang, and Yeon Hee Ryu. 2013. "50 Years of Bong-Han Theory and 10 Years of Primo Vascular System." *Evidence-Based Complementary and Alternative Medicine* 2013.

Sommer, Andrei P., Jan Bieschke, Ralf P. Friedrich, Dan Zhu, Erich E. Wanker, H. J. Fecht, Derliz Mereles, and Werner Hunstein. 2012. "670 nm Laser Light and EGCG Complementarily Reduce Amyloid-β Aggregates in Human Neuroblastoma Cells: Basis for Treatment of Alzheimer's Disease?" *Photomedicine and Laser Surgery* 30 (1): 54–605d

Sommer, Andrei P., Arnaud Caron, and H. J. Fecht. 2008. "Tuning Nanoscopic Water Layers on Hydrophobic and Hydrophilic Surfaces with Laser Light." *Langmuir* 24 (3): 635–36.

Sommer, Andrei P., Mike K. Haddad, and Hans-Jörg Fecht. 2015. "Light Effect on Water Viscosity: Implication for ATP Biosynthesis." *Scientific Reports* 5: 12029.

Spitler, Harry Riley. 2011. *The Syntonic Principle: In Relation to Health and Ocular Problems.* Eugene, Ore: Resource Publications.

Stevens, Larry, Zach Haga , Brandy Queen, Brian Brady, Deanna Adams, Jaime Gilbert, Emily Vaughan, Cathy Leach, Paul Nockels, and Patrick McManus. 2003. "Binaural Beat Induced Theta EEG Activity and Hypnotic Susceptibility: Contradictory Results and Technical Considerations." *American Journal of Clinical Hypnosis* Apr 45(4): 295–309.

Straubinger, P. A. 2010. *In the Beginning There Was Light.* www.lightdocumentary.com.

Strehl, Ute, and Niels Birbaumer. 2006. "Self-Regulation of Slow Cortical Potentials: A New Treatment for Children with Attention-Deficit/Hyperactivity Disorder." *Pediatrics* 118 (5): e1530–40.

Strogatz, Steven. 2003. *Sync: How Order Emerges from Chaos in the Universe, Nature, and Daily Life.* New York: Hyperion Books.

Szent-Györgyi, Albert. 1960. *Introduction to a Submolecular Biology.* New York: Academic Press.

Takeda, Motohiro, Masaki Kobayashi, Mariko Takayama, Satoshi Suzuki, Takanori Irhida, Kohji Ohnuki, Takura Moriya, and Noriaki Ohuchi. 2004. "Biophoton Detection as a Novel Technique for Cancer Imaging." *Cancer Science* 95 (8): 656–661.

Tamietto, Marco, and Beatrice de Gelder. 2010. "Neural Bases of the Non-Conscious Perception of Emotional Signals." *Nature Reviews Neuroscience* 11 (10): 697–709.

Terman, Michael, Jiuan Su Terman, F. M. Quitkin, T. B. Cooper, E. S. Lo, J. M. Gorman, Jonathan W. Stewart, and Patrick J. McGrath. 1988. "Response of the Melatonin Cycle to Phototherapy for Seasonal Affective Disorder." *Journal of Neural Transmission.* 72 (2): 147–65.

Thapan, Kavita, Jo Arendt, and Debra J. Skene. 2001. "An Action Spectrum for Melatonin Suppression: Evidence of a Novel Non-rod, Non-cone Photoreceptor System in Humans." *Journal of Physiology* 535 (pt. 1): 261–67.

Tianhong, Dai, and Michael R. Hamblin. 2014. "Ultraviolet C Therapy for Infections," chap. 21 in *Handbook of Photomedicine*, ed. Michael R. Hamblin and Ying-Ying Huang. Boca Raton, Fla.: CRC Press.

United States Department of Energy (DOE). 2014. "True Colors, LEDs and the Relationship between CCT, CRI, Optical Safety, Material Degradation, and Photobiological Stimulation." https://www1.eere.energy.gov/buildings/ssl/pdfs/true-colors.pdf.

Valdimarsdottir, Heiddis B., Lisa Maria Wu, Susan Lugendorf, Sonia Ancoli-Israel, Gary Winkel, Redd C. William, et al. 2016. "Systematic Light Exposure Improves Depression Among Cancer Survivors." Poster presented at: American Psychosomatic Society 74th Annual Meeting, Denver, Co.. Abstract 1586; March 9–12. https://www.psychosomatic.org/AnMeeting/PDF/APS_Meeting_Abstracts.pdf.

Vanderwalle, Gilles, Pierre Maquet, and Derk-Jan Dijk. 2009. "Light as a Modulator of Cognitive Brain Function." *Trends in Cognitive Sciences* 13 (10): 429–38.

Vanderwalle, Gilles, Christina Schmidt, Geneviève Albouy, Virginie Sterpenich, Anabelle Darsaud, Géraline Rauchs, Pierre-Yves Berken, et al. 2007. "Brain Responses to Violet, Blue, and Green Monochromatic Light Exposures in Humans: Prominent Role of Blue Light and the Brainstem." *PLoS ONE* 2 (11): e1247.

Van Maanen, Annette, Anne Marie Meijer, Kristiaan B. van der Heijden, and Frans J. Oort. 2016. "The Effects of Light Therapy on Sleep Problems: A Systematic Review and Meta-Analysis." *Sleep Medicine Reviews* 29: 52–62.

Van Obberghen, Pierre. 2014. *Traité de Couleur Thérapie Pratique.* Paris: Guy Trédaniel Éditeur.

Van Wijk, Eduard P., Heike Koch, Saskia Bosman, and Roeland van Wijk. 2006. "Anatomic Characterization of Human Ultra-Weak Photon Emission in Practitioners of Transcendental Meditation™ and Control Subjects." *The Journal of Alternative and Complementary* Medicine (12) 1: 31–8.

Van Wijk, Eduard P., Roeland van Wijk, and Rajendra Bajpai. 2008. "Quantum Squeezed State Analysis of Spontaneous Ultra-Weak Light Photon Emission of Practitioners of Meditation and Control Subjects." *Indian Journal of Experimental Biology* 46 (5): 345–52.

Van Wijk, Roeland. 2014. *Light in Shaping Life: Biophotons in Biology and Medicine.* Meluna.

Vazquez, Steven. 2014. *Emotional Transformation Therapy: An Interactive Ecological Psychotherapy.* Lanham, Md.: Rowman & Littlefield Publishers.

———. 2015. *Accelerated Ecological Psychotherapy: ETT Applications for Sleep Disorders, Pain, and Addiction.* Lanham, Md.: Rowman & Littlefield Publishers.

———. 2016. *Spiritually Transformative Psychotherapy: Repairing Spiritual Damage and Facilitating Extreme Wellbeing.* Lanham, Md.: Rowman & Littlefield Publishers.

Von Bertalanffy, Ludwig. 1976 revised edition. *General System Theory: Foundations, Development, Applications.* New York: George Braziller.

Wall, Vicky. 2005. *Aura-Soma: Self-Discovery through Color.* Rochester, Vt.: Healing Arts Press.

Webb, A. R. 2006. "Ultraviolet Benefits and Risks—the Evolving Debate." (Presented at the 2nd CIE Expert Symposium on Lighting and Health.Ottawa, Ontario, Canada, September 7–8, 2006). CIE X031-2006 is available at https://www.techstreet.com/cie/standards/cie-x031-2006?product_id=1371325.

Webb, S. J., and M. E. Stoneham. 1977. "Resonance between 10^{11} and 10^{12} Hz in Active Bacterial Cells as Seen by Laser Raman Spectroscopy." *Physics Letters A* 60 (3): 267–68.

Wiederman, Michael. 2015. "Thinking about Death Can Make Life Better." *Scientific American* March 5.

Wilkins, Arnold J., Ian Nimmo-Smith, A. I. Slater, and L. Bedocs. 1989. "Fluorescent Lighting, Headaches and Eye-Strain." *Lighting Research and Technology* 21 (1): 11–18.

Winkler, Barry S., Michael E. Boulton, John D. Gottsch, and Paul Sternberg. 2007. "Oxidative Damage and Age-Related Macular Degeneration." *Molecular Vision* 5: 32.

Wood, Brittany, Mark S. Rea, Barbara Plitnick, and Mariana G. Figueiro. 2013. "Light Level and Duration of Exposure Determine the Impact of Self-Luminous Tablets on Melatonin Suppression." *Applied Ergonomics* 44 (2): 237–40.

Wright, Kenneth P., Jr., and Charles A. Czeisler. 2002. "Absence of Circadian Phase Resetting in Response to Bright Light behind the Knees." *Science* 297 (5581): 571.

Wright, Kenneth P., Jr., Rod J. Hughes, Richard E. Kronauer, Derk-Jan Dijk, and Charles A. Czeisler. 2001. "Intrinsic Near-24-h Pacemaker Period Determines Limits of Circadian Entrainment to a Weak Synchronizer in Humans." *Proceedings of the National Academy of Science* 98 (24): 14027–32.

Wu, Qiuhe, Ying-Ying Huang, Saphala Dhital, Sulbha K. Sharma, Aaron C.-H. Chen, Michael J. Whalen, and Michael R. Hamblin. 2010. "Low Level Laser Therapy for Traumatic Brain Injury." Proceedings of SPIE–The International Society for Optical Engineering 7552: 6-8. https://dspace.mit.edu/handle/1721.1/58575.

Wunsch, Alexander. 2016. "Potential Relevance of Near Infrared Radiation for Ocular and Dermal Health" (video format). https://vimeo.com/184495934.

Yan, Zhiqiang, Yuro Ng Chi, Pujing Wang, Jing Cheng, Yizhong Wang, Qi Shu, and Guiyu Huang. 1992. "Studies on the Luminescence of Channels in Rats and Its Law of Changes with 'Syndrome' and Treatment of Acupuncture and Moxibustion." *Journal of Traditional Chinese Medicine* 12 (4): 283–87.

Yomiuri Shimbun. 1997. "TV Tokyo to Investigate 'Pocket Monster' Panic." December 18.

Zajonc, Arthur. 1993. *Catching the Light: The Entwined History of Light and Mind.* New York: Oxford University Press.

Zhang, Chang Lin. 2008. "Background of Electronic Measurement on Skin." *International Journal of Modelling, Identification and Control* 5 (3): 181–90.

Zhang, Ray, Nicholas F. Lahens, Heather I. Balance, Michael E. Hughes, and John B. Hogenesch. 2014. "A Circadian Gene Expression Atlas in Mammals: Implications for Biology and Medicine." *Proceedings of the National Academy of Sciences* 111 (45): 16219–24.

Ziemssen, Tjalf, and Simone Kern. 2007. "Psychoneuroimmunology—Cross-Talk between the Immune and Nervous Systems." *Journal of Neurology* 255 (2): 118–21.

Zubidat, Abed Elsalam, Basem Fares, F. Fares, and Abraham Haim. 2015. "Melatonin Functioning through DNA Methylation Constricts Breast Cancer Growth Accelerated by Blue LED Light-At-Night in 4T1 Tumor-Bearing Mice." *Gratis Journal of Cancer Biology and Therapeutics* 1 (2): 57–73.

INDEX

Numbers in *italics* indicate illustrations.